Ethical Conundrums, Quandaries, and Predicaments in Mental Health Practice

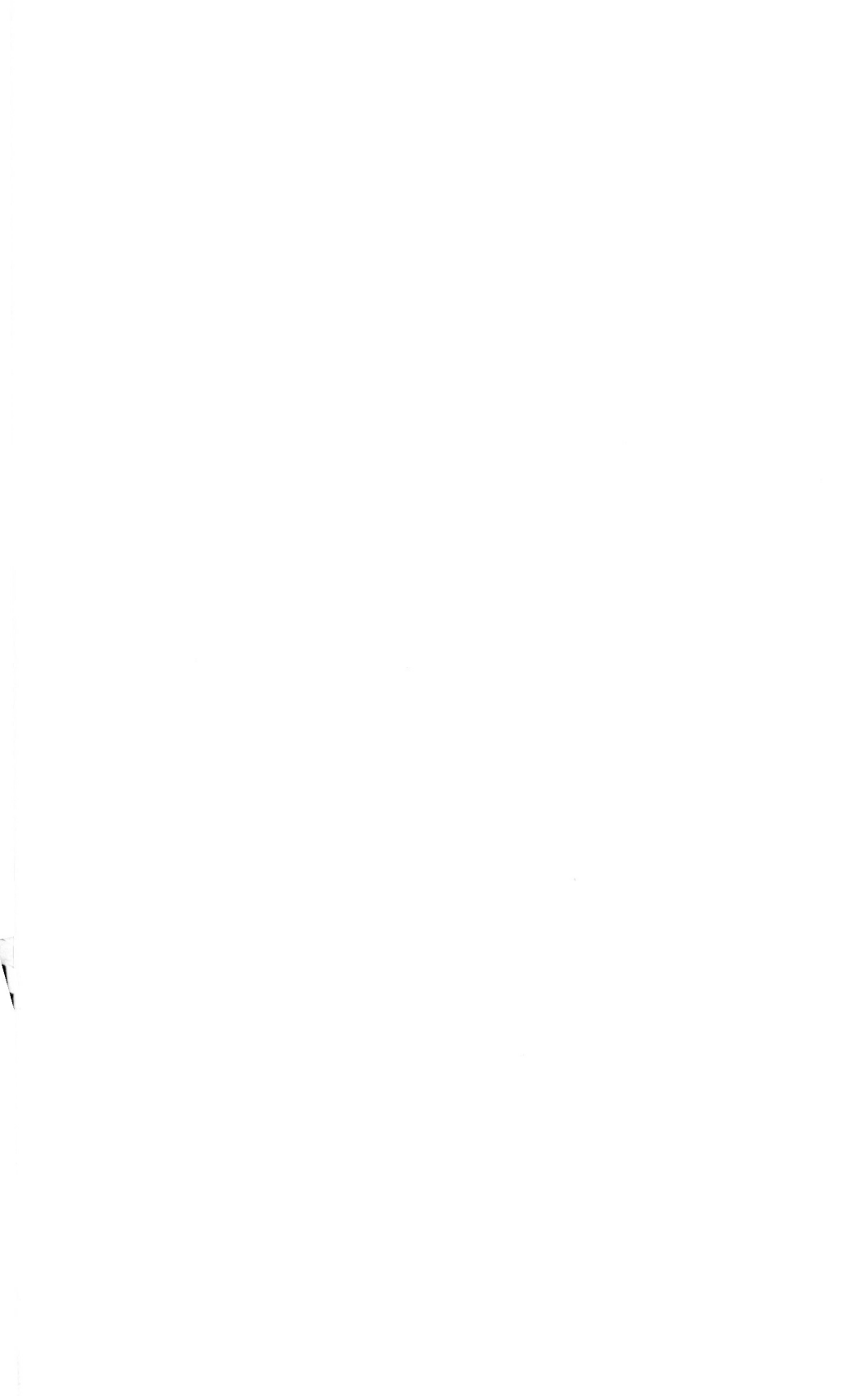

Ethical Conundrums, Quandaries, and Predicaments in Mental Health Practice

A Casebook from the Files of Experts

Edited by
W. Brad Johnson
Gerald P. Koocher

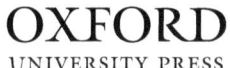

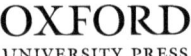
UNIVERSITY PRESS

Oxford University Press, Inc, publishes works that further
Oxford University's objective of excellence
in research, scholarship, and education.

Oxford   New York
Auckland   Cape Town   Dar es Salaam   Hong Kong   Karachi
Kuala Lumpur   Madrid   Melbourne   Mexico City   Nairobi
New Delhi   Shanghai   Taipei   Toronto

With offices in
Argentina   Austria   Brazil   Chile   Czech Republic   France   Greece
Guatemala   Hungary   Italy   Japan   Poland   Portugal   Singapore
South Korea   Switzerland   Thailand   Turkey   Ukraine   Vietnam

Copyright © 2011 by W. Brad Johnson & Gerald P. Koocher

Published by Oxford University Press, Inc
198 Madison Avenue, New York, NY 10016
www.oup.com

Oxford is a registered trademark of Oxford University Press.

All rights reserved. No part of this publication may be reproduced,
stored in a retrieval system, or transmitted, in any form or by any means,
electronic, mechanical, photocopying, recording, or otherwise,
without the prior permission of Oxford University Press.

Library of Congress Cataloging-in-Publication Data
Ethical Conundrums, Quandaries, and Predicaments in Mental Health Practice:
A Casebook from the Files of Experts / [edited by] W. Brad Johnson, Gerald P. Koocher.
   p. ; cm.
Includes bibliographical references.
ISBN 978-0-19-538529-8
 1. Mental health services—Moral and ethical aspects—Case studies. 2. Mental health personnel—Professional
ethics—Case studies. 3. Psychiatric ethics—Cases studies. I. Johnson, W. Brad. II. Koocher, Gerald P.
 [DNLM: 1. Mental Health Services—ethics—Case Reports. 2. Ethics, Professional—Case Reports.
3. Psychiatry—ethics—Case Reports. 4. Psychotherapy—ethics—Case Reports. WM 40 J93 2011]
 RC455.2.E8J84 2011
 174.2'9689—dc22

2010025253

Contents

Contributors, xi

Juggling Porcupines: Being Ethical in Challenging Roles
and Work Settings, 1
W. Brad Johnson and Gerald P. Koocher

PART I: In the Psychotherapist's Office

1. But It's a Really Nice Gift! Ethical Challenges in Responding to Offers of Gifts From Clients, 9
   Jeffrey E. Barnett

2. Everyone I Know Knows Everyone I Know: Boundary Overlap in the Life of One Lesbian Psychotherapist, 17
   Laura S. Brown

3. Hitler Should Have Finished the Job: Countertransference, Anti-Semitism, Abandonment, and Termination, 25
   Michael A. Grodin

4. Suicidal Blackmail: Ethical and Risk Management Issues in Contemporary Clinical Care, 33
   David Jobes

5. An Affair to Remember: Protecting Vulnerable Clients and Confidentiality When Spouses Cheat, 41
   Mary Ann McCabe

6. Trapped by Trauma: When Clients Cannot or Will Not Protect Themselves From Harm, 49
   John Peteet

7. To Warn or Not to Warn: That Is the Question, 55
   David L. Shapiro

8. What Would She Think? Disclosure of Therapy Details After Death, 63
   Dan Shapiro

9. It's My Right! Working With a Terminally (or Chronically) Ill, Persistently Suicidal Client, 71
   James L. Werth Jr.

PART II: In the Forensic World

10. High Stakes Indeed: Forensic Psychology in Death Penalty Litigation, 83
    Richart L. DeMier

11. Is That What I Said? Ethical Challenges When Parents Divorce During Treatment, 93
    Robin M. Deutsch

12. Now You See It, Now You Don't: When Releases of Information Are Rescinded, 101
    John C. Gonsiorek

13. The Siren Song of Silence: Ensuring a Basis for Professional Judgments, 111
    Robert Kinscherff

14. "Thera-mail" for a Quarter Century: Managing Complex Boundaries With a Former Client, 119
    Frederic G. Reamer

15. Jonas and His Protective, Delusional, or Alienating Mother: Advocacy, Forensics, and Boundaries With Battered Women, 127
    Lenore E. Walker

PART III: In Medical Center Corridors

16. Determining a Patient's Capacity to Refuse Dialysis and Die: When Professional Competence and Credentials Do Not Overlap, 141
    James DuBois

17. When Boundaries Intersect in Cyberspace: Facebook, Multiple Relationships, and Confidentiality in a Hospital, 149
    Nabil Hassan El-Ghoroury

18. Second Chances: Decision Making in Pediatric Transplantation, 157
    Lisa M. Farley

19. On Being There: Boundaries in Emotionally Intense Contexts, 167
    Gerald P. Koocher

PART IV: In National Security Settings

20. "I've Got This Friend": Multiple Roles, Informed Consent, and Friendship in the Military, 175
    W. Brad Johnson

21. Establishing Rapport With an "Enemy Combatant": Cultural Competency in Guantanamo Bay, 183
    Carrie H. Kennedy

22. Psychotic, Homicidal, and Armed: The Delicate Balance Between Personal Safety and Effectiveness in a Combat Environment, 189
    Heidi S. Kraft

23. "What Do You Know That Can Help Us?" Behavioral Science in National Security Settings, 197
    Susan E. Brandon

PART V: In Organizations

24. A Disaster in a Suit and Tie: When Organizational Policies Undermine Ethical Obligations, 207
    Charles A. Morgan III

25. Risking Your Job: On Striving to be an Ethical Leader in Difficult Organizational Circumstances, 215
Rodney L. Lowman

26. When Bad Things Happen to People Who Try Really Hard: Ethical Quandaries in Test Validation, 223
Nancy T. Tippins

PART VI: In Schools and Colleges

27. When in Doubt, Pull Them Out? Ethical Issues Related to Decisions on Child Removal From the Home, 233
Lyvia Chriki

28. A Near Fall: The Multifaceted Challenges to Work in Sport Psychology and Intercollegiate Athletics, 241
Edward F. Etzel

29. Doing Good Versus Avoiding Harm: Resolving Situational Contradictions, 249
Alan G. Green

PART VII: Supervising or Assisting Colleagues

30. The Wink: Ethical Aspects of Encountering Clients in Unexpected Places, 261
Stephen H. Behnke

31. Can You Help Us? Supervising Graduate Students in a Crisis Situation, 269
Clark D. Campbell

32. Doing It by the Book: Ethical Issues in Teaching a Group Didactically and Experientially, 277
Gerald Corey

33. So, How *Exactly* Did You Get Interested in Eating Disorders? Confronting a Colleague's Unhealthy Behaviors, 287
Jennifer L. Derenne

34. Knocked Off Kilter: Supervising in the Wake of Sexual Boundary Violations, 297
Janet T. Thomas

PART VIII: Religious Concerns and Settings

35. Of Course It's Confidential—Only the Community Knows: Mental Health Services With the Old Order Amish, 309

    James A. Cates

36. Working Out One's Salvation in Fear and Trembling: Ethical and Spiritual Dilemmas Around Therapeutic Boundaries, 317

    Andrew Michel

PART IX: In the Public Arena

37. A Psychologist in Congress: Ethics, the Constitution, Politics, Clinical Judgment, and the Case of Terri Schiavo, 327

    Brian Baird

38. Isn't This Against the Law? Boundary Problems in Police Psychology, 335

    Gerald Sweet

    Index, 345

Contributors

Brian Baird, PhD
United States House of Representatives
Washington, DC

Jeffrey E. Barnett, PsyD, ABPP
Department of Psychology
Loyola University Maryland
Baltimore, Maryland

Stephen H. Behnke, JD, PhD
American Psychological Association
Washington, DC

Susan E. Brandon, PhD
Department of Defense
Washington, DC

Laura S. Brown, PhD
Fremont Community Therapy
   Project Seattle, Washington

Clark D. Campbell, PhD
Rosemead School of Psychology
Biola University
La Mirada, California

James A. Cates, PhD
Amish Youth Vision
   Project, Inc
Fort Wayne, Indiana

Lyvia Chriki, BA
Clinical Psychology Program
Ohio State University

Gerald Corey, EdD, ABPP
California State University,
   Fullerton
Fullerton, California

Richart L. DeMier, PhD
US Medical Center for Federal
   Prisoners
Federal Bureau of Prisons
Springfield, Missouri

Jennifer L. Derenne, MD
Department of Psychiatry and
   Behavioral Medicine
Medical College of Wisconsin
Milwaukee, Wisconsin

Robin M. Deutsch, PhD
Department of Psychiatry
Massachusetts General Hospital
Harvard Medical School
Boston, Massachusetts

James DuBois, PhD
Albert Gnaegi Center for Health Care
    Ethics
Saint Louis University
Saint Louis, Missouri

Nabil Hassan El-Ghoroury, PhD
American Psychological Association
Washington, DC

Edward F. Etzel, PhD
Department of Sport and Exercise
    Psychology
West Virginia University
Morgantown, West Virginia

Lisa M. Farley, PhD
Children's Hospital of Boston
Harvard Medical School
Boston, Massachusetts

John C. Gonsiorek, PhD
Argosy University
Eagan, Minnesota

Alan G. Green, PhD
Rossier School of Education
University of Southern California
Los Angeles, California

Michael A. Grodin, MD
Department of Health Law, Bioethics
    and Human Rights
Boston University School of Medicine
Boston, MA

David Jobes, PhD
Department of Psychology
Catholic University
Washington, DC

W. Brad Johnson, PhD
Department of Leadership, Ethics,
    and Law
United States Naval Academy
Annapolis, Maryland

Carrie H. Kennedy, PhD
Naval Aerospace Medical Institute
Pensacola, Florida

Robert Kinscherff, PhD, Esq
Forensic Concentration, Doctoral
    Psychology Program
Massachussetts School of
    Professional Psychology
Boston, Massachusetts

Gerald P. Koocher, PhD
Simmons College
Boston, Massachusetts

Heidi S. Kraft, PhD
Naval Health Research Center
San Diego, California

Rodney L. Lowman, PhD
School of Management
Alliant International
    University
San Diego, California

Mary Ann McCabe, PhD
Department of Pediatrics
George Washington University
    School of Medicine
Washington, DC

Andrew Michel, MD
Department of Psychiatry
Vanderbilt University School of Medicine
Nashville, Tennessee

Charles A. Morgan III, MD
Department of Psychiatry
Yale University
New Haven, Connecticut

John Peteet, MD
Department of Psychiatry
Brigham and Women's Hospital
Boston, Massachusetts

Frederic G. Reamer, PhD
School of Social Work
Rhode Island College
Providence, Rhode Island

Dan Shapiro, PhD
Humanities Department
Penn State College of Medicine
Hershey, Pennsylvania

David L. Shapiro, PhD
Center for Psychological Studies
Nova Southeastern University
Fort Lauderdale, Florida

Gerald Sweet, PhD
Los Angeles Police Department
Los Angeles, California

Janet T. Thomas, PsyD
Independent Practice
Saint Paul, Minnesota

Nancy T. Tippins, PhD
Valtera Corporation
Greenville, South Carolina

Lenore E. Walker, PhD
Walker and Associates
Hollywood, Florida

James L. Werth Jr., PhD
Radford University
Radford, Virginia

Juggling Porcupines: Being Ethical in Challenging Roles and Work Settings

W. Brad Johnson and Gerald P. Koocher

Behaving ethically is hard work. Mental health professionals (MHPs) of all stripes struggle to do the right thing in their day-to-day interactions with individual clients, groups, and organizations. Quite often, MHPs encounter *mixed-agency* dilemmas involving the simultaneous commitment to two or more entities; most often, these present as conflicts between loyalties to individual clients and those to an organization. In mixed-agency situations, ethical professionals must carefully identify sometimes competing obligations to clients, organizations, and society while seeking to resolve them responsibly and without causing harm (Johnson & Ridley, 2008; Kennedy & Johnson, 2009; Koocher, 2009). As a group, MHPs tend to have high levels of loyalty and concern for others, which often lead them to feel highly stressed when faced with mixed-agency dilemmas. Although such dilemmas require significant forethought and deft management, they are not insurmountable.

Certain professional roles and work settings in mental health prove especially likely to evoke mixed-agency and other ethical quandaries (Koocher & Keith-Spiegel, 2008). In such settings, client needs may be incongruent with those of the agency, the institution, or the public, placing the MHP in a particularly vexing ethical predicament. For instance, psychologists, psychiatrists, social workers, and counselors working in schools, medical centers, prisons, national security agencies, and even in some independent practice settings may find themselves consistently wrestling with mixed-agency conflicts. What's more, some MHPs live their daily lives as embedded or fully integrated members of the small communities (e.g., cultural, military, religious, rural) they serve; in such contexts, multiple roles with clients become ubiquitous and relational expectations constantly shift. Furthermore, MHPs in many work settings must frequently render high-stakes or "go–no-go" decisions that can have dramatic consequences on the lives of individuals. For example, should a medical patient receive a scarce organ transplant? Can a clinician serving in the military function effectively when deployed to a combat zone? Does a convicted prisoner have sufficient mental competence to face execution? Should the courts remove a child from his parents' home? Must I report a client's suicidal intent to the authorities? These questions, and many like them, can provoke anxiety, insomnia, and worse among MHPs.

The classic ethics text of Koocher and Keith-Spiegel (2008), *Ethics in Psychology and the Mental Health Professions,* contains a chapter on challenging work settings aptly titled "Juggling Porcupines." We think this notion nicely captures the sense of risk and feelings of stress that can accompany operating in certain mental health work roles and contexts. Koocher and Keith-Spiegel identify three components of these settings that make ethical practice more challenging, including the following: (1) the nature and demands of the agency, organization, or special context; (2) issues related to the specific nature of the clients and their problems; and (3) specific skills and competencies needed by MHPs who wish to work effectively with these clients in these settings. With more MHPs entering a wider array of nontraditional roles and atypical work settings, it becomes essential to think about how to behave ethically in these contexts. Most contemporary ethics texts emphasize ethical decision making in traditional counseling and psychotherapy relationships. In our view, standard texts and courses give insufficient attention to juggling such ethical *porcupines*.

The genesis for this casebook on ethically challenging jobs and work settings grew from our own work as clinicians in challenging settings (e.g., medical center, military, forensics) and as educators in training programs in which bright students often ask the difficult "what if. . ." questions, questions that defy boiler plate answers. Knowing that students and professionals alike learn best when applying ethical principles and standards to a specific scenario, we set about devising a case-driven text on challenging work roles and settings. Early on, we realized that the best ethics lessons would come from the real-life experiences of seasoned mental health professionals working on the front line—professionals who could teach through the medium of salient personal experiences. We invited mental health providers with demonstrated expertise in challenging roles and settings to contribute short manuscripts highlighting the ethical challenges germane to their work by using a highly representative case example. Although we asked contributors to carefully protect client identities by changing demographic details or combining elements of multiple cases, each case represents an actual ethical predicament in the work life of the author. Many of the cases in this collection are typical of day-to-day practice, whereas others reflect an exceptionally memorable case in the author's experience.

Each of the 38 case studies in this book is authored by an expert in psychology, psychiatry, social work, or counseling. We have clustered the cases by work setting under the general headings of psychotherapy, forensics, medical centers, national security, organizations, schools, supervision, religious settings, and public service. Each manuscript follows a similar format; it begins with a case, followed by the author's discussion of the key ethical issues evoked, a summary of the primary ethical conundrums prevalent in the work setting, and a final personal reflection in retrospect regarding how he or she handled the ethical quandary. Each contribution concludes with a summary of salient ethical principles and standards as well as a list of resources for further reading.

A quick glance at the primary ethical quandaries our contributors report reveals some consistent themes. First, the authors often wrestle with identifying their obligations to the client(s) in the case and work to clarify their clinical and ethical responsibilities to the various entities involved. Determining the identity of primary and tertiary clients is a first step in sorting one's duties to multiple parties. Second, the authors often worry about avoiding or minimizing harm. In some settings, MHPs may feel compelled to limit the freedom or overlook the best interests of one person in order to promote or safeguard the best interests of a larger group of people, or even society as a whole. Third, our authors struggle with managing multiple relationships. Many work settings create dual identities for MHPs, who sometimes must occupy more than one role vis-à-vis clients or colleagues. Contributors to this volume are acutely aware that multiple roles may compromise professional boundaries, create conflicts of interest, and generate unfair power dynamics. Fourth, authors wrestle with anticipating, identifying, and responding to conflicts between their ethical obligations and both legal requirements and organizational demands. Some of the cases in this volume highlight the risks associated with adhering exclusively to ethical standards or legal statutes while ignoring the other. Other cases focus on the conflicts that arise when the best interests of an individual client are not served by the best interests of the sponsoring or employing organization. Finally, many of the authors in this volume feel concerned about competence. Many of the work roles and contexts they describe involve unique or emerging areas of mental health practice. With little in the way of guidelines, protocols, or even precedent, our pioneering experts worry about their ability to perform with sensitivity and expertise in these unique contexts; in some cases, our contributors are helping to set the clinical and ethical standards in their practice arenas. Of course, the authors touch on other key ethical concerns as these intriguing cases unfold. Readers will find discussions of exploitation, personal problems and conflicts, conflicts of interest, maintaining confidentiality, making disclosures, providing informed consent, and ensuring that the bases of one's assessments are valid.

In the end, contributors to this volume recognize that being ethical in these challenging work roles and settings requires much more than the rote application of objective ethical standards. Although *principle ethics*—the use of rationale, universal principles or standards—constitutes an important facet of professional ethical behavior, the principle-driven MHP tends to become preoccupied with dilemmas and crises. Thus, a practitioner operating exclusively from a principle perspective waits for an ethical problem to emerge and then uses ethical rules and standards to answer the question, "What shall I do?" But are principles enough? It is clear that contributors to this volume also highlight the salience of virtue ethics when thinking about how to be ethical as an MHP. *Virtue ethics* emphasizes the internal qualities or character of the MHP. From the perspective of virtue ethics, professionals who are competent, mature, and defined by character virtues such as fidelity, prudence, humility, and integrity often prove most likely to achieve ethically satisfying outcomes. The virtue-driven MHP always remembers to ask, "Who shall I be" (Jordan & Meara, 1990) when thinking about the best way forward with a client or conflict. Although character virtues alone do not ensure effective ethical decision making, when combined with principles, virtues may help to reduce individual inconsistencies and missteps in the application of ethical principles (Jordan & Meara, 1990). Thus, the authors in this collection recognize the importance of both principles and virtues to good decision making.

We hope that you enjoy reading these masterful reflections on difficult ethical cases as much as we have. In our view, the most compelling aspect of these cases is the fact that the authors are imperfect. Although many are seasoned luminaries in the mental health field, these contributors acknowledge distress and admit errors along the road to resolving quandaries and making decisions. These experts are human; readers will learn as much from the authors' missteps as they will from their elegant solutions.

REFERENCES

Johnson, W. B., & Ridley, C. R. (2008). *The elements of ethics*. New York: Palgrave-Macmillan.

Jordan, A. E., & Meara, N. M. (1990). Ethics and the professional practice of psychologists: The role of virtues and principles. *Professional Psychology: Research and Practice*, 21, 107–114.

Kennedy, C. H., & Johnson, W. B. (2009). Mixed agency in military psychology: Applying the American Psychological Association Ethics Code. *Psychological Services*, 6, 22–31.

Koocher, G. P. (2009). Ethics and the invisible psychologist. *Psychological Services*, 6, 97–107.

Koocher, G. P., & Keith-Spiegel, P. (2008). *Ethics in psychology and the mental health professions: Standards and cases*. 3rd ed. New York: Oxford University Press.

PART I

In the Psychotherapist's Office

I

But It's a Really Nice Gift! Ethical Challenges in Responding to Offers of Gifts From Clients

Jeffrey E. Barnett

A number of years ago, I began work with a new client in outpatient psychotherapy. This woman, whom I will call Sally[1], was an adult who was experiencing difficulties concerning her family of origin. She had harbored great resentment toward her parents because of being abandoned emotionally by them. Her father had been a very successful business executive who consulted internationally. Her mother joined him on most of his trips, and Sally was raised by a series of housekeepers and nannies. As an only child, Sally realized that she felt very alone and had ongoing fears of abandonment. This had adversely impacted her relationship with her husband and her own only child, of whom she was extremely possessive. This caused numerous difficulties in her relationships with them.

Treatment progressed well over time, and she was able to work through and resolve a number of significant conflicts and issues that had been holding her back in her current relationships. Sally's functioning with her husband, with her own child, and

---

[1] The client's name, identifying information, and a number of aspects of her history were changed to help preserve her privacy. The basic issues and dilemmas remain intact.

with friends improved significantly during the course of treatment as she was able to understand these issues and resolve the significant anger, resentment, and fear of abandonment she had been harboring.

Sally's psychotherapy had progressed well, and although issues of termination had not yet been discussed with her, in my mind we were approaching the point in time when that would be appropriate. At the next session, seemingly out of nowhere, Sally asked me if I liked cameras. Taken aback by this apparent non sequitur, I inquired why she asked. Sally informed me that her husband had told her that all men like cameras, and they wanted to make sure I didn't already have one because they wanted to give me a gift to thank me for all the help I had provided to them. Although I had never met with her husband, apparently he was appreciative of Sally's progress as well. I thanked Sally for this kind thought and informed her that I am paid for the assistance I provide and that nothing further was needed, although I very much appreciated the kindness of her gesture. We then moved on to other topics in our session, and I assumed that we had left that topic behind us.

The next session began uneventfully, and we focused on changes in the relationships in her life and on reinforcing the progress she had made thus far. Sally then informed me that she had thought about it further and decided that she still wanted to give me a gift. She asked me if I had heard of a certain inn on Maryland's Eastern Shore. It is a famous inn that is very exclusive, and I had certainly heard of it. Again, I asked her why she was asking. She shared that she and her husband wanted to give my wife and me a weekend there. She said that my wife and I would really enjoy a weekend away and that I certainly deserved the break, having worked so hard and helped so many people. Although I readily acknowledge that the thought of spending a weekend all expenses paid at this exclusive resort crossed my mind, after approximately two seconds the pristine mental image was altered by the thought of being at dinner there one evening and then looking up to see Sally and her husband at the next table. I could imagine her saying, "Oh, what a surprise seeing you here. Why don't we join you?" I again attempted to share with Sally my now-tired rationale for why I could not accept a gift from her. I even discussed boundaries, ethics, the focus on her needs and not mine, and the like. She clearly was not convinced. I also tried to explore with her why this was so important to her and why it was coming up at this particular point in time. Unfortunately, this approach yielded no results. So, I thanked her again and tried to have us move on to what I thought were more relevant treatment issues.

At this time, I was receiving weekly clinical supervision from the psychiatrist in my practice, a very senior and skilled clinician. We discussed these issues in detail, and he reinforced my commitment to not accept any gifts from Sally. At the following session, these issues came up again, and I decided to use a strategy that my colleague and I came up with in supervision. I told Sally that if she felt so strongly about giving me a gift to show her appreciation to me, then I hoped that she would give a gift that I felt comfortable receiving. I was hoping that a compromise on the issue of a gift would be acceptable to her. I suggested that Sally make a donation in my name to the charity of my choice, a community mental health center that provided mental health services to needy individuals. I explained how this would be quite meaningful to me because I knew of the good it would do. I thought I had brilliantly resolved our dilemma. I quickly learned that I was mistaken. Sally informed me that that was definitely not what she had in mind; although it certainly was a nice idea to help others, her interest was in doing something specifically for me.

The issue of the gift had quickly become a major focus of our clinical work together. Although I knew I could easily just accept a gift and get it over with, something felt very uncomfortable about this. Also, I became increasingly aware of a part of me that would be very happy to receive a nice gift from her. Yet, my understanding of ethical practice made me very circumspect about this.

I continued to address these issues in supervision. I had not previously been confronted with such a challenge. The extent of clients offering me gifts up to that point in time had been limited to a plate of homemade cookies around the holidays in December. Clearly, this was a very different situation.

Then, several weeks later, Sally came to a session with a gift-wrapped box and a card for me. The card included an expression of thanks from both Sally and her husband for all my assistance over the time I had worked with her. Sally also wrote in the card that she knew she could always count on me. I opened the gift box and found a very nice watch in it. I was taken aback by this and apparently sat there in stunned silence for a few moments. Sally then said, "Read the inscription on the back." I took the watch out of the case, turned it over, and read the inscription. It said, "To Jeff, I know you'll always be there for me. With appreciation, Sally."

I found myself in a very difficult position. Should I hand it back to her and refuse to accept it? What impact would that have on the psychotherapy relationship and on the psychotherapy process? Also, I doubted she could return it because she had had it inscribed. Maybe that was part of her plan; how could I decline to accept it now? I also knew that she and her husband were quite affluent, so this gift didn't cause any financial hardship for them. Yet, I was well aware of how nice I thought the watch was and of feeling manipulated.

Having to think rather quickly about all this there in the session, I thanked her for her generosity and kindness. I also asked her why she decided to do this after I had repeatedly expressed my discomfort with her giving me a gift and had repeatedly requested that she not do so. She minimized these concerns and moved on to other topics.

As will come as no surprise by now, I continued to give all this great thought and consideration, and continued to address it in supervision. In thinking about the inscription and her family history, I decided to interpret the apparent meaning of this and to confront her on it. I did so at the next session, and after some initial avoidance of the topic, Sally then shared that she knew that treatment was coming to an end, her husband had a heart condition, and her son was leaving for college soon. She feared being left alone and acknowledged a desire to not lose me too. We addressed these issues in treatment and did not immediately terminate our work together, and I informed her that although we would need to end our work together at some point in time, she would always be welcome to contact me in the future if the need ever arose. I informed her that clients are always welcome to come back to treatment as needed in the future, and that I hoped that she would do so as well.

With some trepidation, we were then able to move forward with Sally's psychotherapy, and she successfully completed her treatment. Since that time, she has sent me a holiday card each year and has twice contacted me by phone for a brief conversation. We met for one additional session several years after termination when she was making a significant life change and wanted to discuss it with me. It seemed like a successful session, and from her annual cards it sounds as if Sally has done very well.

I didn't return the watch to Sally, even though I was quite tempted to do so. But, I've never worn the watch. I still have it in its original box in a drawer in my desk.

Discussion

Key ethical issues

A significant issue in this case is that of boundaries. Boundaries exist regarding psychotherapy issues such as the use of touch, self-disclosure, personal space, gift giving, time and location of treatment, and the like. It is widely accepted that these ground rules of the professional relationship are important to be aware of and to respect, that they should not be viewed rigidly but rather as permeable, and that a crucial distinction exists that differentiates boundary crossings from boundary violations.

The crossing of boundaries involves eschewing a strict avoidance of boundaries, but the actions by the psychotherapist are done with careful forethought and with consideration of the client's best interests; they are motivated by the client's treatment needs, not by the psychotherapist's own needs and interests, and the actions are documented as part of an agreed-upon treatment plan. Boundary violations, on the other hand, tend to be motivated more by the clinician's needs and interests, are not consistent with the client's treatment needs or treatment plan, and invariably are harmful to the client.

Although an absolute adherence to strictly enforced boundaries should be avoided, knowing when and how to cross boundaries and just where the dividing line between boundary crossings and boundary violations may be is a significant challenge for psychotherapists.

Additional ethical principles relevant to the case of Sally include beneficence and autonomy. It is important that all actions by a psychotherapist be motivated by the client's best interests and that actions be taken to not promote the client's dependence on the clinician.

Work setting

Mental health professionals in private practice may find themselves facing a wide range of ethically challenging situations. Unless one is a member of a group practice, this may be a very isolating environment in which to work. It is therefore very important that psychotherapists regularly seek out supervision and consultation from experienced colleagues. Additionally, participating in a peer consultation and support group can help by combating professional isolation and by providing trusted colleagues with whom one can openly discuss challenges and dilemmas.

Clinicians in a private practice setting generally spend much of their workday focusing on and addressing the needs of their clients. Other than documentation, returning telephone calls, and other administrative work, much of the clinician's time is spent working with clients. Over time, this may prove to be very challenging and taxing. Mental health practitioners need to engage in ongoing self-care and be sure to strike an appropriate balance among various work-related activities as well as between work and personal activities. The demands of the psychotherapy profession are great. Those who do not pay adequate attention to this balance and their needed self-care may be at risk for burnout and impaired professional competence. Clinicians experiencing these difficulties may be prone to seeking gratification of their own needs through their clients. Blurred boundaries and other potentially harmful behaviors are risks for private practitioners who do not adequately address their ongoing self-care needs.

Reflection

This case presented significant challenges despite my reviewing my profession's ethics code and relevant state laws, consulting with colleagues and discussing the case in ongoing supervision, and attempting to use a structured decision-making model. There were a number of significant challenges for me in this case. I had not initiated the possible boundary crossing or violation. Sally initiated it, and she clearly was not in any way coerced by me to offer a gift; she wanted to give the gift and saw nothing inappropriate about it. Sally did not feel exploited or harmed, did not perceive me as abusing my influence or power in the professional relationship, did not see any conflict of interest, and did not see this as an ethics issue. After all, a gift is just a gift!

On the other hand, I was very concerned about my profession's code of ethics, was aware that accepting a gift worth more than just a few dollars could possibly impact my objectivity and judgment in the future, and generally felt uncomfortable about accepting the gift. But, I consulted with colleagues, addressed the issues openly in ongoing supervision, repeatedly declined gifts from her and explained to her why accepting the gift was inappropriate for me, and even offered a more comfortable alternative to accepting a personal gift in an effort to meet her need to show her thanks to me. This final point seemed important to me because I was trying to be sensitive to her stated need to give me a gift. I didn't necessarily see her gift giving as an attempt to manipulate or control me, and this was a single gift (albeit one that we needed to discuss over an extended period of time), not part of an ongoing pattern.

In the end, I had to consider which course of action would do more harm than good. I also had to confront my own discomfort with accepting the gift and what that meant to me. As Sally suggested at one point in our discussions, perhaps my discomfort with accepting the gift was more of an issue than was her desire to give me a gift. I do know that I have been sensitized over the years about preventing exploitation and harm to clients, to focus on their needs over my own, and to act only in ways consistent with their best interests. Perhaps my great desire to not be seen as taking advantage of a client or as seeking to have my own needs met by a client (regardless of who initiated it) got in the way of seeing that sometimes a gift from a client is just an expression of thanks for meaningful assistance provided over time. Of course, the nature of the gift, how expensive it is, and how intimate and personal it is, are all relevant factors to consider. Additionally, the meaning of the giving *and* receiving of the gift should be considered as well.

In the years that have passed, I have reflected on Sally and the gift-giving situation. Each time, I have questioned myself and thought of things I could have done differently. Perhaps I should have been firmer with her when the issue of the gift first came up; perhaps I should have focused more on the meaning of the gift to her and pushed her harder here with my confrontations and interpretations; perhaps I should have refused the gift of the watch despite the inscription and the clear thought and care that went into its selection. I even questioned if I should have told her that if she insisted on giving me a gift, then I would have to end our work together in psychotherapy.

I also questioned my own motivations and wondered if I was doing anything to stimulate the gift giving, and I questioned my focus on ethical practice and wondered if I was overdoing it in an effort to not appear unethical (even to myself). As a former ethics committee member in my profession, I had prided myself on my adherence to the highest ethical standards. But, was I overdoing it? When deciding on a course of action, I had always considered how it might be seen by my colleagues. I never wanted to engage in any behaviors that would reflect poorly upon me or my profession if others were to learn about them. But, I did have to question if I was struggling with an overly strict adherence to ethical precepts that was more a reflection of my own protective stance and less a focus on what was best for Sally.

In the end, I decided against refusing or giving back the gift. I thought that would do more harm than good. I also believed that the motivations for giving the gift were sincere and that they were clearly relevant to issues being addressed in treatment. Although my own discomfort has prevented me from ever wearing the watch (a too intimate connection to a client? a too visible sign of benefiting from a client beyond the payment of my fee?), the psychotherapy relationship with Sally progressed well, her treatment was a great success, and she has moved forward with her life very positively. I'm always happy to receive her annual card and hear about how she is doing. For me, that's really gift enough.

Key ethical principles and standards

APA (2002): Principle A (Beneficence and Nonmaleficence), Principle B (Fidelity and Responsibility), Principle E (Respect for People's Rights and Dignity), Principle D (Justice), Standard 3.04 (Avoiding Harm), Standard 3.05 (Multiple Relationships), and Standard 3.08 (Exploitative Relationships).

REFERENCES AND FURTHER READING

Barnett, J. E., Lazarus, A. A., Vasquez, M. J. T., Morehead-Slaughter, O., & Johnson, W.B. (2007). Boundary issues and multiple relationships: Fantasy and reality. *Professional Psychology: Research and Practice, 38,* 401–410.

Gutheil, T. G., & Gabbard, G. O. (1993). The concept of boundaries in clinical practice: Theoretical and risk management dimensions. *American Journal of Psychiatry, 150,* 188–196.

Smith, D., & Fitzpatrick, M. (1995). Patient-therapist boundary issues: An integrative review of theory and research. *Professional Psychology: Research and Practice, 26,* 499–506.

Zur, O. (2001). Out-of-office experience: When crossing office boundaries and engaging in dual relationships are clinically beneficial and ethically sound. *The Independent Practitioner, 21*(2), 96–98.

2

Everyone I Know Knows Everyone I Know: Boundary Overlap in the Life of One Lesbian Psychotherapist

Laura S. Brown

Noreen, a mid-50s European-American woman, entered therapy to deal with her attractions to women in the context of her long-standing heterosexual marriage. Our work had been rocky. What she wanted most, and complained about getting not enough of from me, focused on mirroring and validation. When I asked her to take more responsibility for her own decisions, she got mad.

Noreen had joined a number of different support groups in the lesbian community—for lesbians over 40, for fat lesbians, for lesbian artists. Other clients of mine populated each of these groups, and because discussion of one's therapy and one's therapist commonly takes place in the culture of several of these groups, it did not take long for Noreen to ascertain the identities of six other women who were in therapy with me. I knew this because she would often make an angry point of saying, "I know you don't do this with Becky (or Georgia, or Alix, or Zoe), do you? I know you're not as hard on her as on me." My default response, "I'm wondering why you think that you're treated differently than other people, even in therapy," infuriated her, and it nicely skirted the topic of whether the other woman in question was in therapy with me, much less whether or not she was getting nicer treatment.

Noreen then began to complain about me to one of the most vulnerable of my other clients in her social networks. Zoe was struggling with the legacy of multiple real experiences of abandonment and abuse. Fearful of being kicked out of therapy because of her history, she seemed highly attuned to the possibility that a therapist, any therapist, might behave in an unjust manner toward any client. Noreen honed in on Zoe's vulnerability, and soon Zoe's therapy sessions became litanies of her worries about Noreen and how she believed I was treating Noreen, with the theme, "If you can be mean to her, you could do that to me, too. How do I know that you really care about me?" Behind my own mounting irritation with Noreen, I kept the boundaries firm, refocusing Zoe's sessions on her own terrors that I might prove as deceptive in my kindness and compassion as had some of her childhood tormentors. I sought consultation from a colleague who has similar challenges in her work life—not so much for advice, more to keep myself honest in my dealings with Noreen. I worried about how these unavoidable, and for me uncontrollable, overlaps between the lives of two clients could put each one of them at risk for harm.

I found myself steeling physically and emotionally for my sessions with Noreen. I realized that I didn't like her very much, which I could deal with. I've recited the study of Pope and Tabachnick about therapists' dislike and disgust for clients to many a trainee, and I regularly sought consultation to have another eye on my risk for counter-transference acting out. But I also realized, in my discussions with my consultant, that my work with her did not seem very effective. She seemed to mark time rather than work in therapy, and I passively colluded with her in marking time. Because of the boundaries of confidentiality, I never confronted her about how her actions undermined the welfare of another vulnerable human being. In her therapy, she replicated what she had done for 30 years in her marriage: complaining, using the relationship as a rationale for acting out, never moving forward or changing. As with her husband, she had begun to act out against me, creating a relationship in which she could experience herself as the victim while engaging in minor acts of aggression. I began to think that I had a client for whom I was not doing good, but rather had the potential to do harm, and that I might need to initiate the end of our work together because I could foresee that harm and wanted to forestall it.

My consultant agreed with my perception that Noreen's behavior constituted a parallel dance with me as it had within the relationship with her husband. She challenged me, however, on my plans to initiate termination and suggested, accurately, that I seemed prepared to banish Noreen so as to rescue Zoe from the wiles of her erstwhile friend. I felt stunned by this feedback, and I knew it was right. I felt incredibly protective of Zoe in what someone who knows me well calls my "mother bear" counter-transference stance. But that protectiveness could ultimately prove infantilizing, as my consultant pointed out. Noreen's behavior had the effect of undermining Zoe's treatment and left me unable to do as much good as I could with her. If I truly wanted to empower Zoe, it would not happen by my firing Noreen.

So I hung in with Noreen. After a while, Zoe ceased acting as her messenger, in part because she came to feel used by Noreen. I continued to maintain the fiction that I had no idea about the other woman's identity when outside her therapy session. Noreen appointed various other messengers over time. Apparently, none of them succeeded in getting the message to me.

The following spring, Noreen began to come to her sessions drenched in perfume. For many therapists this would merely prove annoying. However, anyone who has more than a casual acquaintance with me knows well that I am chemically sensitive. Perfumes have the effect of lowering my cognitive capacities by several standard deviations and increasing my irritability to well above 8 on a 10-point scale. I tell clients about my sensitivities during the first phone call, ask that they not wear scents to our sessions, and then rarely have to deal with the issue again. Noreen apologized, she had forgotten. She "forgot" the next week, and the next. The fourth week I sent her home at the beginning of her session. Back to my consultant I went. Feeling ill courtesy of Noreen at the beginning of my working day did not simply affect me, nor did it only interfere with her session. Now, five other people each week suffered aftereffects.

My consultant suggested that I give Noreen the choice of remembering that she needed to come scent-free, or treating a scented appearance as a late cancellation for which she would pay and then leave. "No scents" was a personal boundary of mine, in place for reasons of my health and capacity to function.

When I presented this proposal to Noreen, she became enraged. "I'm in menopause, how can you expect me to remember things?" she cried. "You're punishing me for being older than you. You're ageist." She stormed out, calling later that day to say that she wanted to cancel next week's session and would call me when and if she decided to come back. The subsequent month saw several "messengers" from the group for older lesbians raising concerns about my ageism. With each one, I carefully monitored the boundaries of privacy and confidentiality, respectfully explored their worries, and appreciated their willingness to bring a difficult topic into our work. Privately, I felt anger seething at Noreen's latest round of what was feeling like abuse of other vulnerable people, and I spent a number of meetings with my consultant ventilating. It seemed as if Noreen's work with me had become more about how to "get" me than about making changes, and I no longer trusted her not to make me sick.

In consultation, I came to the decision that if and when she called me back, I would decline to continue our work together, offering one closing session and several referrals to excellent colleagues.

I heard nothing directly from Noreen for about six months. Then, her voice on my voicemail: "I'd like to start seeing you again." I waited a day and called her back. "Noreen, I've done a lot of thinking and consulting about our work together. I've come to the conclusion that what we're doing isn't helpful to you, and that it's becoming more difficult for me to maintain caring and connection with you. So I'm not willing to keep working with you." I told her that we could have a final session for closure, and that I had some referrals for her that I had also carefully considered.

Predictably, she became upset. Her anger vanished, replaced by pleading. I *had* helped her, I was the only therapist who had helped her, she really needed to see me, no one else.... I held firm, knowing that I would no longer have to fear having my brain taken down by her "forgetting" or spend another client's therapy hour indirectly addressing her needs instead of those of the immediate client. She declined the final session and the referrals; I reiterated the offer and gave her the names and phone numbers of my colleagues in the letter I sent the next day.

Two days later, Zoe stormed into my office weeping. "How could you do that to Noreen? You terminated her! How can I ever trust you not to abandon me?" Now what was I going to do? I continued to owe Noreen the duty of confidentiality. I could not reassure Zoe that she had nothing to fear by telling her my rationale for my decision. I felt hugely tempted just then to rationalize that because Noreen was no longer my client, and hadn't *really* been for the 6 months that she hadn't been seeing me, I could let a little bit of detail slip about what had happened. I caught that piece of my own hostility quickly enough to keep it in check. Whatever Noreen had done, it had happened in the context of her true terror of change. I owed it to her to keep things clean, and even more, I owed it to Zoe to do that. I also owed it to myself; violating a boundary in therapy diminishes its violator, the therapist.

So I dug in for a stormy passage of work with Zoe in which she and I made use of the painful gift given us by Noreen. Zoe grieved a terrible childhood loss. She got to see me remain resolute about the privacy of everyone's therapy. Eventually, she heard more of the story from Noreen, which evoked *her* protectiveness of me: "She wore perfume to her sessions with you? No wonder you kicked her out," which then allowed Zoe to see that I would not take the invitation to demonize someone else, and that I could appreciate her care for my welfare without then sliding into a role reversal. She also found out, as did the rest of the messengers, that I took confidentiality very seriously.

Discussion

Key ethical issues

All psychotherapists must confront challenges to the boundaries of psychotherapy, and each one of us must sometimes straddle the delicate line between doing things that feel painful to our clients while doing our best to avoid harm. Maintaining confidentiality remains one of the most important boundaries of any therapist. Keeping that boundary and doing no harm when the lives of clients overlap, and the communities of the therapist and the client lead to unavoidable multiple roles, constitute the key ethical issues in this case.

Work setting

The truism (which I helped to invent) is that therapists who are lesbian, gay, bisexual, and transgendered live in a small town no matter how large the metropolitan area of their zip code. The visible lesbian psychotherapist who writes books, gives lectures, trains other psychotherapists, and has a life in which normal life events occur lives in a particularly small town. Enter your author, who fulfills all of these criteria. Having spent my entire professional career and most of my adult life living and working in the same 20-block radius geographically, and in the heart of one of this country's most open, vital, and active lesbian communities socially and politically, it has become one of my facts of life that everyone I know will eventually know everyone else I know.

My clients will know who has called me to try to get an initial appointment with me and discuss my response to that call in their sessions. My friends will know my clients, and my friends and trainees will be other friends' clients, despite my best efforts to make referrals outside my friendship network. It's a bit like living on an aircraft carrier, but with no ranks or hierarchies to create order, no rules against fraternization (except, of course, between therapist and client), and plenty of emotional distress engendered by life-long encounters with, at a minimum, sexism and heterosexism. Oh yes, and no commander of the ship who can require people to behave in a certain way.

I have navigated in these interesting waters for upward of 30 years now. Along the way I have learned some important lessons, not all of them acquired with ease and grace. My understanding of what constitutes the best interest of my clients has at times expanded as a result of their input to me about ways in which my doing the correct thing seemed mainly about covering my behind and avoiding risk. I have had to learn how to live and work effectively as a therapist practicing ethically with *this* group of people, distinct from my work with generic clients.

I do not often initiate the termination of therapy. As a feminist therapist, I tend to err in the direction of assuming that clients know when it's time to go. Many of the people I have seen over the years have needed to feel as in charge as possible of the circumstances of their comings and goings in relationship to me because of early attachment losses and severe childhood abuse. But on the very few occasions when I have exercised my unilateral judgment about when therapy needed to end, the "everyone I know knows everyone I know" phenomenon complicated the process in ways that I had not initially foreseen.

Reflection

Noreen became a teacher to whom I feel grateful. She invited me to think hard about just what confidentiality means, and how the subtleties of insuring that nothing leaks out of a therapy session are as important as avoiding blatant gossip. Interestingly, although confidentiality remains a central concern in this case, self-care is another core construct that I have come to see as I have reflected on my work with her. Seeing a consultant is a form of self-care. A consultant means that someone has my back. Psychotherapy in private practice can become lonely; with my consultant in the symbolic room with me, I had support in soothing and settling myself at those moments when Noreen acted out at her most effectively provocative.

Self-care also stood at the heart of my decision to terminate, although not perhaps in the way that would immediately spring to mind. I did in fact need to stop feeling sickened and disabled weekly. I also, and as importantly, needed not to allow myself to become a therapist who allowed herself to play first the victim of a challenging client, and then the aggressor against her in the name of interpretation or confrontation. Avoiding harm to Norine, Zoe, and all of the other women whose lives played out in that overlap meant caring for my therapist-ideal self. I could not avoid pain for Noreen unless I avoided harm to all of the people in this story, myself included. Too often, therapists stay in therapy relationships in which they allow the client to behave abusively; then they act out, abruptly terminating care or, worse, use their power to "pathologize" and shame that client's behavior after months or years of tolerating it. That does harm to the client. That harms the therapist as well.

As I wrestled with how to be a good enough therapist for Noreen, I also had to confront the responsibility inherent in my role as a therapist whose behaviors affected an entire vulnerable population, the lesbian community in Seattle. This is not my grandiosity speaking; when small community therapists transgress, the toxicity trickles into many segments of those communities, and in a community where upward of 80% of its citizens will likely enter therapy at some time in their life, it's not hard for a little trickle to get to a lot of people. Living and working in this fishbowl provides an ethics class in action almost every day.

Key ethical principles and standards

APA (2002): Principle A (Beneficence and Nonmaleficence), Principle E (Respect for People's Rights and Dignity), Standard 2.01 (Boundaries of Competence), Standard 2.06 (Personal Problems and Conflicts), Standard 3.04 (Avoiding Harm), Standard 3.06 (Multiple Relationships), Standard 4.01 (Maintaining Confidentiality), Standard 4.06 (Consultations), Standard 10.10 (Terminating Therapy). Feminist Therapy Institute (1999): Guideline 3 (Multiple Relationships), Guideline 4E (Self-Care).

REFERENCES AND FURTHER READING

Brabeck, M. M. (Ed.). (2000). *Practicing feminist ethics in psychology*. Washington DC: American Psychological Association.
Brown, L. S. (1994). Boundaries in feminist therapy: A theoretical formulation. *Women and Therapy*, 13, 29–36.
Feminist Therapy Institute. (1999). *Feminist Therapy Institute Code of Ethics*. Retrieved October 23, 2008 from http://www.feminist-therapy-institute.org/ethics.htm.
Lerman, H., & Porter, N. (Eds.). (1990). *Feminist ethics in psychotherapy*. New York: Springer.
Pope, K. S., & Tabachnick, B. G. (1993). Therapists' anger, hate, fear, and sexual feelings: National survey of therapist responses, client characteristics, critical events, formal complaints, and training. *Professional Psychology: Research and Practice*, 24, 142–152.

3

Hitler Should Have Finished the Job: Countertransference, Anti-Semitism, Abandonment, and Termination

Michael A. Grodin

First, I have an important self-disclosure to make to you, the reader. I am an observant Jew, but I do not wear a kippah (skull cap) at work. I come from four generations of rabbis. As the only son of my generation, I was expected to become a rabbi. My father, who died 20 years ago, often stated, half in jest (but there is truth to all jokes) "Had my son studied *properly,* he could have become a rabbi and wouldn't have had to go into medicine . . . psychiatry, no less." One of my past relatives was the great Rabbi Hayyim Ozer Grodzinsky, a Talmudic scholar from Vilna, Lithuania. While my grandfather left Lithuania before the Second World War, most of my family remained in Eastern Europe, and many died in the Holocaust. I began doing psychotherapy with Holocaust survivors and their children 30 years ago. Finally, I direct a program on medicine and the Holocaust at the Elie Wiesel Center for Judaic Studies at Boston University, where I also teach Jewish bioethics and Holocaust studies.

It is important to know that I did not disclose my Jewish identity to the patient in this case. I do not know if the patient had any prior information about my background, experience, or therapeutic style. There is information about me on the Boston Medical Center and Boston University Medical School Web site, and the clinic from which the patient was referred also had information about my psychotherapy practice and interests. In addition, I have published five books and hundreds of articles, and have done countless media interviews.

Ten years ago, I founded a center for the care of contemporary survivors of torture and refugee trauma. Over these past 10 years, in addition to continuing to see Holocaust survivors, I have cared for more than 250 survivors of torture from 37 countries, including many Arabic patients from Iran, Iraq, Syria, Egypt, Sudan, Saudi Arabia, and Lebanon.

I often wonder why my career has focused on studying the Holocaust and caring for survivors. Perhaps I have a need to appease my father. I may have a conscious or unconscious need to "repair" the world. I often feel the moral duty to serve as a witness. Perhaps my care for survivors fulfils a kind of rescue fantasy. After 30 years of my own therapy and analysis, I thought I was familiar with my own transferences and countertransferences. It is this background that frames the nature, context, and conflicts in the case.

Eight months ago, I received a referral from the Boston Center for Refugee Health and Human Rights to treat a Palestinian man (I will call him Abdul, not his real name). Abdul was 27 years old. Upon entering my office, I noted that he was tall, imposing, and neatly dressed, with dark skin and a heavy beard (I had a quick fantasy of an Arab perpetrator). I wondered what had brought him to therapy at this time. Upon asking what he knew about me, he related some knowledge of my experience in the care of trauma and torture victims, and in the care of refugees. I asked if he had any questions about me. Had he asked if I was Jewish, I would have explored the meaning and significance that such information would have on the therapy. If pushed, I was prepared to have responded truthfully. He did not ask, and although I had thoughts of self-disclosure, I did not pursue the issue.

Abdul was born after the 1967 Arab-Israeli Six-Day War and thus had spent his entire life in the West Bank under Israeli "occupation." Abdul came from a large family of seven brothers and sisters. His father owned a tomato farm, and his mother helped with the farm and cared for the children. Abdul often heard his father complain about the frequent boycotts in the West Bank and problems with Israeli border crossings.

Abdul's childhood was marked by extensive exposure to violence. He stated that he had begun to "hate" the Israeli soldiers. During his adolescence, he became more politically active and often had skirmishes with the Israelis. This escalated into stone throwing and physical altercations. In his mid-20s, Abdul joined Hamas and at one point considered becoming a suicide bomber. About a year before treatment, after the Second Intifada (Palestinian uprising), he was arrested by Israeli security forces and detained in prison for 2 months. While incarcerated in Israel, he was interrogated, beaten, and tortured.

Following Abdul's release from prison, he was able to get a visa and travel to the United States to visit an uncle living in Boston. He needed to get out of the Middle East and let things "cool down." It was at his uncle's recommendation that Abdul was referred to the refugee center for evaluation and treatment. Abdul wanted an older male therapist, and as the most senior member of the center and the only male therapist, I agreed to see him. I initially had reservations about working with a Palestinian tortured in Israel. It stirred up feelings of betrayal, aggression, and embarrassment. I was challenged by the blurring of the victim and perpetrator roles between Palestinians and Israelis.

Abdul complained of problems initiating and maintaining sleep, of nightmares, and of flashbacks, especially at the sound of sirens or the sight of police. He had difficulty concentrating, hypervigilance, and anhedonia. At times he had bursts of uncontrollable anger, and at other times he felt disconnected, emotionally numb, and depressed. After four sessions of "getting to know" Abdul, I explained that he clearly had signs and symptoms of post-traumatic stress syndrome and major depressive disorder. I recommended treatment with a selective serotonin reuptake inhibitor and ongoing psychotherapy.

My goal for therapy was to help the patient understand the psychological and biological reaction to trauma. This included the goals of fostering better communication, establishing a safe, nonthreatening environment, and promoting a holding environment in which he could slowly re-experience his trauma in a controlled, supportive setting. He also needed the opportunity to process his anger and hostility.

Initially, therapy progressed, with a great decrease in Abdul's symptoms. His sleep improved as a result of a combination of medication, relaxation exercises, and therapy. We talked about his childhood and family life. Abdul began to tell me about the trauma he had suffered and started to talk about his torture. He repeatedly talked about Israel and the plight of the Palestinians. He reported that he frequently got into arguments with the uncle in whose house he was staying. The fights focused on the Palestinian cause and the role of armed resistance.

After 5 months of weekly therapy with Abdul, I went on a previously planned 3-week trip to Israel to visit Yad Vashem (the Holocaust museum and archives), where I planned to teach and conduct research on a new book about the care of aging Holocaust survivors. I told all of my patients that I was going on sabbatical, would be "out of the country," and would be available by phone and e-mail; I also indicated who would be covering for me in my absence. During these 3 weeks, Abdul had no apparent problems and did not contact my office or see the covering therapist.

Upon my return, Abdul missed his first appointment (I, of course, thought of resistance, anger, and abandonment). On Abdul's next visit, he talked about feelings of anger toward the uncle with whom he was staying. Abdul felt that his uncle was "rigid" and an apologist for the Israelis. His speech was pressured, and he spoke nonstop for 45 minutes. Then, at the end of this session, Abdul exclaimed, "You know the Palestinians have suffered a holocaust, and the Israelis are the present-day Nazis." He then handed me a cartoon, clipped without attribution from an Arab newspaper. The cartoon depicts the railway to the Nazi death camp at Auschwitz-Birkenau. The Arabic sign in the foreground reads, "Gaza Strip or the Israeli annihilation camp," and the Israeli flag appears over the entrance way. Abdul then looked me straight in the eye and said, "You know, Hitler should have finished the job and killed all the Jews." I was stunned by the statement and felt violated. At the time I only listened and did not respond, choosing to remain silent and neutral. As it was the end of our time, I thought of extending the session to explore this issue further but decided to stick to the time limits of the session. I decided we could discuss this more at our next meeting.

After Abdul's statement, I became uncomfortable. I subsequently sought supervision and discussed the issue with colleagues and with my former analyst. As Abdul's next appointment approached, I planned to bring up the missed appointment and the issue of his powerful and provocative statements at end of the last session. At the next session, Abdul immediately began by talking about his anger toward his uncle and a fight over recent terrorist acts in Israel and the Israeli retaliation. I thought about interrupting him and redirecting the conversation toward his statements of the previous session. I decided against this, feeling it would eventually come up again on its own. It felt intrusive to interrupt Abdul because his flow of feelings was intense, and I felt it premature to interpret the transference. The session ended and Abdul left my office.

Abdul subsequently missed his next scheduled appointment. After 2 weeks, I called him to follow up on this missed session. He said he was "feeling better" and thanked me, but said he wouldn't be coming anymore. I encouraged him to at least attend a final session to wrap things up and to wean him from the medicine. He declined.

Discussion

Key ethical issues

Should I have accepted this patient? Should I have initially self-disclosed my Jewish background? Should I have worried about items in my office that send a message? Should I have told this patient that I was going to Israel? Should I have responded immediately to his offensive comments and printed material? Should I have extended the session to discuss his statements? Should I have insisted on discussing his statements at our next session? How long should I have waited after his missed appointments to follow up?

In my work with Abdul, I was keenly aware of clear ethical obligations, such as doing no harm, protecting my patient's best interests, respecting his rights and human dignity, and ensuring that I did not exploit or undermine him in any way. But beyond these global principles, more specific ethical considerations defied simple answers. For instance, at what point does a therapist have to place self-care above the value of continuity in the therapy relationship? Was I competent to work with Abdul in light of our stark cultural differences? Did Abdul have adequate informed consent regarding psychotherapy with a clearly Jewish psychiatrist? In light of my Jewish identity and experience with Holocaust survivors, did my personal concerns hinder clinical care? Finally, termination of therapy relationships requires considerable care and effort to further the patient's interests. The abrupt nature of our termination prevented the sort of closure and transfer that I would have preferred.

Work setting

At the office where I conduct a private practice, I have a small mezuzah (ornamental Jewish case) affixed to the outer door frame of my office. Most people do not notice it, and I have never had anyone comment on it. In my office, I have many posters, pictures, photos, and artifacts from around the world. These objects include African masks and drums, Tibetan flags, Buddha statues, a lamp from Lebanon, a box from Syria, and one poster in Hebrew. In addition to my diplomas and medical licenses displayed on the wall, there are several honorary awards for teaching and humanitarian service. One such award is a photo of the United States Holocaust Memorial Museum with an inscription citing my "profound contribution to Holocaust study and remembrance."

Reflection

Are there patients the therapist should initially decline to see, predicting an unsuccessful therapeutic encounter? And if so, who, when, and why? When, if ever, should therapists disclose facts about themselves before commencing therapy, and if so, what should be disclosed? What decorations, diplomas, or certificates should a therapist have in his or her office, realizing that all such objects may send a message to clients and are forms of self-disclosure regarding tastes, interests, and attitudes? What should clients be told about the therapist's plans of absence or vacation? How and when should therapists respond to disturbing clinical material? When, if ever, is it appropriate or even therapeutic to extend a session? Are any types of threats made directly or indirectly to the therapist unacceptable? What is appropriate follow-up for premature termination of a patient's therapy? All of these issues arose in the context of treating a patient in my psychotherapy practice. I am still working through and processing what happened and what I might have done differently.

Was this case a failure or a success? I am aware of the phenomena of transference and countertransference, which most certainly occurred here. But our final sessions gnawed at me. Why did he say, "Hitler should have finished the job"? Was he trying to provoke me? What should I have said? Was he detecting unconscious hostility, vulnerability? Was he angry at my leaving? Had he somehow found out that I had visited Israel? Perhaps he was testing me to see if I would be able to care for him, if I would be able to maintain a neutral, nonjudgmental stance, or if I would abandon him.

In looking back on this interaction, I believe I made an error in not addressing the patient's anti-Semitic statement at the outset. By not addressing this statement, I lost a critical opportunity in the therapy to explore important associations, fantasies, defenses, aggression, transference, conflicts, anger, trust, ambivalence, and issues of self-worth. These areas were left unanalyzed. Instead, at the patient's expense, I rationalized, intellectualized, and justified my oversensitivity and defense in order to avoid addressing the statement. Under the guise of neutrality, I became paralyzed. Racial, religious, ethnic, and social stereotypes are means of expressing inner conflict. Abdul's anti-Semitic statement came up at a crucial time in therapy, after my return from Israel, and my "silence" may have led to escalation and premature termination.

Final thoughts

What have I learned and what would I do differently? I am still unsure. But this case did gave me the opportunity to learn once again how important good supervision and ongoing therapy are, no matter how seasoned and experienced the psychotherapist. Through this case I became a better therapist, more sensitive and more aware of the power of transference and countertransference. As I concluded the initial draft of this case history, I left the final thoughts section with a note in the margin to myself stating "expand, elaborate, complete." After the second and third drafts, I realized that I still had not finished my final thoughts. It was at that point that I realized the parallel process of my unconscious relationship with you, the reader. I had ended my essay abruptly perhaps as a way to leave the reader unsatisfied and to mirror the premature termination I experienced with my patient Abdul.

Key ethical principles and standards

The Principles of Medical Ethics With Annotations Especially Applicable to Psychiatry (American Psychiatric Association 2008): Section 1 states, "A physician shall be dedicated to providing competent medical care, with compassion and respect for human dignity and rights," and it annotates, "A psychiatrist shall not gratify his or her own needs by exploiting the patient. The psychiatrist shall be ever vigilant about the impact that his or her conduct has upon the boundaries of the doctor-patient relationship, and thus upon the well-being of the patient. These requirements become particularly important because of the essentially private, highly personal, and sometimes intensely emotional nature of the relationship established with the psychiatrist."

REFERENCES AND FURTHER READING

American Psychiatric Association. Principles of medical ethics with annotations especially for psychiatry. Retrieved January 6, 2008 from http://www.psych.org/MainMenu/PsychiatricPractice/Ethics/ResourcesStandards/PrinciplesofMedicalEthics.aspx.

Dwairy, M. (2006). *Counseling and psychotherapy with Arabs and Muslims: A culturally sensitive approach*. New York: Teachers College Press.

Gelso, C. J., & Hayes, J. (2007). *Transference and the therapist's inner experience: Perils and possibilities*. Mahwah, NJ: Lawrence Erlbaum Associates.

Grodin, M. A., & Annas, G. J. (2007). Physicians and torture: Lessons from the Nazi doctors. *International Review of the Red Cross*, 89: 635–654.

Knafo, D. (1999). Anti-Semitism in the clinical setting: Transference and countertransference dimensions. *Journal of the American Psychoanalytic Association*, 47: 35–63.

Laqueur, W. (2008). *The changing face of anti-semitism: From ancient times to present day*. New York: Oxford University Press.

4

Suicidal Blackmail: Ethical and Risk Management Issues in Contemporary Clinical Care

David Jobes

Sheila, an attractive 24-year-old physical therapist, had an extensive history of sexual, physical, and psychological abuse and a remarkably complex set of psychological issues. She originally presented for psychotherapy with a long history of bulimia, severe depressive episodes, various acting-out behaviors, and polysubstance use and abuse. Sheila also had a significant history of suicidal thoughts and attempt behaviors. For Sheila, suicide had become a constant companion; the idea of not "having" suicide as a focal option for coping with her pain seemed simply unthinkable. In other words, the prospect of suicide became an organizing focus of Sheila's psychological world—it *comforted* her. Although suicide played a central role in Sheila's life, she willingly sought mental health care, and to that end I had worked with her for 4 years in ongoing psychotherapy. In the course of this treatment, Sheila had made three suicide attempts by medication overdoses and a harrowing near-attempt off her 17th-story apartment balcony (her boyfriend barely grabbed her at the last moment as she went over the railing). She required hospitalization on three separate occasions, and frankly, her situation had deteriorated significantly over the course of our work together.

At the year mark, Sheila again required psychiatric hospitalization for a fourth time following her fourth medication overdose of her antidepressants. At this point in her life, Sheila had become psychiatrically disabled, and she received a modest level of support from disability insurance. Her boyfriend, with whom she had lived for two years, had become completely fed up and seemed poised to end their relationship; her larger nuclear family had all but abandoned her. The situation appeared bleak, and Sheila's eventual suicide seemed only a matter of time.

As her outpatient psychotherapist, I was at my wits end. I cared deeply for Sheila and felt committed to her care, but I had also become overwhelmed and was at a loss for what to do next. We had tried every psychotherapy approach I could imagine. Sheila had undergone many trials on various medications—antidepressants, mood stabilizers, and anti-anxiety drugs—which yielded minimal results. She tried group therapy, herbs, and acupuncture; her psychiatrist considered electroconvulsive therapy as the only other option not tried, but that prospect frightened her. Thus, we had pursued multiple tried-and-true conventional approaches and various and alternative and holistic approaches. But the situation remained desperate. In truth, we both felt desperate and scared.

As I reflect back on this case now, our treatment had gone off the rails. My work with Sheila had turned into a therapeutic free fall; I felt constantly in a reactive mode and in a continuous state of anxiety and worry. By our fourth year, I found myself on the phone with Sheila almost daily, helping her get through sometimes hour-to-hour crises that she somehow managed to barely survive every day. Worst of all, I felt as though I were a prisoner within this case. Although I cared for Sheila, I also resented her. I felt blackmailed by her constant verbal threats of suicide, her obsessive suicidal thinking, and her repeated suicidal behaviors. On the one hand, I felt as if I had to do everything I could to ensure that she would not take her own life (which had come to mean over-functioning and burning myself out). On the other hand, I believed that if I backed off in any way, Sheila would undoubtedly take her own life.

As a career suicidologist, I found the prospect of a suicide outcome utterly and entirely unacceptable. At the time, I deemed that a patient's suicide would (1) completely undermine my credibility in the field, (2) render my research and professional publications bankrupt, (3) ultimately *out* me as an incompetent imposter-clinician, and (4) somehow *define* me as a professional and a person. Beyond this uncharacteristic self-doubt and castigation, I can now see that I had become personally at risk. This complex case had moved to the verge of consuming me and all that I most care for in life—my professional self, my marriage, even my sanity. Fortunately, supportive colleagues, key clinical consultants, and a remarkably patient and supportive wife all offered variations of the same theme: this cannot go on, you must make a radical change in the patient's care, to continue to work with this troubled patient in this fashion is simply not acceptable. Indeed, one particularly treasured friend and colleague looked me in the eye and said, "To knowingly continue as you are would be unprofessional—without some sort of major therapeutic change, continuing in this way would be *unethical*."

Unethical? The word stung me like a slap in the face. At first, I felt ashamed and embarrassed in the eyes of my colleague and friend; he had obviously seen that I had somehow let this complex case get out of control. But as we consulted further, he gently pointed out that I had actually done nothing wrong. He noted that the case had evolved—and unraveled—incrementally over years, with both of us (clinician and patient) doing everything we knew how to do as best we could—earnestly and in good faith. He further pointed out that I had always behaved appropriately with her and remained true in my therapeutic intent; my only "failing" involved perhaps caring too much and trying too hard. He said, "At the end of the day, her life needs to matter more to *her* than it does to *you* . . . right now that is not the case." In turn, he pointed out that my patient—whom he had seen in group treatment—was unusually and deeply disturbed. Then he said the unspeakable: "Perhaps she is simply beyond your, or anyone's, therapeutic reach; all you can do is all you can do." Reflecting on this point, I knew that he was 100% correct.

Armed with his support and insightful feedback, I began a new process of picking myself up and dusting myself off, with new clinical resolve and determination. With my patient recently transferred from the inpatient psychiatric unit to a substance abuse residential treatment setting for six weeks, I felt poised to either chart a whole new course in our work together or discontinue therapy with her. Thus, I told her the first week in the residential center that I planned to "clear the deck" and completely "reboot" our treatment plan during her stay in the residential program. After much consideration, and additional professional consultations, I wrote an extensive 12-page evaluation report describing our work together and what we had learned. Moreover, I explained that I would present a completely new treatment plan for her to consider at the end of this evaluation process. At this crucial juncture, she would then have the following options: (1) embracing the new, finite treatment plan that we could extend in the event of therapeutic progress, (2) accepting a referral to another clinician for a different course of care, or (3) taking a break from treatment altogether. Whereas I had been previously reluctant to take such a firm position, fearing it would provoke her suicide, I now plainly saw the need to render my best possible clinical judgment and recommendations for prospective care, which she could ultimately take or leave.

Naturally, Sheila responded warily—even fearfully—to my new clarity, firmness, and resolve. Frankly, the initial weeks of this new effort became quite rocky; she felt quite confused, even betrayed, by this approach. But she did find my thorough evaluation report both accurate and remarkably helpful. I believe that Sheila eventually understood that my therapeutic change of course was motivated by concern for her best interests. The previous treatment plan had become a bust. In turn, Sheila began to see and appreciate that it would in fact be " . . . unethical to knowingly continue in a treatment plan that is plainly not working."

The busted treatment plan? For four years we had largely focused directly on her painful memories of past trauma, working through feelings of betrayal, vulnerability, and terror. Without delving into the contentious debate that plagues discussions of clinical treatments for victims of trauma, let me simply say that for Sheila, "abreactive" therapy, working through her trauma history and memories of abuse, proved utterly iatrogenic (although for the record, I have many times seen this exact kind of work help other trauma victims). Plainly, we know that profound individual differences exist in how people cope and what works for whom; we intuitively know that one treatment size cannot fit all. In Sheila's case, a highly structured treatment plan that focused on "therapeutic" repression, avoidance, and containment of traumatic material proved extraordinarily helpful. We also developed a singular and intense focus on behavioral functioning and concrete goals. Although this approach would not work with every trauma victim, it helped Sheila to stabilize and then improve.

At the start of our fifth year together, we turned an imperceptible therapeutic corner and never looked back. Six months later, Sheila had gone off disability and begun working part time; still later that year, she returned to her old job and functioned remarkably well. At the six-year mark, we began a gradual process of mutually terminating our work together. After termination, Sheila relocated and soon met and then married a loving and supportive man. Today, some 12 years since we finished our work, Sheila has become an award-winning health professional, working in a large urban hospital. She is happily married and has been sober for 14 years. Finally, and most critically from my view of these things, she feels extremely grateful to be *alive*.

Discussion

Key ethical issues

As a trainer of mental health professionals, I know firsthand that many clinicians have harrowing cases, cases like Sheila's. Relevant to this particular saga, I can further attest that many professionals feel similarly "blackmailed" by a patient's suicidal thoughts, verbal threats, possible attempts, and related behaviors. The anxiety of clinical work with suicidal patients is palpable. One can easily come to feel utterly responsible for another's life, with all the accompanying convoluted clinical, moral, legal, and personal implications. The sheer weight of this life-versus-death sense of responsibility can insidiously distort a clinician's judgment, which can then lead to enmeshment and clinical over-involvement, with the clinician feeling compelled to do too much. Alternatively, the weight of responsibility can lead to abject clinical paralysis.

Ethical issues related to the prospect of clinical abandonment also lurk in this discussion. Truthfully, many clinicians understandably fear and frankly resent patients with suicide risk behaviors. They naturally want to rid themselves of the worries, hassles, and anxieties incumbent on psychotherapists who care for a patient standing on the ledge of suicide. The temptation to rid oneself of the burdensome suicidal patient can lead to acting out by the clinician, perhaps most commonly manifested as clinician-imposed hospitalizations that may prove fruitless and even unhelpful to the situation at hand. Although I believe that certain hospitalizations can save lives, I also believe that some hospitalizations have more to do with the clinician's desire for riddance (or what he or she perceives as legally protective) than with purely clinical motives.

Beyond these perhaps provocative musings, I would further contend that suicidal risk in a patient can potentially adversely affect other ethically relevant practices related to the central ethical consideration: professional *competency*. In my view, ethical and competent care of a suicidal patient involves a number of critical clinical activities, including thorough informed consent, competent clinical assessment, competent (ideally, evidence-based) clinical treatments, and appropriate risk management.

Having said this, I do fear that in general practice many clinicians often fail in these areas when working with suicidal patients. For example, clinicians too often fail to provide sufficient informed consent as to what they can do and, more critically, cannot do when helping a high-risk suicidal person and his or her family. In turn, I fear that the thorough and comprehensive assessments that suicidal states require remain rare because clinicians may fear a deeper level of inquiry. I further worry that many clinicians succumb to temptation and rely too much on inpatient hospitalizations, which often prove too brief to help. In lieu of an inpatient admission, too many clinicians I encounter still rely on utterly inadequate "no suicide" or "no harm" contracts, which protect neither the patient nor the practitioner should malpractice litigation occur. I regret that too many clinicians do not use empirically supported interventions that emphasize coping and the development of new skill sets—particularly in a suicidal crisis. Finally, I find that too many clinicians do not use sufficient risk management techniques; they often fail to embrace the use of consultations with key colleagues and fail to carefully document assessment material and a suicide-specific treatment plan within a well-maintained medical record.

I recognize that the preceding discussion reflects a rather bleak view of how clinicians in general practice commonly work with suicidal patients; I say it with no sense of superiority or relish. I do not mean to preach. But let us be plain: working with suicidal patients is scary. It is inherently challenging work, both professionally and personally. Just to clarify, my rather harsh views and genuine concerns and fears about our field in relation to suicide risk are based on four main sources: my clinical experiences, my research of 25 years in clinical suicidology, my experiences of training mental health professionals in clinical suicidology, and my work as a plaintiff and defense expert in malpractice tort litigation cases of wrongful death. Based on these varied perspectives, I have come to a rather stark and unpleasant conclusion—we have a major professional and *ethical* crisis in relation to the standard clinical care of suicidal people within the United States. It is my unvarnished view that significant changes are needed in routine clinical mental health practice if we are to have any genuine ambitions of meaningfully impacting this leading cause of premature death.

Work setting

I believe that the vast majority of suicidal patients can be appropriately and safely treated on an outpatient basis. There will always be a need for inpatient care, and I am an ardent proponent of such care for a certain subset of high-risk suicidal patients. But the reality these days is that inpatient care is severely limited by insurance constraints, and inpatient psychiatric stays are now remarkably short. Nevertheless, I hope that in coming years we may see new models of care and coverage, particularly in light of the recent passage of mental parity within the U.S. Congress.

Reflection

As I reflect on my work with Sheila, I arrive at a rather blunt and unpleasant truth. Even when a clinician provides stellar assessment and clinical interventions, and even with spectacular consultation and inspired clinical competence, determined suicidal persons can and sometimes do take their own life. It is, of course, *their* life, no matter what we think, wish, or do. This central consideration is obviously not trivial. My core struggle with Sheila was inextricably wrapped up in this consideration. I simply could not accept the prospect of her suicidal death; I could not go there. But my absolute insistence on her living, no matter what, got me (and us) into clinical trouble over time. In hindsight, much of what came to ultimately plague my treatment of Sheila directly followed from my dogmatic, if unconscious, insistence that suicide was an absolute non-option.

Herein lies a reflective paradox at the heart of the matter: *suicide is always an option*. What I have now come to appreciate (at least intellectually) since my work with Sheila is that even expert professional competence in clinical suicidology will never *guarantee* that I will never lose a patient to suicide. Herein lies another paradox: this realization is simultaneously grim and also quite liberating. As my dear friend and consultant noted, I can do what I can do . . . but what I can do is a lot! This pragmatic truth was crucial in my ability to re-engage Sheila in a whole new line of treatment.

Thus, the central clinical question is not whether a patient *can* take her own life; she most certainly can on a daily basis. Rather, the central question is whether the patient *should* take her own life while engaged in a mental health treatment designed to save her life. This is not a mere ploy or a play on words, it is central to my thesis. The central clinical question at hand for patients is whether they are willing to seek a clinical treatment that potentially renders suicidal coping obsolete. One can readily argue to the patient that he or she has everything to gain and nothing to lose by engaging in a life-saving treatment over a finite period of time. If the treatment does not work, the patient is free to pursue other "options" for dealing with his or her pain and suffering.

I fully appreciate that these arguments may seem quite provocative, but I contend that we communicate an empathic respect of the patient's pain and struggle when we take this position properly. From Sheila, I learned to disengage from the power struggle of *whether suicide* to more properly focus on *if not suicide, then what instead and for how long?* To be clear, I am a passionate suicide preventionist, but I am also a student of suffering, human nature, paradox, pragmatism, and the importance of hope in dealing with suicidality. Indeed, there is something quite powerful in offering a potentially life-saving treatment that can be juxtaposed with other possible options, which of course include *not being in treatment*. The unique and skillful interplay of clinical empathy, respect, autonomy, and the presentation of alternative prospects for coping can become a compelling recipe for instilling the seeds of hope in a suicidal person. The goal is to raise in the patient the following considerations: maybe there is a way out of this hell; I guess I can give this treatment to save my life a try; there is no downside to trying this for now because I always have the option of suicide *later*.

The above observations are just some of the things that Sheila helped me to understand about the effective care of suicidal people. In the case of Sheila, I visited the limits of my clinical endurance, influence, and ability to care for another person. All these years later, I am so grateful to Sheila for putting up with my earnest—yet largely unhelpful—clinical efforts. The irony that I came to appreciate (and now fully embrace) was that my hard-earned ability to recognize my clinical limits, and contemplate the loss of my patient to suicide, created a crucial turning point in what proved to be a potentially life-saving treatment. Let us thus face the facts: we no longer have the luxury of simply locking up suicidal persons in an inpatient setting until they come to their senses. But here is the final paradox: when a clinician perseveres and finds a way to be forthright and honest, and to disengage from the suicidal power struggle with the patient, the prospect for pursuing a truly life-saving course of care can be created and clinically realized.

Key ethical principles and standards

APA (2002): Standard 2.01 (Boundaries of Competence), Standard 2.06 (Personal Problems and Conflicts), Standard 3.04 (Avoiding Harm), Standard 10.01 (Informed Consent to Therapy), Standard 9.02 (Use of Assessments), Standard 10.10 (Terminating Therapy).

REFERENCES AND FURTHER READING

Jobes, D. A. (2006). *Managing suicidal risk: A Collaborative approach.* New York: The Guilford Press.

Jobes, D. A., Rudd, M. D., Overholser, J. C., Joiner, T. E. (2008). Ethical and competent care of suicidal patients: Contemporary challenges, new developments, and considerations for clinical practice. *Professional Psychology: Research and Practice,* 39: 405–413.

Rudd, M. D., Joiner, T., Brown, G. K., Cukrowicz, K., Jobes, D. A., Silverman, et al. (in press). Informed consent with suicidal patients: Rethinking risks in (and out of) treatment. *Psychotherapy.*

Werth, J., Welfel, E., & Benjamin, G. (2009). *The duty to protect: Ethical, legal, and professional considerations in risk assessment and intervention.* Washington DC: American Psychological Association.

5

An Affair to Remember: Protecting Vulnerable Clients and Confidentiality When Spouses Cheat

Mary Ann McCabe

Family A. John's parents consulted me when he was seven years old for help with early academic problems, tantrums, inflexibility, and problems with peers. Psychological testing confirmed a diagnosis of attention-deficit disorder and additional anxiety. John had a younger sister who was three years old at the time. John's parents requested assistance with managing his challenging behavior and helping him adjust to school. However, after only two sessions, Dad reported that he planned to move out of the family home, owing to dissatisfaction that had grown over the years. John's mother accused her husband of having an extramarital affair, which he adamantly denied. The parents asked that the focus of therapy turn to helping them inform the two children that Dad would be moving out, and to advise them about the developmental and emotional best interests of the children as they moved toward divorce. Because they also entered mediation, I could truly focus on consultation regarding the children's best interests.

I split the sessions between individual time with John and consultation with his parents. Time with John was focused on helping him manage the anxiety, sadness, confusion, and self-reproach that resulted from his Dad leaving home. Time with the parents included discussion of the full range of issues that emerge as parents of young children separate: visitation schedules and how these might vary according to the children's ages; whether to hold visitation in the family home, with the other parent leaving; establishing a second "home" environment that is beneficial for young children, with new traditions; maintaining consistency and routines; managing challenging behavior, made worse by the emotional turmoil surrounding the parents' separation; and minimizing conflict and criticism of the other parent in front of the children. Fortunately, the parents had minimal conflict *during* the sessions, although John's mother periodically reiterated her accusation that her husband had left the marital relationship for an affair, which he continued to deny. In one session, she raised the fact that John had told her he had spent time with his dad and a female friend (and her children) during one visit, which John insisted was just a work gathering with a number of colleagues.

Family B. Eight months after I began seeing John and his parents, Joy's parents were referred by a co-worker of Mom's. Joy was 4 years old, and she had a younger brother age 14 months. Joy had begun showing signs of extreme anxiety and sadness at home, at preschool, and in child care. She had particularly dramatic struggles with her mom, including difficulty separating. Mom also reported having significant depression, for which she had started to see a therapist. Extended family members had begun weighing in with advice, adding to the stress in the family. The parents requested help in teaching Joy more effective skills for coping with anxiety and building her self-esteem. They also reported significant marital conflict, including many disagreements about parenting, and they requested assistance in becoming more consistent with Joy. After only four sessions, the parents asked for a "different kind of session," reporting that Mom had revealed an extramarital affair with a co-worker of one year's duration. Dad was devastated, and Mom felt very guilty and depressed. They asked to shift the focus of therapy to how to manage their emotional turmoil with the children, and they also wondered if I would see them for marital therapy. I suggested that the children's best interests and both of their individual best interests might no longer prove fully congruent, so I referred them elsewhere for marital therapy.

Immediately after the infidelity revelation, I suspected that Family B's initial referral to me had actually come from the father in Family A, who may well have been the "co-worker" engaged in the affair with Joy's mom over the last year. I felt certain when I confirmed that both worked in the same department, not merely the same large company, and put the timing together in the case history. I wondered about any potential conflicts in my continuing to see both families for parent consultation about issues for their children related to separation and divorce. I could not reveal or discuss these conflicts without revealing to all four spouses that both families had entered treatment, thereby breaching confidentiality. I could not even reveal to the referring partner, or the referred partner, that I had become aware of the source of the referral between them without compromising confidentiality that treatment had begun with the second family. In a sense, it felt as if the therapeutic relationship with me was being brought into the affair, rather than that the affair was being brought into the therapy sessions. I worried about the practicalities of ensuring that the two couples would never meet in my waiting room.

All four spouses appeared vulnerable: the two spouses who had been deceived about the affair were already harmed by the betrayal and breach of trust, yet still unsure about permanently ending their marriages, and the two spouses engaged in the affair were vulnerable to losing their spouse and/or their lover. Despite these realities, the children in these two families appeared to be the *most vulnerable*. In addition to the preexisting difficulties for which they had been referred in the first place, they now exhibited worsened behavior and emotional concerns while their parents were in various stages of emotional crisis (and unavailability). At the same time, these families were undergoing inevitable changes in their physical and financial stability that also affected the children.

The clinical dynamics changed immediately in both cases because I had become privy to possible "secrets" with an unknown number of keepers of secrets: the affair was confirmed (while Dad in Family A continued to deny it to his wife); the referral to me had come from *within* this affair; both couples and their children were seeing the same therapist regarding recent or impending separation. I had been deceived by the two parties in the affair and wondered about the meaning of this power and deception for them. I wondered if they were discussing therapy sessions outside their own family. Yet, if I were to speak with either of them about this situation, it would create a troubling clinical dynamic of my entering into private conversation with them without their spouse—whereas my therapeutic relationships involved the two sets of spouses/parents about their unique goals and struggles of shared parenting. If during the course of this work I were to inadvertently "help" either marriage, it would be at the expense of the affair, or if I were to inadvertently help to sustain the affair, it would be at the expense of one or both marriages; I would thereby be contributing to harm for someone with whom I had a therapeutic relationship.

My work with each family was made more stressful by the concurrence of the two cases. Clearly the most comfortable solution for me would have been to end my work with both families and refer them to separate therapists. However, I worried that these two children seen individually and any or all of these parents would experience this as abandonment. I wondered if perhaps the two involved in the affair would experience it as a moral judgment or "punishment" of sorts, when what they needed was therapeutic stability for their children and their parenting in a very complex, high-stakes situation. Although not the focus of my work, it was clear that these two individuals had significant emotional and attachment difficulties that were contributing to their relationship decisions, and that might heighten their sense of abandonment with therapy termination. These same underlying difficulties were making shared parenting difficult, yet each of these parents was committed to therapy with this goal.

After seeking consultation about the decision, I agreed to continue to advise the parents in Family B regarding the children and parenting decisions. Mom reported seeking a new therapist for herself, and I gave Dad some recommendations for his own individual therapy to help him through this period of crisis. However, shortly thereafter, these parents decided to focus their energy on individual and marital work in order to determine whether to remain married. They called six months later to request another consultation about the children. They had decided to separate because Mom had resumed the affair. At this time, Dad revealed that he had learned over the ensuing time that they had actually been referred to me by his wife's lover, who had brought his son for therapy. However, he did not feel this presented an obstacle to my helping them concerning their children, and he thanked me for having referred them to someone else for marital therapy. I acknowledged to Dad that indeed it had been important for me to protect confidentiality but did *not* acknowledge to him that I, too, had been deceived about the source of referral—suspecting it on my own only after some time. This felt like an unnecessary disclosure that would have stemmed from my own feelings and would compromise my therapeutic neutrality by my joining him in our mutual experience of having been lied to. I did, however, reinforce that it had been, and continued to be, important for me to maintain the children's best interests as the focus of my work with them. The couple met for two additional sessions to discuss considerations regarding telling the children about impending separation and shared parenting. Once again, they discontinued parenting work and resumed marital therapy when Mom promised to end the affair for good.

Discussion

Key ethical issues

This pair of cases brought to life several ethical issues, which together generated one of the most unusual dilemmas I have faced in my clinical practice.

A primary ethical consideration for me was clarifying who was my primary client/patient in each case, and the relationship I should have with each of the four parents and the children. As is often true in clinical work with children, I felt a professional duty to each child *and* both of the parents in both cases. And, as is common in work with couples and families, particularly parents undergoing separation and divorce, the "best interests" of one member of a family did not necessarily agree with the best interests of another. Therefore, in weighing the decision about continuing treatment, I emphasized consideration not merely of "Who is the client?" but also of "Who is the most vulnerable client?" In both cases, I determined it to be the children, and this was the basis for my decision to continue the professional relationship with these two families. It was crucial that I maintain a focus on the children's well-being and the parenting, and try to avoid discussions related to the parents' relationship. The reasoning and decision in these cases would have been different had the primary client, or even the most vulnerable client, been one of the spouses rather than their children.

The ethical issues involved with working with couples and families were still relevant here. For example, it is often difficult for the therapist to maintain a nonjudgmental stance in working with separating or high-conflict couples when the parents' own needs cloud their judgment about their children. It was that much harder in this pair of cases, in which one of the two parents was more overtly the "bad guy." It required a weighty and continuous process of checking myself to ensure that I was maintaining therapeutic neutrality.

Perhaps one of the most complex ethical considerations in working with couples and families pertains to confidentiality, and that was a cornerstone of my decision making in these cases. In beginning work with Family A, I clarified my obligation to maintain confidentiality, as I typically do with cases concerning children and their parents. First, I reassured them that their work with me was of a confidential nature. Furthermore, I advised these parents that although they maintained legal privilege, under ordinary circumstances I do not share information from individual meetings with children unless I deem it particularly important for their safety or well-being. (I also reassured them that there is rarely information in these sessions that parents do not know about; rather, this protection is a vehicle for the therapy relationship with children.) I did *not* promise the parents in either case that I would keep information confidential from their spouse.

This became quite murky in this pair of cases as information became available that would be of interest within the couple, but it emerged in psychotherapy sessions with a separate family. For example, when the affair was confirmed for the dad in Family A (who continued to deny it to his wife), it was not his revelation that could be shared, or encouraged to be shared, but a revelation in Family B. I was never able to acknowledge to either couple whether the other was or was not in treatment; indeed, both families took "breaks" from treatment. Ironically, my knowledge of the affair and the overlap was confined by confidentiality but caused me to be an unwilling participant in the deception—however ethically justifiable. Although I could not make these disclosures myself, I longed for everyone to know the same amount of information as the other parties involved. I prepared myself to manage any resultant mistrust.

A related ethical issue that required careful thought involved the multiple relationships, and possible conflicts among my obligations, in these concurrent cases. When the issue of marital separation arose in each case, I did clarify that my therapeutic relationship prohibited me from assuming a conflicting role, such as that involved in legal determinations about custody. I recommended in advance that they pursue an independent professional for that work should it become necessary. I also advised them that the therapeutic work needed to remain confidential in order for it to be effective and for them to feel safe going forward. With these clarifications, a therapeutic focus on the children, and clear boundaries regarding the parents' relationships, I felt that it was possible to maintain my objectivity and effectiveness and avoid exploitation or harm to the parents or children. Helping the children and assisting parenting in one family did not conflict with similar goals for the second family.

However, I found that I entered each session aware of the possibility that my relationship with these two families might *become* problematic at any time. For example, had the parents involved the children in keeping secrets, or had the affair evolved toward a new marriage, I would have felt that my therapeutic efficacy was more compromised. Therefore, I remained vigilant to the possibility of needing to refer one or both families to other therapists if they ceased to benefit or if I found it too difficult to remain objective.

Both families—children and parents—were struggling with issues of attachment and loss as they underwent, or were threatened with, separation. This gave heightened salience to their ability to trust the therapy relationship and its continuity, which contributed to my decision to continue working with them. However, I would have made a different decision if a psychotherapy relationship had not already been formed when I learned of the connection between these two families. In that situation, I could end my professional obligations to the second family without considerations of abandonment.

Interestingly enough, I encountered a *second* pair of cases in the same year in which this was indeed the case. As with the first pair of cases, marital infidelity and deception about the source of referral linked the second pair.

However, this time I was better prepared. The first family in the pair was referred by a colleague but attended only a few sessions. A few years later, the family returned for help for their daughter's heightened anxiety after the dad left the family home for an extramarital affair. At the end of one session, Dad mentioned in passing that he had given my name to a friend. This is commonplace, so it did not raise any red flags. However, a few months later, a new family called for a single consultation session to discuss preparing their four young children for an impending separation. Mom had recently revealed she was having an extramarital affair and wanted to leave the marriage. Dad, who called to make the appointment, stated that his wife had my name from her individual therapist, so all seemed well. The parents requested advice regarding informing the children about the separation and tailoring visitation to each child's developmental needs. Their immediate needs were satisfied with the initial consultation session. Yet, upon meeting the family, I became suspicious that this mom and the dad in the other family were romantically involved, and that this mom was the "friend" whom the other dad had referred.

Had I not had recent experience with the pair of families previously described, I might not have become suspicious. It undoubtedly helped me to prepare to handle this second pair of cases differently. In this instance, I suspected the relationship (and potential conflict) *in advance* of entering a therapeutic relationship with the second family, having completed a consultation with them. Some months later, as the marital separation and visitation decisions progressed, Dad called back to request additional sessions. Dad reported having learned from his wife that she had lied about the source of the referral, that she had actually been referred by her lover, who was seeing me for help with his daughter. Dad stated that he had carefully considered this and still wanted to proceed with further sessions because he trusted that my professionalism and ethics would prohibit me from having a conflict. However, I declined to see the parents again. I reinforced his sense that careful ethical practice made it possible to maintain therapeutic focus on his children and parenting in this situation. Yet I recommended that *clinically* it was in his best interests not to be encumbered by wondering if my advice was at all influenced by the other family. He should simply not have to share the same therapist in this situation. I referred these parents to another therapist for work to resolve conflict about shared parenting.

Work setting

My private clinical practice is in a major metropolitan area, with an abundance of highly skilled therapists. I remain surprised that not one but two pairs of cases with these ethical issues appeared in my practice in the same time frame. This situation may be more common than realized, particularly in communities with fewer mental health resources.

Reflection

I found the process of seeking consultation essential in thinking through the ethical issues and decisions in these cases. Furthermore, although ethical considerations may have led to the consultation, the process was also very helpful for my clinical work because it afforded me an enhanced opportunity to pay special attention to my countertransference with the two spouses/parents involved in the extramarital affair, their varying stages of deception to their families and to me, and my wish to extricate myself from the situation. For the duration of my work with these two cases, I wished that all of the parents knew of the affair and the overlap in therapy relationships, and I agreed to continue under these circumstances. I would have felt more respectful of each, of their dignity and self-determination.

Key ethical principles and standards

APA (2002): Principle A (Beneficence and Nonmaleficence), Principle B (Fidelity and Responsibility), Principle C (Integrity), Principle E (Respect for People's Rights and Dignity), Standard 3.04 (Avoiding Harm), 3.05 (Multiple Relationships), 3.06 (Conflict of Interest), 4.01 (Maintaining Confidentiality), 10.02 (Therapy Involving Couples or Families), and 10.10 (Terminating Therapy).

REFERENCES AND FURTHER READING

American Psychological Association. (2002). Ethical principles of psychologists and code of conduct. *American Psychologist, 57,* 1060–1073.

Hodges, W. (1991). *Interventions for children of divorce: Custody, access, and psychotherapy.* New York: Wiley.

Imber-Black, E. (1999). *The secret life of families: Making decisions about secrets.* New York: Bantam.

6

Trapped by Trauma: When Clients Cannot or Will Not Protect Themselves From Harm

John Peteet

I first saw Gail in her early 20s. She was referred by a church leader for anxiety that interfered with her sleep and ability to work. She reported growing up as a "sensitive" child in a fundamentalist Christian family and feeling most anxious when expected to attend family functions; she explained that she could not refuse, both because she felt obligated ("Children obey your parents") and because she feared that the consequences of refusal would likely prove harsh. Many years before, her mother had threatened to leave her father unless he stopped drinking. Ever after that, her mother had supported his "strict" disciplinary practices, which included lining the children up, stripped to their underwear, for beatings.

Gail initially presented as very neat, mildly overweight, and engaging but anxious, with an evident desire to please and a clear preference for asking about me rather than talking about herself.

Several weeks into weekly therapy, I found her after a session sobbing in the stairwell. She admitted to feeling overwhelmed and suicidal; shortly thereafter, she told me that her father had sexually assaulted her, beating her when she resisted, and that this represented only one more incident in a pattern that had begun in childhood. She had managed to move away from her parents and achieve months of relative stability, but she never felt safe or able to refuse invitations to return home. Each incident of abuse left her apprehensive, ashamed, at times suicidal, at times dissociating for hours, and afraid of letting anyone know what her life really felt like. Her closest male friend broke off contact with her when she would not report her father's behavior to authorities.

Fearful of my rejecting her as well, she nevertheless became more open with me over time. At least every few months, she would call me at home when feeling overwhelmed and suicidal, fearful of talking with anyone else, who might take control away from her by committing her to a hospital. At these times I felt torn. On the one hand, I hoped to strengthen her trust in me and her ability to manage her feelings by talking them through. On the other hand, I feared that allowing her to rely on my availability to do so was supporting an unrealistic dependence on me, at the expense of her learning other strategies, including being proactive to protect herself. In time, we agreed that to avoid hospitalization, Gail had to agree to stay in close contact with me and/or have a friend with her until she felt in more control. At times, I would insist on speaking with the friend to ensure that she understood my concern for Gail's safety, even though this threatened confidentiality.

Over the next several years, this pattern intensified her dependence on me and heightened her anxiety about what I thought, or might do. It also seemed to provide some leverage to encourage steps that she could take toward independence and safety. I was encouraged that she ultimately confided in some friends and her brother, avoided overnight stays at family events, and found an apartment some distance away. At one point, she also spoke with her father's pastor, who met with him for a time and obtained a promise to continue meeting, until her father found another church. However, her father's anger at these steps led him to continue to pursue and beat her, and on one particularly brutal occasion, when he was impotent, he penetrated her with a screwdriver. Afterward, she was shaken, shocked, hurt, and (uncharacteristically for her) briefly angry toward him. She expected me to be angry, both with him and with her, but was touched by my horror and sadness and agreed to go to an emergency department for an evaluation, where the staff were horrified as well. They collected forensic evidence and told her they had no choice but to file a police report, given the evidence they had for rape. This led to her father's arrest and the convening of a grand jury. The district attorney obtained a written statement from her and pressed her to testify as well. Her father's attorney arranged for his transfer to a psychiatric unit, and when Gail ultimately could not bring herself to testify against him ("I don't want to see him in jail—I just want him to get help"), the authorities released him. During this process,

I felt torn, on the one hand wanting her to follow through with what seemed to me the only realistic way to stop his abuse, and on the other to continue functioning as a therapist by enhancing her ability to think through for herself the decision with which she and her family would forever have to live.

Meanwhile, under the strain, Gail became less able to continue her work as a nanny, lost contact with concerned friends, and became insistent that she needed more of the benzodiazepine medication that I had prescribed for use on an "only as needed basis" rather than on a daily basis. I persuaded her to attend a partial hospital program, where she met a fellow patient, an abuser of prescription medications, and moved in with him. I learned through a call from a pharmacist that she had crudely altered a prescription of mine to supply both of them. In the next session, I confronted her with this, trying to make clear that I was not interested in punishing her but needed to be able to trust her in order to remain her prescriber. She was initially apologetic and had her boyfriend come in to explain that he had been responsible for asking her to help him out. However, she continued to insist that she needed more anti-anxiety medication, and for the first time, she became angry with me in a sustained way for refusing to give her more than small amounts on a frequent basis. When she appeared at sessions seeming intoxicated, I refused to prescribe more, and she found another psychiatrist who would. I was not surprised that she would not allow him to contact me, and I was very frustrated and sad to learn later that she had sustained major injuries in an automobile accident after falling asleep at the wheel. Eventually she returned, physically disabled, to live with her family, now in another state. From there, she gave me permission to release information about her treatment to her new psychiatric providers, and thanked me.

Discussion

Key ethical issues

Several related questions—raised by the ongoing damage that Gail was suffering at the hands of her father—caused me considerable angst. First, how could I help her to protect herself? She trusted me with her story only after deciding I shared her faith and would remain available in her crises. This gave me a special, privileged role, but I struggled to find the optimal balance between its risks and benefits. On the one hand, I had therapeutic influence to use in helping her make some changes and to learn strategies for coping when she became suicidal. On the other hand, I ultimately failed to help her change enough to stop the pattern, and her dependence on me became an obstacle to widening her circle of therapeutic supports; she consistently took my encouragement to do so as rejection.

I had hoped to be able to draw on our shared faith in helping her to respect and protect herself, but the differences in our theological perspectives and spiritual experience raised the issue of whether I was acting in a pastoral or a traditional psychiatric role, and of how to think about the boundaries between these. Her insistence on seeing only a Christian therapist seemed to reflect a fear that an outsider might unfairly judge her family's authoritarian system of belief, and also some wish that I could help her enlist her faith in moving forward. Although I initially hoped that a church community could help support her in re-evaluating the primitive and rigid aspects of her experience of God, her anxiety and shame prevented her from even attending services. And when her questions of me uncovered differences in our view of God (e.g., loving, punitive, indifferent), she became more anxious. Even my efforts to explore her faith-based ideas about the meaning and consequences of suicide proved disappointing. She acknowledged that God did not favor suicide but also felt strongly at times that she would feel better off in his presence. The rigidity of her religious beliefs and practices made it difficult for me to demonstrate respect for them; I struggled to remain culturally sensitive to her religious stance. I ultimately decided to accept whatever positive transference and trust my faith engendered, without confronting her beliefs unless they seemed to be life-threatening (when she used them to rationalize suicide) or expecting that she would let a faith-based resource speak to her core difficulties.

Second, what was my obligation to protect her if she was incapable of protecting herself? Because she was a legally competent adult, her abuse did not fall into any category of reportable offenses that would mandate disclosure to an outside state agency. From an ethical perspective, I wanted to promote her autonomy, independence, and confidentiality, but this came into conflict with my duty to protect. At times, I pushed the limits of respect for her privacy by insisting that she let me talk with a friend who could stay with her to help her avoid hospitalization, or take her to an emergency department for evaluation. Should I have done more, such as insist that a family meeting, a domestic violence referral, or a restraining order be a condition of my continuing to treat her? Ultimately, I decided no. I made this decision both because her parents had made it very clear that they opposed her treatment, and also because she would need to tolerate seeing her father jailed if any legal intervention had a hope of success.

Complicating my struggles with these questions were feelings that Gail and her situation evoked in me; at times, these feelings were intense.

In sequence, they included first protectiveness, then frustration and anger, and finally helplessness. Not surprisingly, she proved quite attuned to whether I felt angry and acknowledged feeling paralyzed when she sensed that I had become angry with her. Aware of how much deception, collusion, and manipulation marked her family life, I tried to respond with honesty to her questions. Yes, I did feel angry at times with her, but because she had not called me sooner, and I felt more sad than angry that she yet again found herself in so much pain. I also downplayed how angry I felt with her father and mother out of concern that Gail would feel even more need to protect them.

Work setting

I saw Gail in an outpatient setting within the general hospital where she received her medical care. This had the advantage of being a familiar, trusted place but the major disadvantage of lacking an inpatient partial group or dialectical behavior therapy (DBT) program as part of a continuum of care. When she eventually accepted a partial program, I did not work on site and thus could not completely support her full participation. Although my hospital does have an active domestic violence program, she successfully resisted involvement.

Reflection

In important respects, Gail's trapped state seemed to resemble that of many severely addicted individuals and adults subject to violence and/or intimidation (e.g., cult members, victims of domestic violence) who require a period of physical separation and intensive intervention in order to recover. Their treatment can seem similarly frustrating and uncertain, given that the process of bringing such individuals to readiness for change can take years and may never succeed. Treatment with a patient such as Gail risks the acting out of countertransference wishes either to rescue or to disengage from the patient. Of course, at times disengaging until an individual "hits bottom" provides the only effective way to avoid enabling continuation of a destructive pattern. At other times, coercion has a legitimate role, as in the court commitment with family support of addicts who endanger their own health. Yet disengaging can also feel tantamount to premature abandonment, and well-intended coercion can itself become abusive. Exit counseling has largely replaced the forcible deprogramming of cult victims.

One principle helpful to me in negotiating these potentially treacherous waters was to *never worry alone*. Discussion of Gail's case with colleagues over the years both evoked a fuller awareness of my own feelings (often in response to theirs) and provided opportunities to see my options in a new light.

Key ethical principles and standards

Relevant documents for dealing with the ethical issues raised by this case include the chapters on boundary violations and confidentiality in *Ethics Primer of the American Psychiatric Association* (2001) and the American Psychiatric Association resource document entitled "Religious/Spiritual Commitments and Psychiatric Practice" (2006).

REFERENCES AND FURTHER READING

Glick, S. M. (2000). The morality of coercion. *Journal of Medical Ethics*, 26, 393–395.

Kinzie, J. D., & Boehnlein, J. K. (1993). Psychotherapy of the victims of massive violence: Countertransference and ethical issues. *American Journal Psychotherapy*, 47, 90–102.

Peteet, J. R. (1994). Approaching spiritual issues in psychotherapy: A conceptual framework. *Psychotherapy Practice and Research*, 3, 237–245.

Peteet, J. R. (2004). *Doing the right thing: An approach to moral issues in mental health treatment*. Washington DC: American Psychiatric Publishing.

Willbach, D. (1989). Ethics and family therapy: The case management of family violence. *Journal of Marital and Family Therapy*, 15, 43–52.

7

To Warn or Not to Warn: That Is the Question

David L. Shapiro

Most mental health professionals will recognize the case of *Tarasoff v. Regents of the University of California* (1976). In this case, the court ruled that when the therapist believed that his client posed a threat of imminent harm to an identifiable third party, he had the obligation to take some action to protect that third party. Many states followed California's lead and, through either statute or common law, added some language to the body of state law dealing with a duty to warn or protect third parties under such circumstances.

In the early 1980s, I practiced in a state (Maryland) where no such case law or statute then existed. In fact, the only case addressing the issue noted, "The lips of the therapist are sealed shut by statute, subject to being unsealed only by the patient or the patient's authorized representative" (*Shaw v. Glickman*, 1980). In other words, in Maryland at that time, breaching confidentiality under such circumstances would have violated the law. Nevertheless, the *Ethical Principles of Psychologists and Code of Conduct* of the American Psychological Association in effect at that time permitted such disclosure in cases involving imminent danger of harm to self or others. In short, although the law said do not disclose, this was incongruent with my ethical obligations.

Against this background, I began seeing for individual psychotherapy a man referred to me by his urologist. While on the job, he had entered an elevator, which then plunged 10 floors. Remarkably, he survived the fall but consulted the urologist because of some injuries that had led to blood in his urine. The urologist referred him because he recognized that the man had serious depression, in addition to kidney problems. I conducted an intake assessment, along with a battery of psychological tests; these led me to conclude that the man clearly needed psychotherapy. At that time, he thanked me politely but said that he thought he could take care of his problems by himself.

About eight months later, he called me, sounding quite distraught on the telephone. He reported having increasing problems controlling his anger. He recounted an incident in which he became furious about a minor situation and punched a hole in the wall of his apartment. He also stated that he had almost run down a motorcyclist with his car when the motorcyclist cut him off and seemed "rude" to him. His live-in girlfriend regarded this as a dramatic change in his behavior and insisted that he call me to make an appointment. The client had always regarded himself as "in total control" while in his previous occupation (serving on the county police force) and as "never losing my cool," even in some very dangerous situations. His loss of control of his anger in these two situations, therefore, became of major concern to him. He also described some unusual dissociative-like experiences, some associated with the violent behavior and some that occurred quite independently of them. At the time of some of the episodes of violence, he said that he had a feeling of depersonalization, as if he were standing off and looking at someone else performing the acts.

History revealed that he grew up in an intact family, although he described his father as an alcoholic. He said, however, that his father never behaved abusively to either him, his younger sister, or his mother. He described his father as "a happy drunk" who died when the client finished college in his early twenties. His mother had not remarried. The client had married once and by that union had a 14-year-old son who currently lived in another state with his mother; the client saw him on vacations for a few weeks at a time. As previously noted, the client had served as a county police officer, had skill in weapon use, and had charge of the K-9 squad. He had retired from the police and set up his own business selling automotive parts. He described himself as somewhat of a "risk taker" and getting a "rush" out of doing "dangerous things," such as climbing mountains and racing cars. As noted earlier, he lived with a woman whom he had known for about two years. At the end of the first session, I provided him with an informed consent form, which among other things detailed possible limits of confidentiality in the event I became concerned that he posed an imminent danger to some identified third party. This practice derived from the APA *Ethics Code* because no applicable case law existed and the Health Insurance Portability and Accountability Act (HIPAA) did not exist. He understood this and readily accepted it.

I soon became concerned, given the nature of his symptoms, with some possible neurological involvement (e.g., sudden explosive rages, disorientation, depersonalization), as well as the need to help provide him with some immediate symptom relief. I therefore referred him both to a psychiatrist for a medication evaluation and to a neurologist for a neurological evaluation.

The psychiatrist initially treated him with both a mild anxiety agent (Ativan) and an antidepressant (Elavil) and later altered the medications several times during the course of the treatment. The neurologist had the opinion that the client's rages did flow, at least in part, from some damage sustained in the course of the fall and prescribed Tegretol for him.

This client's treatment therefore became a team effort, with me seeing him twice weekly for psychotherapy and the psychiatrist and neurologist each seeing him on a monthly basis. I remained in frequent contact with both of them. Payment for the client's treatment came from his worker's compensation insurance carrier because his injury had occurred while he was on the job making deliveries to some customers. This carrier required periodic treatment summaries, which I provided with the client's consent approximately every three months.

After approximately 12 years of treatment, the insurance carrier requested an independent medical evaluation (IME) to evaluate the client's need for continued treatment. The client reported to me that he had seen a psychiatrist for the IME, thought it had gone well, and especially commented on the psychiatrist telling him that the experience of falling in an elevator "must have been terrible" and that some subsequent chest pains the client experienced almost certainly represented "a manifestation of your overwhelming anxiety." The client therefore became very distressed when his attorney sent him a copy of a letter from the psychiatrist rendering the opinion that the client was malingering. A hearing followed, during which the attorney for the insurance company reiterated the opinion about malingering and indicated that the company would immediately terminate the client's benefit.

The client came to his next session enraged, not only by the fact that his benefits would cease but also with what he perceived as the duplicity of the psychiatrist, who sounded so empathic and then "stabbed me in the back." At that time, the client announced to me that he planned to kill both the psychiatrist and the lawyer. The threat did not seem imminent, as the client announced to me that he intended to "stake out" his two potential victims. In addition to trying to dissuade him from acting out, I began a detailed risk assessment. I considered his past history of violent behavior, the fact that the violence seemed associated with his mental disorder, the degree of his preoccupation with his plan, the extent of his anger and impulsivity, his skills with weapons, and his inability to consider alternative ways of handling the situation, to name a few factors. My thinking flowed largely from clinical factors, as structured standardized interviews to assess violent behavior had not yet been developed. I became particularly concerned when the client came to a session with diagrams of his two intended victims' homes and a time schedule of when they left for work, when their families seemed to be in the house alone, the routes they took to and from work, and the times they arrived home. My assessment led me to conclude that this client posed a definite threat to these two individuals. I still believed that breaking of confidentiality should come only as a last resort and attempted to deal with the issues clinically.

I contacted the psychiatrist and neurologist, apprised them of the threats, and asked that they see him for emergency consultations to evaluate the efficacy of their current regimen of medication. I provided the client with my pager number and my home telephone number, with instructions to call me if he felt as though he might lose control and his fantasies might spill over into actions. I discussed voluntary hospitalization with the client and he agreed to go, but as soon as the hospital discovered that he no longer had insurance in force, they discharged him. I told the client that I would need to file for involuntary commitment, and he replied that if I did so, he would merely deny to the hospital staff that he had ever made any such threats, would behave as a model patient, would soon be discharged, and would not return to treatment. Considering the length of the treatment thus far, and the strength of the therapeutic alliance, I decided not to proceed with seeking commitment. I felt left with the one alternative I did not want to confront: breaching confidentiality and warning the intended victims.

With some trepidation, I planned for the next session; I told the client that I saw him as a serious threat, that I believed I had exhausted more traditional clinical means of handling the problem, and that the only thing I could now do involved notifying the intended victims. I knew that in doing so, I would be breaking the law as it existed at that time, but I preferred to take that chance rather than not take protective action. I reminded the client of the informed consent that he had signed giving me that option. What happened next still amazes me to this day. Rather than becoming distressed about a breach of confidentiality, the client stated, "That's a great idea! Then they will be terrified and never know whether I will strike or not! I will keep them permanently off guard!"

In the client's presence, I then made both telephone calls. The psychiatrist became very concerned and asked me if I thought he should re-evaluate the client. It was remarkable the lack of insight the psychiatrist seemed to have into his own conflict of interest when considering whether he should re-evaluate the person now threatening him. The attorney acted in a somewhat more brusque manner, telling me that he would swear out a warrant against my client and subpoena me to testify against my own client.

The remarkable change that occurred following this encounter was that the act of notifying the endangered third parties in the client's presence seemed to "take the edge off" the feelings. The client stopped talking about plans to kill these two individuals. His anger against them began to take more indirect forms. For instance, during one subsequent session, the client told me of a colleague who owned a printing company and described a plan to go into partnership with this man, print bogus stock certificates, get another friend to convince the psychiatrist and the lawyer of the value of this bogus stock, and sit by and wait for them to lose their fortunes. (This scheme predated the Bernard Madoff financial scam by about 25 years.)

Discussion

Key ethical issues

The first of the ethical issues involved here is the conflict between ethics and law. This ethical standard directs us to make consumers of our services aware of any ethical conflicts that might arise between our obligations under the *Ethics Code* and certain laws and regulations and take responsible steps to resolve the conflict. It is noteworthy that the *Ethics Code* states that if the psychologist is unable to resolve the issue, he or she "may follow the law." It does not say that the psychologist *must* follow the law. In this case, even though I was breaking the law, I felt that the acting out could in fact harm all involved, the client and his two victims, and in my mind, this harm outweighed the fact that I "may" follow the law. It interfaces with another ethical standard stating that the psychologist takes reasonable steps to avoid or prevent harm.

Another key ethical issue had to do with the basis for scientific and professional judgment. Ethically, of course, one needs to have a basis in some literature or research for the decisions that one makes in clinical practice. As noted earlier, formal risk assessment procedures had not yet been developed at the time of this case, but one tries to structure an assessment based on the available information, and the intervention should logically derive from it.

Another issue, of course, had to do with the limits of confidentiality. I had clearly spelled out these limits of confidentiality in the informed consent document, even though the law at that time did not require it. The *Ethics Code* did speak about the necessity of informing the client about possible limits of confidentiality. Disclosures, according to the *Ethics Code*, also had to be the minimum necessary to accomplish a particular end. It had occurred to me, had this situation progressed and the lawyer sent me a subpoena, what I would have done. It did not take too much effort to conclude that I would have filed a motion to quash the subpoena and indicate to a judge that great harm could be done to the therapeutic relationship by my testifying against my own client.

Work setting

This was a private practice setting. The danger in working in such a setting is that the practitioner can be isolated from colleagues and not utilize available consultation. In this case, it was essential to work along with the psychiatrist and neurologist as essential adjuncts because the client was in need of both immediate symptom relief for his anxiety and depression and the anticonvulsant medication used to control his explosive rages.

Reflection

One should never break confidentiality without careful consideration of the consequences. The APA *Ethics Code* does allow for breaches when an imminent danger to self or others arises. However, we have few guidelines available for determining when the threat is imminent or for the appropriate parameters of the assessment. This remains a matter of clinical judgment, and despite the advances in evidence-based treatments, the responses to such emergency situations are generally not found in manual-driven treatments. Although one would ideally conduct a comprehensive risk assessment, this may prove unrealistic if the client seems poised to act out. In general, one's actions should align with the assessment data. Assessments also change over time, as may the intervention, including careful documentation of the reasons behind the change. In the case discussed here, breaking confidence came only as a last resort, not as the first line of action.

Clinically, I have often wondered about this case and my client's surprising response. It appears that having some sense of control over the lives of other persons rather than actually harming them could have been the underlying motivation. Also, I took the client seriously, all the time maintaining the therapeutic alliance. I did not minimize the threat, nor did I panic and go through actions attempting to terminate the relationship and avoid the responsibility of dealing with the situation. I passed on my concern to the client and acted as a kind of validating proxy, letting those who angered him hear the follow-up from an independent clinical source. In so doing, I allowed the client the goal of communicating his anger by proxy, and that apparently satisfied a critical emotional need. This suggests another cautionary note: when a client threatens violence, it may not reflect his or her true intent, and the clinician needs to inquire further before deciding on a course of action.

Relevant ethical principles and standards

APA (2002): Principle A (Beneficence and Nonmaleficence), Standard 1.02 (Conflict Between Ethics and Law), Standard 2.04 (Bases for Scientific And Professional Judgment), Standard 3.04 (avoiding Harm), Standard 3.09 (Cooperative with Other Professionals), Standard 3.10 (Informed Consent), Standard 4.02 (Discussing Limits of Confidentiality), Standard 4.05 (Disclosures), Standard 10.01 (Informed Consent to Psychotherapy).

REFERENCES AND FURTHER READING

Shaw v. Glickman, 415 A2nd 625 (Md. Ct. Spec. A.P., 1980).
Tarasoff v. Regents of the University of California, 551 P2nd 334 (Calif. Sup. Ct., 1976).
Tarasoff Duty to Warn Discussed in Three Cases: No Such Duty Found in Maryland (1980), *Mental Disability Law Reporter*, 4, 313–315.

8

What Would She Think? Disclosure of Therapy Details After Death

Dan Shapiro

Here's a little secret that all of us in mental health know.

We like some of our patients more than others. Julie was one such patient. A woman in her early sixties, she was Jewish like me, roughly my mother's age, and vivacious. That's an understatement. She had too much personality for one body and filled my office with broad statements and gestures. An exercise expert and fanatic, she'd helped start a new nutrition craze and was independently wealthy from her success. She asked about my eating habits, and although I avoided answering, I enjoyed it when she said, "You look like you're in good shape, but you should try our system."

Her five children and a grandchild were her lifeblood, and she enthusiastically described them in great detail. Her bubbly style was infectious, and I found myself laughing frequently in those early sessions. Having treated my share of patients struggling with depression and anxiety, she was a breath of fresh air. I thought of her as chronically happy and recall looking forward to her sessions.

There was just one problem: she had pancreatic cancer.

At first, she described her illness as an inconvenience; it would be a nuisance, but she would overcome it with will and perseverance. Given her confidence and certainty, I was almost convinced. But having spent time myself fighting lymphoma—a virulent form of cancer that is nonetheless more treatable than pancreatic cancer—I remember thinking ahead that when her illness took its likely course, she might be profoundly saddened.

As the months passed and Julie received a grim trickle of medical information, her mood did change, but she didn't become sad. Instead, she became angry and expressed this frequently to me and apparently to her oncologist, who confided that her rage made their meetings very difficult.

From her perspective, she had always been destined for great things, and the cancer was robbing her and those of us who might benefit from her wisdom and innovations. Although from some patients such statements would sound narcissistic and entitled, in Julie's case, I agreed. She was more full of life than the average person, and it did seem uniquely rotten that cancer had chosen to reside in her pancreas.

Julie wanted to keep the diagnosis and prognosis from her children and husband and tried vigorously to keep things normal when she was with them. She believed that a positive attitude could result in a cure and expressed the opinion that this would likely occur in her case. It was important that they not know the full story and "bring her down." Although they knew she had cancer, they were not aware of the specifics. Despite her attempts at normalcy, her rage leaked out. She had a uniquely short fuse and snapped frequently, most often at the people she loved the most. I encouraged her to be honest with them and explain her circumstances and reasoning more fully, but she would not. Given how different this behavior was from her typically optimistic outlook, her outbursts left her family confused and bewildered. Eventually, one of her children, a daughter, asked if she could meet with us together. My patient consented, saying, "I'm an open book."

I liked her daughter immediately. Like her mother, she was energetic, attractive, and bright. She was taking a job working for *The Washington Post* as a reporter and had a journalist's ear for details and incongruity. She gently asked me questions about her mother, and I answered as best I was able, although her mother interrupted frequently in an effort to keep our conversation "on track." In the end, I realized, her daughter did not grasp how grim her mother's prognosis was, or that her mother was fully aware of the situation and was "pissed off" about it. I did not feel that I should share these details, and in the end the meeting felt strained. I was uncomfortable with the conference. It was as if I had been an accomplice in my patient's ruse. Notably, Julie did say that we could meet and talk anytime we wanted.

Soon after the meeting, Julie fired her oncologist and flew off to Southeast Asia to consult a healer who'd promised a cure. Then she was in Central America and Mexico and eventually returned and rehired her doctor.

A few months after her travels, we moved to phone sessions because she found travel impossible but wanted to continue the therapy. She expressed anger at her husband, her children, and me. All of us had disappointed her in one way or another.

On a cold winter Tuesday, I got a call from her daughter. Julie had died.

Over the next months, I thought of my patient frequently and wondered if I could have done more to ease her suffering. I would have liked to have healed the rifts between Julie and her family and found some way to help Julie see how she'd isolated herself from her family through her attempts to prevent them from "bringing her down."

I eventually stopped seeing as many patients and started spending more time teaching medical students. During this period, I created a program in which medical students visited patients at home and filmed their lives; the project was growing and spreading to other schools.

After a few years, I received an e-mail from my patient's daughter, the reporter. She told me she'd had some success as a reporter and wondered what I was up to. I shared the project I was working on, and she said it sounded intriguing and wondered if she might help me get press about the project in her paper. I was excited by the prospect of getting publicity for the project. She indicated that she had some questions about her mother, and then she said, "Let's get together. I'm going to be in town."

Her words were breezy, and there was a hint of something flirtatious there too; I felt a quickening, like when I was 20 and an attractive, smart girl wanted my attention. I knew what she wanted, and in an instant, I wanted to give it to her. Here was my chance to let her know what her mother felt and thought about her, how she knew all along that her illness was serious but that she'd tried, erroneously, to protect her from it, and how her anger had leaked out indirectly and caused a great deal of unhappiness.

But my feeling of excitement quickly gave way to something else, like when, as a child, I was taken to a deep pool by friends of my parents and wandered out onto the high diving board and glanced over. *I'm not supposed to be here.* It's a physical thing, and I've learned over the years to trust it. When I traced the feeling back, I realized I was considering breaching my patient's trust. Her confidentiality. There was an ethics issue here.

On the one hand, I wanted to try to heal a rift my patient had created during the course of our treatment when she took a common pop culture sentiment to the extreme—namely, that thinking positively at all times and maintaining a sense of normalcy can improve one's health and even lead to cure. But there were also secondary issues at play—my own desire to get publicity and her daughter's attractiveness and role as a reporter.

Discussion

Key ethical issues

The ethical principle of nonmaleficence, avoiding harm, is key to understanding this case, as are the ethical standards bearing on maintaining confidentiality, disclosures (of confidential information), and the maintenance, dissemination, and disposal of confidential records of professional and scientific work.

A patient's right to confidentiality clearly survives death. The notion that a patient cannot be harmed after death is invalid; clearly, great harm can be done to a reputation, memories, and any survivors after death. Disclosing information a patient expected to keep confidential would breach the patient's trust.

In this case, the patient had explicitly given me the right to speak with her daughter. But she'd made that decision in the context of being alive and able to influence both me and, perhaps, her daughter's perceptions after any conversation. Indeed, in the one conversation we all had together, she had managed the conversation carefully. While on the one hand she had said "I'm an open book" and professed an interest in our speaking openly, on the other she had indirectly prevented this communication.

In practice, family members often seek information after a patient's death. Family may seek assistance with clarifying matters related to a will, after a suicide to understand the patient's frame of mind, or to help with grief.

Legal statutes vary by jurisdiction, but one text commonly used by psychiatrists advises clinicians, "Psychiatrists must be careful not to make unauthorized extrajudicial or statutorily prohibited disclosure of patient records unless the disclosure is justified by overriding public interest." Furthermore, they write, "If a psychiatrist feels compelled to reveal confidential information after the patient's death, legal risks may be minimized by providing just enough information for the task at hand. Details of the patient's therapy are rarely, if ever, required. Relevance is the rule" (Simon & Sadoff, 1992, p. 309). Unfortunately, the ethics code governing psychologists does not explicitly describe confidentiality after death.

Fidelity and loyalty are also relevant principles, as is the portion of the psychology ethics code that warns against multiple relationships. In this case, it was important to remember to whom I owed allegiance. Julie's child was not my patient. Julie was my patient. And although I felt I owed the family and could improve the daughter's memories of her mother by explaining her mother's psychological approach to her illness, I had to weigh this against the patient's right to confidentiality.

My personal stake in having a good relationship with the daughter also complicated the discussions. My own fears of using this relationship for my own betterment (publicity for my project) may have interfered with my ability to balance the issues at hand. Looking back, perhaps I shouldn't have responded to her e-mail at all. She wasn't my patient, she wasn't a friend, and I had no justification for chatting with her. Or perhaps I should have said I'd be happy to talk with her, but only on the condition that she not write about my project.

That the patient's daughter was a journalist also complicated the discussion. Having written for *The New York Times* and spent time with journalists myself, I am aware that many are remarkably talented at drawing information from reluctant sources. An attractive, younger journalist would likely have been particularly challenging for me, should issues have come up that I did not want to disclose. On some level, I recognized this, and it certainly influenced my thinking.

Work setting

Working in a medical school with physically ill patients presents challenges for all health professionals. The privilege of working with dying patients also has its burdens. Clearly, one of those burdens is carrying a patient's unfinished business.

The setting is also rife with dual roles. For example, Julie's oncologist was one of my "teammates," and Julie knew we communicated. I learned that she'd fired him before heading off on her trip to find an alternative cure. She would have likely preferred to explain her side of the story first, but my proximity to him resulted in my knowing what had transpired earlier than I would have were I in a private office. In addition, because the hospital allows and invites visitors, family members may feel more able to communicate and participate in patient's therapies, particularly if they occasionally occur when the patient is admitted. In inpatient settings, family members often "chat" with physicians and nurses about issues outside medicine. This is a natural part of the culture that is different from the culture generally encouraged by therapists, in which boundaries are more tightly drawn. In this case, it felt natural, I suspect, for my patient's daughter to come in and meet me—just as she had met the patient's oncologist, radiation oncologist, and potential surgeon. It may have also felt natural for her to contact me later and discuss a wide range of topics, including my professional work.

In addition to the unique elements of the medical setting, I brought to therapy an insider's knowledge of the psychology of cancer. At one point, my illness was quite serious, and an oncologist told me he didn't believe I could be cured, but that he would try. I remember intimately the psychological challenge of living with this fear. I suspect I understood my patient's desires to think positively and even force this attitude in a desperate attempt to survive. I may have initially been slow to respond to the patient's desires to prevent her family from "bringing her down" because I had had similar thoughts at one time.

Reflection

There is a famous case of a psychiatrist disclosing a patient's therapy tapes to a biographer, and the maelstrom that followed is well documented. Martin Orne, a psychiatrist, gave early therapy tapes to Diane Middlebrook, biographer of the poet Anne Sexton. Following the disclosure, William Gaylin, a Columbia University professor, described the disclosures as "a betrayal to his patient and the profession." Orne argued in a subsequent editorial that he had had the permission of Orne's literary executor (Anne Sexton's daughter) and that Sexton herself wanted him to disclose the tapes. The chair of the ethics committee of the American Psychiatric Association commented on the case, saying, "Only a patient can give that release. What the family wants does not matter a whit."

Although surprised by his disclosure, the biographer later wrote, "I don't think Anne Sexton cared what was known about her private life, she just didn't want to be known as a bad artist" (Stanely, 2001).

I believe that my own patient wanted what was best for her family, and this probably would have eclipsed her desire for confidentiality, but there was no way for me to know that for certain. She likely would have embraced an opportunity for me to share with the daughter how much her mother loved her and wanted to be truthful with her, but she was distracted by her desire to always think positively and maintain a sense of normalcy in the face of a dooming diagnosis. I might have also shared that my attempts to encourage more honest discussion were futile, and I blamed myself partially for my inability to help my patient maintain intimacy with her family while fighting her cancer.

On the other hand, there was no way for me to confirm these suppositions, and clearly, a patient's confidentiality survives death.

In the end, I did not agree to meet with the daughter, nor did I disclose any of my patient's information. The daughter did not write about my project in the *Post*, and I haven't heard from her since.

Although I relied on my professional code in formulating my response to this situation, I still wonder if I did the most ethical thing, given the circumstances. In truth, what I would have been disclosing were my own perceptions of the therapy rather than my patient's secrets. The daughter and her family are now well aware of my patient's diagnosis and the course of her illness. They are not aware of how I framed her behavior and its unintended but devastating consequences for them. Given that this information might have been therapeutic for them, and that the patient would have likely encouraged me to reach out to them in this way, I still wonder if not speaking with her was the right thing.

For precedent, I'm glad I did not speak with the daughter. Most patients would likely be reluctant to speak openly with a therapist if they feared that the therapist might decide to disclose sensitive information based on their own decisions about what's right following death (or perhaps only older therapists would have much business). But weighing a concern for the long-term welfare of the profession against what was right in the moment was not particularly on my mind at the time. It's only now, as I write down what happened, that this thought is prominent.

To this day, I don't know if I did the right thing. I can only hope that the daughter and her family found some sense of peace.

Key ethical principles and standards

APA (2002): Principle A (Beneficence and Nonmaleficence), Principle B (Fidelity and Responsibility), Standard 3.05 (Multiple Relationships), Standard 4.01 (Maintaining Confidentiality), Standard 4.05 (Disclosures of Confidential Information), Standard 6.02 (Maintenance, Dissemination, and Disposal of Confidential Records of Professional and Scientific Work).

REFERENCES AND FURTHER READING

Orne, M. T. (1991, July 23). The Sexton tapes. *The New York Times*, Op-Ed.
Simon, R. I., & Sadoff, R. L. (1992). *Psychiatric malpractice*. Washington DC: American Psychiatric Press.
Stanely, A. (1991, July 15). Anne Sexton: Controversy surrounding the biography. *The New York Times*.

9

It's My Right! Working With a Terminally (or Chronically) Ill, Persistently Suicidal Client

James L. Werth Jr.

For many years, I have offered pro bono individual and group psychological services to people with human immunodeficiency virus (HIV) disease, often receiving referrals from local HIV organizations and medical clinics. At one point or another, nearly all of my clients have indicated that they have considered suicide as an option. For the most part, it becomes clear to me fairly quickly that these comments arise as expressions of a need to feel some control over their life and the course of their condition. However, at any point in time, at least one or two people in my caseload express thoughts of suicidality—not as vague and passing remarks, but instead as reflections of constant and sometimes strong beliefs regarding decisions about the length of their life. Given the illness(es) they have, they assert that they have a "right" to consider suicide an option and tell me that when the quality of life has fallen too low, they will then take active measures to end what they perceive as intolerable suffering. Although to my knowledge none of these persistently suicidal clients with HIV have actually committed suicide, I have had to accept that at any point during treatment or after termination I may learn that a client has indeed ended his or her own life. Of all my recent clients, "Pat" best reflects these issues.

Pat came into the waiting room exactly on time and had not even sat down before I came out to meet him for the first time.

He followed closely behind me into my office and selected the chair that would place his back to the door. I had no information other than he had called and asked for an appointment. He appeared thin and breathed with some labor; his eyes darted around the room, starting at the window—with shades drawn—and working back to me. He completed the paperwork quickly, without saying a word. As I moved into the informed consent, he stopped me after I said, "If I am concerned that you might hurt yourself or someone else, then I might need to take some action." He said that he wanted to hear more about what I meant. I explained the duty to protect in principle and under state law. He asked for clarification about why I said I "might" need to do something. Based on my experience, I had a sense that he might feel similarly to other clients who had thought of suicide as an option; although this proved somewhat accurate, I had not correctly gauged the depth of his consideration.

After I spent another few minutes explaining this aspect of the informed consent material, he seemed satisfied. I said I wanted to come back to talk more about his questions but asked permission to finish the informed consent (e.g., talking about reporting child abuse). Upon completion of these aspects, I returned to his concern with the "harm to self or others" component. He said, "Suicide is always an option for me. I think about it all the time, from when I wake up until when I go to bed." Now, although it is not unusual for a client to say that he or she has considered suicide, few have indicated feeling constantly suicidal. Of course, I immediately began mentally reviewing the questions I wanted to ask him.

Pat proceeded to say that he had done a Web search on me and decided to follow up on the referral from both his physician and his case manager after reading an article I wrote that took a contextual view of suicide intervention. He stated that he felt willing to come in and speak honestly about his nearly constant suicidality only because he believed that no immediate attempt to hospitalize him would be made. He asserted that such an action would only make things worse for a variety of reasons (e.g., people would find out about the hospitalization, he would incur charges for the treatment, he believed his family would overreact), and he said he was smart enough to know what to say and what not to say to prevent an involuntary admission or at least having to remain admitted for very long. Pat reported that his suicidal ideation resulted from two concurrent, potentially terminal health conditions, one of them advanced HIV disease. Before these health problems, he indicated that had never considered suicide an option. He said that his suicidality was not the major issue that had brought him in and led to the referrals. He reported some obsessive-compulsive tendencies causing problems in his life and with his partner. He also stated that he had some family concerns.

Once he had gone through these major issues, he said that his confidentiality remained very important to him because he had not informed very many people, including family members, that he was HIV-positive. He knew that I saw only people with HIV and their significant others—as the only mental health provider in town who specialized in HIV, I received the referrals. He indicated that he had waited until his exact appointment time to enter the office so that no one would see him in the waiting room and he would not run into someone leaving the previous appointment. He said he would watch the time and wanted to leave a little earlier than usual, again to reduce the likelihood of being seen by my next appointment. This pattern continued throughout the approximately eight months that I saw him, except that I learned to tell him when I had an appointment after his so that on the days when I was free he could stay the full time. Even on those days, he watched the clock and seemed very conscious of when the allotted time ended and would close the sessions for us.

During the first session, we negotiated how we would work with his suicidal feelings. He understood that we would need to talk about how he was doing each time and he would bring it up at the start of the session. We worked out a self-care plan in case his suicidal thoughts moved beyond ideation to potential action, building on what he had already developed on his own to add some new coping strategies, including calling me and asking for an extra session during the week. I believe he reported honestly when we talked because I recall times when he would tell me he'd had a bad week and had decided not to go into the kitchen on certain days because there were knives in there, or that he had looked at the plastic bags longer than normal. He had told me that if he were to kill himself, he would put plastic bags down so that his blood would stay on the plastic and be easier to clean up. He also said he would place a note by his body warning anyone who might come in contact with his blood of his HIV status.

I always felt relieved when Pat came in for his appointment because although I thought we were doing good work and making progress on his concerns, as well as getting appropriate psychopharmacological treatment for his obsessive-compulsive tendencies and depression, I remained nervous that he would implement one of his suicidal plans. One of the issues we had to negotiate involved recognizing that although it might make sense to consider his constant suicidality as part of the obsessive nature of his condition, he did not consider the persistent suicidal thoughts that way. Rather, he considered these thoughts as an understandable reflection of his physical health status. He also said that his rumination on other things provided a helpful distraction from thinking too much about suicide. So, together we walked a fine line between managing his nonsuicidal obsessive thoughts and compulsive behaviors and not eliminating them because he saw them as a coping mechanism that kept him alive. For example, he would spend hours many days during the week engaging in searches for items (e.g., pop bottle tops) he could exchange for things he could not otherwise afford, such as soda or movie tickets. Although he certainly recognized that this activity did not make efficient use of his time, he indicated that he couldn't work because of his disabilities, so instead of sitting at home thinking about killing himself, he went out searching and had something to look forward to.

By the time I started seeing Pat, I had worked with HIV-positive and suicidal clients for many years. I had somewhat resolved that people would do what they wished to do and that I, as a psychologist who saw them only for about one hour a week (leaving them 167 hours away from my presence), had no real control over them. Furthermore, because of my thinking about suicide, my reading of the ethics code and laws/regulations, and my review of the literature, I believed I stood on solid ethical, legal, and standard-of-care ground in working with Pat, with the understanding that he might decide to kill himself. However, I still felt nervous about becoming a "test case" if he did die and his partner or family decided that I had not done enough to try to save him or had not informed them of the depths of his suicidality.

During the time I worked with Pat, I had another eight or nine people in my caseload, all HIV-positive and seen every week or every other week. I also led a support group for HIV-positive gay or bisexual men. About half of these individual and group clients also had some suicidal ideation, but I did not feel concerned that they would act on their thoughts, so I rarely got to the point of thinking about doing more than continuing to meet with them. However, during this time I did intervene with two people by calling their psychiatrist directly and getting them in immediately for crisis appointments. I also worked with one client to disclose to a family member the fact that he felt in crisis. If necessary, I think I would have taken some action even if any of these clients had objected. Yet with Pat, I recall feeling both more nervous about what would happen and less convinced that I would take some action to intervene over his objections. My struggle revolved around what I believed would be in Pat's best interests (in the short and long term) and would minimize harm to him (in the short and long term). I regularly reflected upon and re-evaluated my initial determination that violating confidentiality and pursuing hospitalization, should the need potentially arise, might be more harmful and less beneficial than respecting Pat's right to self-determination and dignity. Naturally, I realized that I was taking a chance that he might injure or kill himself, just as my other suicidal clients might. However, my thoughts seemed to go beyond just rationalizing because I believed that actual differences existed between Pat and these other individuals, but I remained uncertain about how the state licensing board or a family member would have evaluated the situation.

My work with Pat ended when I accepted another job and had to move. Of all the people I had treated individually, I felt most worried about him, how he would react, and what he would do afterward. We saw each other up until the week I left, and even though I tried to find someone else to see him, I could not find another mental health provider to take him on. He could not get community mental health care in the county where he lived, so I felt afraid he would not have any professional support. I do not know whether he is still alive.

Discussion

Key ethical issues

The primary ethical issue in this case, and in general, involves confidentiality. Although most mental health professionals learn about confidentiality, the duty to protect, and working with suicidal clients, the issues in Pat's case present a different twist. Such cases will not typically come up during professional training, except perhaps in programs that have a health emphasis or include some teaching on dying and death. I have attended suicide training sessions, belong to suicide prevention organizations, and collaborate with others on involuntarily hospitalizing clients, so I do not oppose intervening to prevent people from killing themselves. The difference here flows from the fact that Pat had two potentially terminal illnesses that significantly negatively impacted his quality of life. He managed them as well as he could through medication and behaviors, but he still could not work and had no realistic chance to regain his health. He also felt isolated and oppressed, primarily out of fear that others would find out he had HIV. However, even though his perspective was somewhat exaggerated, at least some of his concerns had a legitimate foundation. If others had found out, he might have lost the little support he had. He did have some psychiatric symptoms but could manage them through therapy and with medication. Thus, the issues related to his suicidality focused on whether his quality of life could improve in any way and whether his judgment and decision making had become impaired.

While working with Pat, I felt keenly attuned to these issues. During the whole time that I worked with him, I believe he did the best he could to maintain as high a quality of life as possible by trying the various medical interventions available to him. I also think that his judgment and decision making were not impaired. I believe that he could have prevented himself from being involuntarily hospitalized or could have presented himself in such a way that he would have qualified for release soon after. I am convinced that he would not have returned to therapy with me, or with anyone else, in the future had I attempted to hospitalize him. As a result, I did not focus on trying to take away his suicidal thinking or engage in the standard interventions described in the suicide prevention literature, but I did retain hospitalization as a final option in the event that my analysis of his judgment changed. As I indicated, this seemed correct to me, but if Pat had ended up killing himself, then someone else reviewing the case—say an expert witness called in by the family whose focus involved working with suicide prompted by psychiatric diagnoses or impulsivity—might have come to a different conclusion, which could have led to an adverse licensing board or court decision.

My review of the literature indicates that a patient exhibiting suicidality in the face of terminal physical illness, without comorbid psychiatric conditions that impair judgment and decision making, cannot be equated with the more typical suicidal client. I have found the following: (1) in most states, no legal or regulatory *mandate* exists for mental health professionals to intervene to attempt to prevent all suicides; (2) no clear *mandate* to prevent all suicides exists in mental health professional ethics codes, especially when combined with other public statements by professional organizations regarding terminally ill persons; (3) in most states, when a mental health provider does decide to pursue some sort of intervention, such as psychiatric hospitalization, the commitment must usually specify a clearly diagnosable mental health condition as a cause for the suicidality (i.e., justification for the involuntary hospitalization flows from a presumed need for mental health treatment); and (4) although the standard of care may be to intervene with the typical client who is suicidal and therefore to not do so may lead to a malpractice, licensing, or ethics charge, no officially documented cases exist to demonstrate how a licensing board or court would rule in a case such as Pat's. Thus, although I think that working with Pat the way I did remains ethically and legally justifiable, I still felt concerned that I could end up losing my license, having a negative financial judgment, or facing some other sort of adverse consequence. One thing I could have done (but didn't) to help support my position would have been to ask him for a copy of his living will documenting that he did not want any efforts to prolong his life.

Work setting

I have had the ability to choose to do pro bono work with clients and not have to worry about making ends meet through seeing enough clients every week or dealing with insurance companies and billing and utilization review. Doing pro bono work with HIV-infected people has become important to me as a way of fulfilling what I perceive as my professional obligation to help others, my personal convictions regarding social justice, and the reality that this underserved population often has few mental health resources available to it.

Although the ability to fulfill these drives has proved positive, if I deal honestly with myself, I have to admit that at times I ask myself if the value of the work justifies the angst. This questioning tends to arise when I am wondering whether one or more clients will come in for their next session or will die before I see them again as a result of their medical condition or suicide. In other words, I reflect on whether the positive sense of self sufficiently offsets the stress involved and the concern that someone may die "on my watch." I suppose I could decide not to see anyone who had serious or even remote suicidal ideation, but then I would probably not have many clients, and those who need care the most might remain unserved. The lack of mental health services for this highly stigmatized group in many areas of the country presents another frustration with which I must deal because then I feel my inner voice saying, "If I don't do it, no one will." Although this may not always prove true, it was true at the last place where I lived and worked; once I moved, the mental health care for HIV-positive people disappeared.

Reflection

I have thought about these issues long enough to realize that at least some of my sense of acceptance of the suicidality demonstrated by clients such as Pat reflects my own personality and knowledge that I qualify as a person who needs to feel some sense of control. If I were facing a terminal illness, with a very unpleasant course, I might want to believe that I could decide when and how to die, as opposed to waiting for the disease to take me. Thus, part of my struggle involves determining what constitutes a client's assessment of his or her situation and options and what represents my own beliefs and issues.

Another area on which I have spent much time and energy is the role of fundamental ethical principles (e.g., respect for people's rights and dignity) in situations in which the ethics code and supplementary literature are silent or unsettled. Although some may want to believe that the enforceable sections of professional ethics codes provide firm guidance in situations such as Pat's, they do not. A close reading indicates that nearly everything is left to the professional's judgment. As a result, I have had to move up a level in my analyses in order to find some direction, and the ethical meta-principles (or their operationalization in the aspirational sections of ethics codes), which I discuss briefly below, have provided me with this grounding. Most ethical decision-making models include some reference to these principles in situations in which there is no specific standard addressing the issues at hand, and I have seen and experienced the wisdom of including this analysis in situations such as the one I have described in this chapter.

I also recognize that a client I saw during an early practicum in my doctoral studies has affected how I view suicidality. I thought I was making good progress in helping a female student I saw at a university counseling center deal with her bulimia and interpersonal issues when one week she did not come in. The following week she returned and apologized for missing the session. She said that she had been in the hospital because she had attempted suicide. As in reports in the literature, I immediately blamed myself for her action and wondered whether I should quit the practicum site and resign from the program before being removed. Thanks to supportive faculty, supervisors, and peers, I was able to move past this point, but in the process I had to reflect on how much control I really had with clients. My resolution involved reminding myself that I didn't have a lot of control because clients can decide to act in many ways, regardless of what we have done in session or my beliefs about what they should do. So in some sense, my acceptance of the fact that Pat, or other clients, may decide to die and I cannot really do much to prevent this from happening probably represents a coping mechanism, albeit a rational one (I hope).

One other point of reflection that may deserve mentioning involves the presence of the Internet and how it affected Pat's coming in when he did and what he knew about me. The fact that a savvy client with access to the Internet can obtain information on us as providers becomes an important consideration. Pat found out about, and actually read, my work on "rational suicide," which proved important in this case. However, significant misinformation about me and my beliefs around these issues exists, and I do not know how this has affected other clients or prevented some people from coming in to see me. I can do nothing about this except remain aware that just as clients may have perceptions of therapy based on what they have seen on television when they come in for their first or subsequent sessions, the same may be true about their beliefs regarding me as a therapist.

Key ethical principles and standards

As a psychologist, I follow the American Psychological Association Ethical Principles of Psychologists and Code of Conduct (APA, 2002). I am also a member of the American Counseling Association and therefore need to follow the ACA Code of Ethics. For the most part the two codes are compatible regarding the areas of relevance to this case. Both codes include sections on confidentiality (Standard 4 for the APA and Section B for the ACA). The primary difference is that the section of the ACA Code on exceptions to confidentiality (B.2) includes a statement that "[a]dditional considerations apply when addressing end-of-life issues" (B.2.a. Danger and Legal Requirements, p. 7) and refers the reader to a previous section on end-of-life care for terminally ill clients (A.9). This section includes a statement indicating that "[c]ounselors who provide services to terminally ill individuals who are considering hastening their own deaths have the option of breaking or not breaking confidentiality" (A.9.c. Confidentiality, p. 6). Thus, the ACA Code makes it clear that there is not an ethical obligation to intervene in cases such as Pat's, whereas the APA Code (Standard 4.05[b] on disclosures) uses generic permissive language regarding breaking confidentiality.

There are also meta-principles involved in cases like this. All five apply here: beneficence (What will prove most helpful to the client?), nonmaleficence (How can I do the least amount of harm?), autonomy (How can I act in the most culturally appropriate way to enhance and respect the client's self-determination), fidelity (How do I remain true to the client?), and justice (How do I promote fairness, equity, and equality with this client and others?).

REFERENCES AND FURTHER READING

Kleespies, P. M. (2003). *Life and death decisions: Psychological and ethical considerations in end-of-life care.* Washington DC: American Psychological Association.

Weiner, K. (Ed.). (2005). *Therapeutic and legal issues for therapists who have survived a client suicide: Breaking the silence.* Binghamton, NY: Haworth Press.

Werth, J. L., Jr. (1992). Rational suicide and AIDS: Considerations for the psychotherapist. *The Counseling Psychologist, 20,* 645–659.

Werth, J. L., Jr., & Richmond, J. (2009). End of life decisions and the duty to protect. In J. L. Werth, Jr., E. R. Welfel G. A. H. Benjamin (Eds.), *The duty to protect: Ethical, legal, and professional considerations for mental health professionals* (pp. 195–208). Washington DC: American Psychological Association.

Working Group on Assisted Suicide and End-of-Life Decisions. (2000). *Report to the American Psychological Association's Board of Directors.* Washington DC: American Psychological Association. Retrieved January 16, 2009, from http://www.apa.org/pi/aseolf.html. [Note: See especially Appendix F: Issues to Consider When Exploring End-of-Life Decisions.]

PART II

In the Forensic World

10

High Stakes Indeed: Forensic Psychology in Death Penalty Litigation

Richart L. DeMier[1]

At first, he seemed like any other patient. He was crazy, to be sure, but that was nothing unusual. Our facility evaluates lots of patients with severe mental illness. And this patient fit the bill. His speech was very difficult to follow. His ideas did not seem connected in any way that made sense. He used words in a peculiar manner that sometimes made it impossible to discern any meaning. He seemed focused on some key ideas, but try as I might, I could not seem to make sense of them. Just another day at the office, except for one thing. This man had been sentenced to die.

I work as a forensic psychologist at a federal prison hospital. Most of the forensic work qualifies as fairly routine—lots of evaluations of competency to proceed, as well as assessments of defendants' mental state at the time of an alleged offense. Some pretrial patients arrive committed for treatment in an effort to restore them to legal competency. We endeavor to provide them with the abilities necessary to understand the proceedings, cooperate in their defense, and confront their accusers, rights guaranteed by

---

[1] This chapter represents a combination of cases. Details have been changed to protect the confidentiality of the patients. The views expressed here are those of the author and do not necessarily reflect the views or policies of the Federal Bureau of Prisons or the U.S. Department of Justice.

the Sixth Amendment of the Constitution. Others arrive committed following verdicts of not guilty by reason of insanity. Still other patients have voluntary admission status—as sentenced prisoners who need inpatient mental health treatment and have volunteered for it. And although any of these patients may pose clinical and ethical challenges, few present with such high stakes as a death penalty case.

In this instance, the state prisoner was referred to our facility during the process of federal appeals, and his competency to proceed with the appellate process was called into question. He faced major decisions about his case, such as how (or whether) to proceed with various grounds for appeal. During the proceedings, various parties agreed that a *bona fide* doubt existed regarding whether he could make rational decisions about those issues. If he could not make rational decisions—if he proved unable to think through his decisions in a reasoned manner—profound consequences would follow. If capable of rational decision making, then the time-sensitive nature of certain avenues of appeal demanded that his case move forward with all haste.

Naturally, I determined to exercise particular caution in my approach to "Red," the name he preferred, and the one to which he responded most readily. Early in the case, I sought to identify potential ethical considerations and think them through before they snuck up on me. After considerable thought, I identified five areas that required attention and forethought in order to reach my goal of completing this evaluation in an ethical manner. The first had specific relevance to my unusual work setting and the unique focus of forensic psychology. The others apply as key principles to competent and ethical work generally.

Discussion

Key ethical issues

My work was informed by my consideration of four key ethical issues. Although not exhaustive, these key areas required special attention. First, I needed to explore my personal values regarding capital punishment and assess any effect those values might have on the outcome of the evaluation. Second, I had to carefully consider technical issues related to diagnoses and competencies in order to perform the evaluation ethically. Third, I would have to recognize my vulnerability to confirmatory bias, by considering data that supported or refuted key hypotheses equally. Finally, when ultimately providing testimony in court,

I would need to remain cognizant of and focused on my limited role in the proceedings.

PERSONAL VALUES REGARDING CAPITAL PUNISHMENT. For some time, I felt quite conflicted regarding my own views about the death penalty. To accomplish the task before me, it seemed imperative that I recognize any personal qualms about capital punishment and examine whether my beliefs about this decidedly emotional issue would bias my professional work.

At one point, I supported the use of the death penalty. But as I learned more and thought more, my position shifted to a moderate one, and ultimately, I became an opponent of the death penalty. In the most heinous cases, that option still holds a visceral appeal, of course, but I developed a personal belief that capital punishment is not applied fairly in the United States and, as a practical matter, will not ever be fairly applied.

Given this personal position, I needed to determine whether I could reconcile my opposition to the death penalty with the task of evaluating Red. If I could not, then I would have to withdraw from the case. And to my employer's credit, I had that option. The Federal Bureau of Prisons has a policy that allows staff members to refrain from participation in any phase of a death penalty case, and I assume this applies to evaluations such as the one required for Red.

One can easily perceive an evaluator working for the Federal Bureau of Prisons as an arm of the prosecutor. It's a natural mistake to make. In fact, over my career, I have had to disabuse dozens of people of this notion. However, the nature of forensic work demands that an evaluator remain scrupulously neutral. Such a stance does not serve the prosecution or the defense; it serves justice. In this case, I recognized that the prosecution had an interest in resolving all issues that could lead to an appeal and in proceeding to the imposition of the death sentence sanctioned by a jury of Red's peers. I recognized that the defense attorney had a duty to make certain her client had the necessary cognitive abilities, and that his thoughts and behaviors had a rational basis and did not result from a thought disorder or mood disorder.

As I pondered this dilemma, I reached the conclusion that to best serve the court, I needed to perceive myself as more than a simple cog in the machine. The court needed a thorough and careful evaluation of the defendant's mental state and his competency-related abilities in order to proceed in a manner that would afford the defendant every opportunity to make decisions in his own best interest. Conducting the evaluation was not tantamount to participating in the imposition of the death penalty. A fair and accurate assessment of the defendant's competency-related abilities would serve all parties and prove essential to a just outcome.

LEGAL CONTOURS RELATED TO MENTAL RETARDATION AND MENTAL ILLNESS. Numerous issues remained active in Red's case, and two of them specifically focused on whether he legally qualified for execution. First, his level of intelligence stood at issue. In 2003, the U.S. Supreme Court ruled in *Atkins v. Virginia* that execution of a person with mental retardation is unconstitutional. Second, some concerns suggested that mental illness had left Red too impaired to truly understand what execution meant. The U.S. Supreme Court had also addressed this issue. The 1986 case of *Ford v. Wainwright* established a standard for competency to be executed: a person facing execution must understand the penalty about to be imposed and the reasons for its imposition. Not only did I need to understand each of these complex issues to proceed in an ethical manner, I also had to conduct a valid evaluation focused on these issues, and I needed to convey my understanding in a transparent manner, so that legal decision makers could properly understand the basis for my opinions.

The issue of mental retardation raises several thorny issues. Graduate students in intellectual assessment classes understand the imprecise basis of IQ testing. Those classes teach about error, "standard" deviations, confidence intervals, and assorted other ways to quantify ambiguity. Students learn to couch their conclusions in an appropriately fuzzy manner because they know that no bright line separates the IQ scores of 69 and 71. All psychologists should know that a diagnosis of mental retardation requires more than just a substandard IQ score; deficits in adaptive functioning represent equally essential criteria. And to add more complications, what of the ramifications of the Flynn effect, which refers to changes in the average IQ of a population over time and may cast doubt on one's ability to accurately interpret IQ scores from many years ago? Clearly, I would have to pay particularly close attention to the interpretation of any testing data.

In the case of *Ford v. Wainwright*, Justice Lewis Powell's concurring opinion argued that "the Eighth Amendment forbids the execution only of those who are unaware of the punishment they are about to suffer and why they are to suffer it." Much has been written about the *Ford* criteria and their application. I had to become familiar with that literature, so that competent practices would form the bases for my opinions.

My report, I determined, must clearly indicate the way I understood the *Atkins* and *Ford* standards, and it would need to provide ample evidence upon which I would base my conclusions. I would want to quote Red's statements and describe his behaviors, and I would want to explain how those statements and behaviors informed my opinion. Similarly, I would reference relevant documents in Red's records and relate their importance to the issues at hand.

Simply stating my opinion would not prove sufficient; I resolved to include a careful explanation of its basis, so that the court could weigh its value based on all the relevant information.

CONFIRMATORY BIAS. Before Red's arrival, I had access to records from the state where his trial took place and where execution might await him. I knew that I would see him for only a period of a few weeks, and I already had access to records from clinicians who saw him over a period of years. This provided an important advantage insofar as I could give the patient a "fresh look." It could also prove difficult, I realized, if my opinion differed from the opinions of clinicians who had known Red for much longer.

What those records showed surprised me. They included indications that Red had engaged in malingering shortly after his incarceration. In other words, he had feigned or exaggerated symptoms of mental illness for some secondary gain. Even though I became convinced during my first interview that he had a legitimate mental illness, strong evidence in the record demonstrated that he had engaged in faking shortly after his arrest. Over time, he began to exhibit more significant symptoms. My interpretation of the records suggested that psychotic symptoms emerged following his arrest, and they became gradually more severe over a period of years.

The clinicians who interacted with him during that time did not share that interpretation. As he exhibited symptoms that became progressively more severe, the record reflected a belief that he had simply gotten better and better at feigning. What I interpreted as the emergence of illness, they interpreted as increased efficacy in presenting convincing symptoms of mental illness. One note actually said, "He's getting very good at looking sick!"

So, what was going on here? It certainly seemed possible that the clinicians who had interacted with Red for several years had formed an initial opinion that colored all their future interactions with him. Given their early conclusion regarding faking, during subsequent interactions, they sought information to support that view. They may have ignored, or at least failed to consider, information to the contrary.

Such an adherence to one's initial hypothesis is known as *confirmatory bias*, and I was by no means immune. Because Red had presented with what appeared to be legitimate symptoms of mental illness during the initial interview, I would need to continually challenge my own preconceived notions and to actively seek evidence for alternative hypotheses. Moreover, in the final report, I would need to discuss data that supported my conclusion *and* data that was contrary to my conclusion.

STAGE FRIGHT. Testifying in any case can provoke anxiety. In Red's case, I was especially concerned that I testify effectively. Although I always have that goal, I felt increased pressure in this case. The reason may seem somewhat paradoxical. My goal, as previously discussed, focused on providing the court with balanced and accurate information that informed my opinion. However, I was afraid I would fall prey to the trap of believing that I knew the answers. I anticipated feeling more tense than usual on the witness stand because I would want the judge to agree with my opinion. It took some reflection to recall that my opinion was only one piece of the puzzle that the judge had the task of solving. (It happened to be the only piece that I had intimate familiarity with.) Although I would seek to present my opinion with appropriate conviction, I had to make a conscious effort to remain cognizant of my limited role. Even if I believed Red competent to be executed, my job did not include hastening the appellate process. Even if I believed Red incompetent to be executed, my role could not involve "saving" him. I derived comfort from the fact that the judge would consider lots of information, including things that I did not know about. If the judge's ruling did not concur with my opinion, that would not mean I had failed. I resolved in advance to find solace in the majesty of the adversarial process, regardless of the outcome. Of course, I would feel better if the judge concurred with my opinion, but that could not be the standard by which I evaluated the quality of my work.

Still, I was anxious about how my words would be heard. For guidance, I relied, broadly, on the *Specialty Guidelines for Forensic Psychologists*. The current guidelines and a proposed revision both address the issue of public statements and testimony. The guidelines indicate, "Forensic psychologists realize that their public role as 'expert to the court' ... confers upon them a special responsibility for fairness and accuracy in their public statements." Moreover, the guidelines discourage out-of-court statements. The record would have to speak for itself.

When Red's day in court arrived, I pledged to approach the task of providing testimony as routine. Of course, I would strive to explain my opinion and its foundations as clearly and persuasively as possible. I would remain aware of my personal beliefs but keep them separate from my professional opinions (to the extent humanly possible, at least). I knew the provision of my testimony would prove easier, and more effective, if I did not accept the undue burden of believing that Red's fate lay in my hands.

Work setting

The distinctive nature of the work setting for this case involved its location within the mental health unit of a federal prison. The unusual nature of the work involved its rarity as a type of evaluation, even among clinicians who practice forensic psychology. The nature of the setting required a careful clarification of roles and examination of boundaries.

All mental health professionals recognize the importance of good rapport in clinical work. Indeed, the nature of the relationship between psychologist and patient is the most important component in a therapeutic relationship. But Red did not come to our hospital for psychotherapy. The referral involved a forensic evaluation. The results of that evaluation could potentially prove beneficial for him, but there was no such guarantee—and no such goal. The purpose of the evaluation was narrowly focused: the judge needed information about Red's competency-related abilities.

In all clinical settings, a critically important step occurs when the mental health professional explains the contours of the clinical relationship, and this includes a discussion of the limits of confidentiality. Especially in a case like this one, it was incumbent on me to educate Red about the nature of our relationship. He needed to know that my job was not to help him. That comes as a shock to many people referred for forensic evaluation; they have come to see a doctor, after all. But in this relationship, my primary client was the court. This involves more than mere semantics. I had a crucial obligation to help Red understand that my job focused on serving the court by providing objective information. Whether that information might prove potentially helpful or harmful could not influence my behavior; the forensic evaluator's responsibility involves giving the court an impartial opinion containing the best information possible.

But there's the rub. To get the best information possible, I would need to forge an alliance with Red. Some have argued that to do so might somehow constitute unethical behavior. Psychologists are so skilled in forming relationships, such critics say, that forensic patients are at a disadvantage. Psychologists may exploit that relationship to gain information that can ultimately become harmful to the patient. Most forensic professionals, particularly in the criminal law arena, have had to grapple with this challenge.

Fortunately, empathy and good clinical practice are not inconsistent with forensic work. The explanation of the nature and purpose of the evaluation forms the basis for an understanding about how the information will be used. I would have to carefully assess Red's ability to understand those issues to ensure an appropriate degree of understanding; simply acquiescing to the evaluation and saying, "I understand," does not satisfy legal standards. Moreover, frequent reminders of the nature of this unique relationship may prove necessary to ensure that the person undergoing evaluation does not forget about the intended uses of the information. When the person under evaluation understands the nature and purpose of the evaluation and clearly recognizes the limits of confidentiality, and when frequent checks indicate that he remains cognizant of the intended uses of the information, only then should the psychologist feel free to use his or her clinical and relationship skills to gain the information necessary to answer the referral question for the court.

Any attempt to deceive the patient or to lull him into a false sense of comfort creates a major ethical problem. Forensic evaluators must scrupulously avoid misleading the patient. Veiled suggestions that the conclusions of the evaluation may prove more beneficial to the patient if he only cooperates are clearly wrong. The reason for the endeavor should remain transparent. Of course, one can show empathy, or build trust, and establish a comfort level in which the patient will easily engage, as long as the limits cited here remain clearly defined, well understood, and routinely reviewed.

Reflection

My approach to this difficult case appeared to rest upon a straightforward conclusion: good practice equals ethical practice. A mentor once told me that forensic work is simple. The forensic clinician's job involves saying "what you think and why you think it." Remaining thoughtful and careful includes an analysis of potential ethical pitfalls.

As I left the initial interview, I found myself in a somber mood, knowing that my work would likely have important repercussions. At the same time, however, I felt excited by the opportunity to serve the court with a carefully reasoned, well-balanced, empirically supported, explicitly articulated, and defensible set of opinions related to the referral questions. Such evaluations are essential in a just system of law. I had met the patient, prepared for the ethical situations that I might face, and developed a clear understanding of my role. I was ready to go to work.

Key ethical principles and standards

APA (2002): Principle C (Integrity), Principle D (Justice), Standard 2.01 (Boundaries of Competence), Standard 3.05 (Multiple Relationships), Standard 3.06 (Conflict of interest), Standard 3.07 (Third-Party Requests for Services), Standard 3.10 (Informed Consent), and Standard 9.01 (Bases for Assessments).

REFERENCES AND FURTHER READING

Bonnie, R. (1990). Dilemmas in administering the death penalty: Conscientious abstention, professional ethics, and the needs of the legal system. *Law and Human Behavior, 14,* 67–90.

Committee on Ethical Guidelines for Forensic Psychologists. (1991). Specialty guidelines for forensic psychologists. *Law and Human Behavior, 15,* 655–665.

Melton, G. B., Petrila, J., Poythress, N. G., & Slobogin, C. (2007). *Psychological evaluations for the courts: Mental health professionals and lawyers* (3rd ed.). New York: The Guilford Press.

Small, M. A., & Otto, R. K. (1991). Evaluations of competency to be executed: Legal contours and implications for assessment. *Criminal Justice and Behavior, 18,* 146–158.

Watt, M. J., & MacLean, W. E. (2003). Competency to be sentenced and executed. *Ethics and Behavior, 13,* 35–41.

11

Is That What I Said? Ethical Challenges When Parents Divorce During Treatment

Robin M. Deutsch

Lily was a 7-year-old child when I began to work with her in psychotherapy. She initially presented with anxiety, resisting going to school, having play dates, or separating from her mother. Her mother had a part-time job teaching at a nursery school, and her father frequently traveled as a part of his sales job. It was not unusual for him to be gone two nights a week. Lily also had an older sister, age 13, who by report functioned well academically, behaviorally, and socially and did not have any emotional problems.

Treatment with Lily progressed well in that she was able to master her separation anxiety enough to go to school without protest and had connected socially to the point that she had some play dates with one of her classmates who lived in the neighborhood. Lily continued to have difficulty separating from her mother; she protested if anyone but her mother attempted to put her to bed, and she wanted her mother to fall asleep with her. Periodically, Lily went to the nurse's office at school complaining of a stomachache requiring her to return home.

I attempted to provide some guidance for the parents regarding techniques such the use of positive reinforcement and self-monitoring at times of separation. Whereas the mother made herself available for such guidance, either after a session with Lily or on the telephone, Lily's father was difficult to engage. He came in for one session at the beginning of treatment with Lily because that is an essential part of my treatment protocol; however, the few times that we scheduled phone contacts, he did not answer his phone at the appointed time.

About six months into treatment with Lily, her mother called to inform me that her husband had filed for divorce. Accompanying the petition was an affidavit including allegations that she was a dysfunctional parent and that her mental health problems had resulted in significant psychological disturbance in their younger daughter; consequently, he was seeking primary custody of Lily.

The mother engaged an attorney, and shortly thereafter that attorney called me. Initially, she wanted to hear about Lily's treatment. I told her I was unable to talk about Lily's treatment without the father's permission as well as the mother's. I did answer her question about who brought the child to treatment and which parent I communicated with. She then wondered if I could provide an affidavit for the court that testified to the mother's good psychological health and parenting skills. I explained that the mother was not my patient; I had never evaluated her in order to be able to speak to that issue. The lawyer followed up that conversation with a letter to me, copied to the father's attorney, thanking me for my observations of the mother's good psychological functioning, my concern about the father's absence in the treatment, and Lily's fear of her father. Once I got over the initial shock of such misrepresentation, I needed to decide what to do, if anything. The next day, before I had framed a response, I received a subpoena duces tecum ordering me to turn over copies of Lily's treatment records and appear for deposition at the father's attorney's offices the following week.

Lily was coming in for her weekly appointment the following day, and I was concerned that her mother would try to engage me in a discussion about the legal proceedings and about how Lily was now going to be in the middle of the conflict between her parents. I sought consultation with a well-respected senior colleague who has a part-time forensic practice. We agreed that I would send an e-mail to Lily's parents stating that although I would be responding to both the letter from the mother's attorney and the subpoena from the father's attorney, I was concerned that Lily might be exposed to anxiety, hostility, or negative comments from either parent. I urged them to be very careful that she did not overhear any telephone calls involving discussion of the litigation, and that though they were both most likely distressed by the current situation, they should keep their communications with each other as cordial as possible. I let them know that the way they now handled themselves in Lily's presence was directly related to whether Lily would maintain the therapeutic gains she had achieved in the past six months. I ended the e-mail by telling them that I knew that they both wanted to be the best parents they could be for Lily and that I was available to provide feedback about how Lily was progressing and what she needed. I also emphasized that I would not be talking to them about the custody dispute.

I then called the legal counsel consultant for our state psychological association and made a telephone appointment. I wanted to be certain that I understood my legal obligations in responding to the subpoena. In my state of Massachusetts, a child's treatment is privileged. When a child is involved in the legal system in any way, the child's psychotherapy is protected so that only the court or its representative, a guardian ad litem, can waive the psychotherapist-patient privilege. Upon consultation, we decided that I would initially write a letter to both attorneys. The letter stated that I first wanted to clarify what in fact I had stated to the mother's lawyer—that is, that I would not comment upon either parent's functioning as I had not evaluated them and that was not my role as Lily's therapist. I would then let them know that I had received the subpoena duces tecum from the father's attorney for a deposition and was very concerned about efforts to bring Lily's treatment into their custody litigation. I opined that it would be very damaging for Lily, that it would compromise our treatment, and that she was a child who needed a safe place where she could share her worries and concerns. Unless I heard from the father's attorney within 48 hours canceling the deposition, I would file a motion for protection with the court seeking protection from the deposition. I added that I knew that I was not legally obligated to provide the records or to testify unless the child's privilege had been waived. The mother's attorney supported my letter and filed a motion for protection. Before the motion was heard, the father's attorney agreed to release me from the subpoena.

I did see Lily one more time, and then the father rescinded his permission for treatment. He stated that Lily was doing better, and that he was concerned that I was biased in favor of the mother and would ultimately perpetuate that bias in my work with Lily. My next contact with the case was from the custody evaluator, who let me know that the court had just appointed a guardian ad litem for the waiver of the psychotherapist-patient privilege and that she hoped that I would support the waiver. It was my intention to let the guardian ad litem know that I felt very strongly that Lily needed to be in treatment and that I was concerned that if her parents were not protecting her from the conflict, her symptoms of anxiety would re-emerge.

Discussion

Key ethical issues

In the following discussion, I refer to the American Psychological Association *Ethical Principles of Psychologists and Code of Conduct* (2002). This was a very challenging case for me in that I believed that Lily was being harmed by the conflict between her parents and I needed to make certain that I did not contribute to that harm (Principle A: beneficence and nonmaleficence). Because we know unequivocally that children are often harmed when they are in the middle of their parents' conflict, I was clear that I needed to stay as objective as possible and not contribute further to the pull for alliance that Lily was now most likely experiencing. It is not uncommon for parenting to be compromised when spouses begin to engage in marital or postmarital conflict. Parents are focused on the significant change they are experiencing and on the emotions attached to change and loss, and their efforts are often focused on reconstituting. They are often less attuned to their children. I was aware that it would be even more harmful for Lily to potentially hear that her therapist was engaged in their conflict as well.

Confidentiality (Ethical Standard 4.02) was a key ethical issue in this case. Beginning any treatment with a discussion of the limits of confidentiality is critical. With children, we tell them that the things that we talk about are confidential unless we are worried about their safety, or if there are things that we think their parents need to know. If we do feel that we need to tell authorities or their parents something, we let them know. A discussion of limits of confidentiality with parents must cover who the client is, the importance of protecting the child's confidentiality, the limits to confidentiality (including any suspicion of abuse or neglect), concerns about the child hurting herself or others, and whether the court has ordered that the treatment be subject to subpoena or testimony. It is prudent to let parents know the potentially negative effect of testimony or release of records on a child's treatment—that is, the child will discover that her confidential disclosures are now the subject of a legal proceeding. This occurrence often compromises the utility of any subsequent psychotherapy; the child will not trust that she has a confidential place where she can share worries or concerns.

The issue of disclosing Lily's treatment records highlights another salient ethical quandary in Lily's case. Ethical Standard 4.05 states that psychologists disclose confidential information with appropriate consent and without the consent of the individual only as mandated by law or where permitted by law for a valid purpose. The first consideration in deciding whether to release treatment records is Lily's minority status. Although Lily is the client, she is a minor, and therefore her parents protect her confidentiality. If both parents are legal custodians, as in Lily's case, her treatment records can be released with their joint consent. However, in states that have psychotherapist-patient privilege laws requiring the court to consent to the release of a minor's treatment records, if the minor is involved in a legal proceeding, the only relevant consent is that mandated by the court.

The issue of identifying the client is also relevant to this scenario. I had not contracted or engaged the parents in family therapy, or in an assessment of parenting capacity. It would have been a conflicting role had I changed roles to assess the mother's parenting (Ethical Standard 10.02b). The mother's attorney wanted me to describe her parenting and reflect on that in relation to Lily's needs. Ethical Standard 9.01b states that psychologists offer opinions about psychological characteristics of individuals only after they have conducted an evaluation sufficient to support their statements or conclusions. I was engaged as Lily's psychotherapist, and I never evaluated the mother's psychological health or parenting. Although I could comment on how often she brought Lily to treatment and whether she reported following through with the strategies and parenting guidance that I provided, I had no basis to comment on anything else regarding the mother's psychological functioning.

Although I was certainly aware that Lily's treatment had been terminated by the father and believed that the father might have been concerned that I was biased, I also knew that I would have done more harm if I had taken a position, relinquished neutrality in the face of the conflict between the parents, and aligned with one of the parents. Doing so would have further polarized Lily in this high-conflict situation. I had an ethical obligation to avoid harm (Standard 3.04), and I believed that aligning myself with anyone other than Lily would have increased the risk of harm to her.

Work setting

Providing psychological services to children usually requires contact with the environments in which they function, including school and home. As legal minors, children constitute a particularly vulnerable population; their brain and emotional development are evolving. Psychologists can provide crucial information and perspective to those people who care for child clients, and who serve as part of the team helping the child to function better. In that role, we do have thoughts about how these environments serve the children and are able to support them. However, in most instances we do not evaluate the teaching style of the teacher or parenting style of the parents and have only hypotheses about how the child is served by these key people. It can be tempting for a psychologist to go beyond his or her role and, in the service of advocating for a child patient, make formal or informal comments that may cast hypotheses as actual findings. Although we are aware of how parents, teachers, and other medical providers respond to our concerns or suggestions, we are not aware of the child's full experience with any of these people.

As child psychologists, we often find ourselves interacting with larger systems, including the social service and legal systems. A change in the parents' marital status is not uncommon, given that the parents of more than a million children each year divorce. We know that marital conflict is a predictor of child maladjustment, so it is not unusual for that to be an environmental stressor when parents bring a child in for treatment. It is sometimes most effective to refer the parents for marital therapy or the family for family therapy. But when we are treating a child, maintaining the boundaries of our role can be challenging, particularly when we are being pulled to protect or advocate for the child.

One of the great challenges of providing child treatment is the frustration that can arise when the environments and systems in which the child exists fail to support the child's best interests. As the child's psychologist, we can educate the people who interact with the child, but in the end, we cannot control whether these entities abide by our recommendations.

Reflection

This case was particularly difficult for me because I lost Lily, my client, at a time when I believed that she needed psychotherapy. I had to struggle with maintaining clinically sound and ethically mandated boundaries, knowing that my client, the most vulnerable member of this family, now had no place where she could share her anxieties and concerns. Fortunately, I had the opportunity to consult with the legal counsel of our state psychological association, who helped me think through my options, ethically and legally. I was able to consider the immediate issue of responding to the subpoena, as well as the potential long-term consequences for my client of the custody dispute.

Considering Lily's clinical needs, the potential long-term effects of violating the boundaries of treatment (i.e., offering an opinion about the mother's psychological functioning and parenting, a clear violation of my ethics code) would have very likely intensified the destructive legal positioning. Lily was now the subject of a custody battle. If I had joined in that battle, I could have predicted further polarization of the family and an increased probability that Lily would be stranded in the middle of her parents' conflict.

Had I shared Lily's treatment records, I would have violated state law. It might have offered data for both of the parents regarding the effectiveness of the treatment and the benefits to Lily, but it was not my place to decide whether the disclosure would be beneficial for her. I had to comply with the law, and I did not know how Lily's trust in the psychotherapy process would be affected by my disclosure.

Had I not followed the APA *Ethics Code* or had I been unaware of the law of my state, I could have compromised Lily's treatment and provided sound grounds for either parent to terminate the treatment. The way the situation played out, I was able to clarify the ethical and legal requirements to which I was bound. I also had to believe that the court system to which Lily was subject would be able to protect her and provide for her best interests. The court would be able to gather the information required to make the best decisions for Lily.

In my work with children, there is often a pull to protect them and, given their vulnerability, to advocate for them. Children are not heard or seen directly in court. It is particularly difficult to maintain my therapeutic boundaries and stay true to my role when I do have thoughts about how each parent interacts with and considers the needs of my child client. Yet, unless I have a reason to suspect that my clients are being abused or neglected by one of their parents, thus triggering a mandated report to social services, I cannot opine upon the parents in any way, nor can I suggest what kind of parenting arrangement is in the child's best interests. For these reasons, it is essential that psychologists who treat children remain aware of their personal biases and issues, so that they do not get pulled into the legal manipulations that so often occur when children are the subject of parental legal wrangling.

Relevant ethical principles and standards

APA (2002): Principle A (Beneficence and Nonmaleficence), Principle B (Fidelity and Responsibility), Standard 3.04 (Avoiding Harm), Standard 4.01 (Maintaining Confidentiality), Standard 4.02 (Discussing the Limits of Confidentiality), Standard 4.05 (Disclosures), Standard 9.01b (Bases for Assessments).

REFERENCES AND FURTHER READING

Doolittle, D., & Deutsch, R. (1999). Children and high-conflict divorce: Theory, research, and intervention. In R. M. Galatzer-Levy & L. Kraus (Eds.), *The scientific basis of child custody decisions.* (pp. 425–440). New York: John Wiley & Sons.

Greenberg, L. R., Gould-Saltman, D. J., & Gottlieb, M. C. (2008). Playing in their sandbox: Professional obligations of mental health professionals in custody cases. *Journal of Child Custody, 5*, 192–217.

Knapp, S., Gottlieb, M., Berman, J., & Handelsman, M. M. (2007). When laws and ethics collide: What should psychologists do? *Professional Psychology: Research and Practice, 38*, 54–59.

Koocher, G. (2008). Ethical challenges in mental health services to children and families. *Journal of Clinical Psychology, 64*, 601–612.

12

Now You See It, Now You Don't: When Releases of Information Are Rescinded

John C. Gonsiorek

The subject of my forensic evaluation was a health care professional whom a state licensing board alleged had engaged in serious professional impropriety of a sexual nature. This type of evaluation may be referred by health care licensing boards, employers, ethics committees, bishops, or ecclesiastical councils, depending on the helping professional involved. This professional understood that the purpose of the evaluation included an assessment of his potential for remediation, a focus central to these evaluations.

After years of conducting evaluations of impaired professionals, I have learned that most impropriety has a pedigree. Intelligent professionals with years of graduate education do not just wake up one morning and decide to commit crimes, violate their clients' trust, damage or destroy their careers, embarrass their associates and professions, imperil their significant relationships, and transfer a good portion of their assets to the legal profession. The misconduct in question has a natural history, and a core function of the impaired professional evaluation is to ascertain the sources of misconduct and estimate if the problems discovered may be remediable.

When I conduct an impaired professional evaluation, anything is fair game in my search for reasonable hypotheses to address those questions, especially any history of other boundary violations or near misses of such. My tediously detailed informed consent document spells this out, and the professional had signed it before I commence the interview.

This professional's story was a common one in its outlines. His marriage of some decades became increasingly estranged, and he and his wife separated. One adult child sided with his wife, and the other supported him but had moved across the country. Then followed the disappointment of not getting a desirable job at a prestigious clinic, which he had hoped would reignite his moribund career.

One day, she appeared in his caseload. He began looking forward to her sessions. He dressed more smartly; his sense of humor returned. Within two months, he felt infatuated with her, in five months they became lovers, and at 11 months she filed a complaint about the relationship with his licensing board.

In interview, he seemed remorseful, self-castigating, worried about the heartache she might be experiencing at the abrupt termination of their relationship and that he had failed her as a professional. He seemed like many other middle-aged professionals who become needy and exercise very poor judgment at low points in their lives, ending up further down the slippery slope of boundary violations with clients than they ever imagined.

His presentation seemed consistent until I asked about earlier boundary violations. I am often apprehensive about this inquiry because it can be difficult to get the interview back on track afterward. The remorseful, guilt-ridden professionals, with no earlier history of serious boundary violations, can go down a rabbit hole of shame as they worry how others may construe their behavior; this echoes their own disapproval. Those who disclose earlier boundary violations often suddenly realize the implications of how this new information will bear adversely on their case. Many have attempted to dissuade me from including it in my report. My response focuses on reviewing the signed informed consent, which clearly indicates that I will make such inquiries, that this information will become a part of my report, and that they have agreed to accept the deleterious risks that all this entails.

Most give up after a while, a few surrender their licenses or resign their ministry, a very few threaten me with legal action or bodily harm. Of course, there are those who have earlier boundary violations and lie about them; I have no way of determining when this occurs. But no matter what is disclosed or not regarding previous transgressions, getting the interview back on track after these inquiries often proves a challenge.

In the current case, earlier boundary violations had occurred like clockwork every few years, involving both patients and supervisees. No complaints related to these boundary violations had come to light. He attributed them situationally to work stress, marital distance—anything but the chronic pattern that stared us both in the face.

From this point, the current case evolved differently. After a few attempts to persuade me why I did not need to include this information in the report, followed by my usual response, he stated that he understood my position. That evening, I received a voice mail message informing me that he had rescinded all releases of information, including the release to the licensing board. He further instructed me to have no contact about him with his licensing board, and that written documentation would follow. The next day, a letter by courier from his legal counsel confirmed this in writing. I telephoned the professional, who again requested that I make no mention of his earlier improprieties in my report. I told him I could not comply; this would be contrary to the informed consent agreement and would require me to knowingly present erroneous conclusions in my report. He stated that on the advice of his legal counsel, his rescission of all releases stood.

In the meantime, my report to the licensing board was due in 10 days. Because the board required verification of the evaluation date—the professional sent them a copy of my scheduling letter—and because the board had provided me with investigatory and background materials related to the case, it was quite clear that the board expected a report. The board's mailing included the due date for the report and a stipulation with the licensee that he was responsible for completing and paying for the evaluation, as well as signing the appropriate releases with me.

I was fairly certain that under Minnesota law, any legally competent adult had the right to rescind any release of information, unless it was overridden by a court order. It was also my understanding that a board stipulation on a licensee fell far short of a court order. To be certain, I consulted a forensic psychologist colleague. He reasoned that I had to produce and disclose a report despite the professional's explicit rescission of permission to do so because the board had ordered him to undergo an evaluation. This made no sense to me; the board placed an order on him, not me, and their order specifically referenced the requirement to obtain appropriate releases of information, underscoring their perception that these were necessary. My problem, I argued, was that the releases were now void, and stipulation on the licensee to sign them did not change that. My colleague responded that he always thought a board stipulation was like a court order. We continued the conversation, but it illuminated or satisfied neither of us.

Next, I called another forensic psychologist colleague, who responded that the rescinded release left me with nothing I could do; I could not legally or ethically release any information whatsoever pertaining to this professional. I explained the other colleague's viewpoint, which the second colleague attributed to a common confusion: some types of criminal law forensic evaluations involve court orders, and one could argue against the necessity of releases in such cases. But, he maintained, these did not occur in civil or administrative law contexts (licensing boards falling in the latter category), where releases were always necessary. Furthermore, he took the position that even in those criminal law contexts in which the evaluations were court-ordered, he still would not conduct the evaluation without releases. Judges and lawyers found this an unnecessary obsession on his part, but he could not feel comfortable with his ethical obligations as a psychologist otherwise.

Next, I called the toll-free hotline of my professional liability insurance carrier and scheduled an appointment with legal staff. No appointment was available until the following week. When I started to explain my dilemma, the attorney abruptly concluded that subjects of forensic evaluations had no confidentiality rights and I had nothing to be concerned about. I explained the lack of a court order, the stipulation referencing the need for releases, and the specifics of my state's data privacy act. He complained that my state had strange laws and had nothing further to offer.

Now I felt thoroughly alarmed, especially as my report now officially stood one day overdue; I already had a voice mail from the board reminding me that my report was due immediately. I then called my attorney. In retrospect, she was probably the first person I should have called; she knew my practice, had helped me finalize my informed consent documents and releases, regularly represented licensees to various boards, and defended professionals in malpractice cases. After I explained my dilemma, she told me my analysis remained essentially correct and that it would be both illegal and unethical to release any information. I then told her I remained concerned based on the discordant opinions I had gathered. She grumbled at the first colleague's opinion, stating it had no legal basis, and made approving noises at the second colleague's opinion. But on hearing the malpractice carrier attorney's opinion, she burst into a tirade, stating that I was the third of her clients to whom that carrier had given erroneous legal advice, and that the carrier had an obligation to consider all relevant laws before giving opinions. In actuality, her phrasing was considerably more tart. She concluded that my analysis was correct and that I should do nothing further.

Over the next few days, the voice messages from the board kept coming, and then arrived a rather acid letter reminding me of the due date. I felt humiliated to be thought irresponsible by the board and continued to worry that I was not fulfilling obligations to this third party. I kept pondering the situation and concluded that I had arrived at a technically correct solution that nonetheless left all parties unsatisfied: me, the professional, and the board. Was there not a better solution?

I called the second colleague and sought his opinion on the wisdom of requesting that the professional provide me with a release of information allowing me to tell the board that he had revoked all releases of information, but nothing else. He saw no fault in this plan. I then ran it by my attorney, who was puzzled why I would bother to do this when I had a legally sound solution. I explained to her that legally sound was necessary, but not sufficient. It was my practice to be transparent about issues of confidentiality and informed consent, and I saw no reason to not do so in this case. I also thought that the best way to not get sued in complex situations like this was to treat all parties with dignity, respect, and transparency. She ultimately thought that the request was legally unnecessary, but perhaps sound risk management.

I called the professional, told him about the contact from the board, and my unresponsiveness to them, as well as my discomfort. He acknowledged that he had received similar contacts and also felt uncomfortable. He agreed to discuss my suggestion with his attorney. He called me shortly thereafter and stated that his attorney had agreed to a release that would allow me to inform the board that the professional had rescinded releases of information, provided that they reviewed my letter in advance. I prepared a letter stating only that the professional had rescinded all releases of information, including the release to the board, and that it was my understanding and my attorney's opinion that I was obliged to honor the professional's revocation. The professional and his attorney agreed to the letter's content, and off it went.

A few months later, the professional contacted me, informing me that his license had been suspended indefinitely, pending receipt of a report from me with accompanying valid releases. He further offered that he initially had felt angry with my stance but recognized that despite our differences I had treated him respectfully, and he appreciated that. I heard nothing from his licensing board. After some time had passed, I realized that they were continuing to refer evaluations to me at a similar pace as before. I suspect, but do not know, that they did not perceive me as ignoring my obligations to them.

Discussion

Key ethical issues

Each domain of psychological practice includes areas of particular ethical vulnerability. This case illustrates that for forensic psychological practice, ethical issues of informed consent and confidentiality are preeminent concerns. These are especially challenging because the informed consent issues tend to be highly specific to the psycho-legal question at hand. One will not lose custody of children in a disability hearing; one will not be executed as a result of a civil lawsuit for damages stemming from sexual harassment. But the former can occur in a child custody evaluation, and the latter in a competency to be executed evaluation. Forensic practice, then, demands informed consent procedures tailored to the particular psycho-legal question at hand, and extra efforts to be certain that the consent is truly informed and real. Similarly, being certain to whom ones owes duties and how to prioritize those duties, although important in all psychological services, is an exquisitely pointed concern in forensic activities. Giving these issues the due diligence they require for a sound resolution can be an inconveniently complex, expensive, cumbersome, and time-consuming process, but the alternatives are ultimately much worse on all these counts.

Ethical concerns become dilemmas when there are multiple competing inconsistent solutions to the issue. In this case, I had a forensic evaluation client who had contracted and paid for psychological services. I accepted him as a client and so incurred primary duties to him; informed consent was given and signed, and I had rendered but not completed psychological services. He then elected only to rescind releases of information, which was his legal prerogative. The complication was that this prevented my satisfying the expectations of the third party that initiated the evaluation. Could my primary duties to him, which included his rights to confidentiality and not being harmed by my actions, be discharged while I was also being responsive to the third party? Making the third party primary was both illegal and unethical; merely following his revocation was legally sound and ethically adequate, but suboptimal.

Work setting

In recent years, I discontinued a long-standing solo clinical and forensic practice. In complex forensic evaluations, my solo status presented positive and negative aspects. Positive aspects included the following: enhanced privacy in sensitive/high-visibility cases; reduced overhead, allowing me to turn away with fewer consequences cases that seemed ethically compromised or high-risk (e.g., attorneys prone to misrepresent facts to their own experts); and intimately knowing all aspects of the practice. The downsides were real, but remediable: lack of in-house colleagues and consultation; greater volatility in income with one practitioner; stress, especially having a monster for a boss and no one to whom one could delegate. I made significant efforts to seek out collegial consultation and legal support, and I operated a fiscally conservative business. Managing stress was the most challenging aspect and included giving significant attention to the quality of my primary relationship, taking regular vacations, engaging in aerobic exercise, and having interests and a real life outside psychology. Despite these efforts, I survived a heart attack at age 51 and learned of the sudden death of two forensic psychologist colleagues from similar cardiovascular events. These experiences persuaded me to end my forensic practice. Now, I teach, write about, and engage in limited consultation in forensic psychology. These activities are almost as much fun as forensic practice, and a great deal less stressful. My income has decreased, but overall, this outcome is considerably better than a body bag.

I am not suggesting that psychologists avoid stressful work in general or stressful forensic work in particular, nor am I suggesting that forensic work leads to an early demise. I am suggesting that we owe it to ourselves and the public to engage stress with hard-headed appraisals of our personal risk factors, be they medical, psychological, fiscal, systemic, or other, and to be willing to make substantive behavioral changes to manage them when the situation calls for it. Protection of our clients and the public is the most commonly articulated reason for this, but of equal primacy is self-protection.

Without thoughtful consideration of the stressors and ethical quandaries associated with independent practice, this case could have easily ended badly. I had already arranged sound legal counsel and had colleagues available for consultation. I used them to manage the stress of a novel conundrum: the revocation of the release of information to the requesting third party in a forensic evaluation. I was distressed at the prospect of alienating a licensing board that referred cases regularly, but with sound fiscal management of my practice, the loss of any referral source was survivable. Although the case was stressful, my life was otherwise not unduly stressed, so I could muster my clearest thinking and judgment. These assets are reliably needed by mental health professionals who engage in a forensic or an independent practice that depends on third-party referrals when a conflict emerges between the demands of a client and those of a referral source.

Reflection

The inconsistent advice from consultants about the proper course of action was probably the most difficult feature of this case—especially the erroneous input from my own malpractice carrier. The situation drives home the admonition that forensic psychologists must be very familiar with the case law, legal concepts, and evidentiary standards in the areas in which they practice—and they should make no assumptions about what these laws and standards may be in areas outside their typical scope of practice. This is likely why forensic practice tends to be so narrow, with most forensic psychologists focusing on a small subset of psycho-legal questions. It is simply too hard and too treacherous to do otherwise. This case highlights the importance of finding an attorney with genuine expertise in forensic work as well as in the laws relevant to your jurisdiction. It also serves as a caution about the importance of obtaining multiple sources of consultation. Although the discordant advice was uncomfortable, it was precisely the effort to resolve inconsistent perspectives that clarified my own perspective.

In this case, the process of obtaining consultation was active, challenging consultant input and obtaining reactions to perspectives contrary to the consultant's. My goal was to emerge as certain as possible about the bases for the opinion I eventually held about the dilemma. I needed to fully understand why I concluded as I did, and to have considered counterarguments. This unabashedly adversarial cognitive style is one of the gifts of the legal profession for forensic psychologists. Although we as behavioral scientists aspire to a similar process of evaluating competing hypotheses, as a profession we have had a hard time resisting the siren call of grand theory, which often attenuates the aggressive questioning of assumptions. I recommend this cognitive habit to all psychologists, forensic or not.

Ethical forensic psychologists often lose referral sources when they call cases as they see them. Attorneys often publicly state preference for experts who testify for both defense and prosecution, plaintiff and defense. But when attorneys expect psychological experts to see things their way, especially if there has been agreement in the past, more than a few hold grudges if disappointed. Similarly, efforts at due diligence with confidentiality and informed consent are often viewed by attorneys as legally irrelevant fussing, or even obstructionistic. Sometimes, explaining the legal and ethical duties of psychologists to them solves the misunderstanding, but other times it does not.

The devil is always in the details, and the details always matter. Other licensing boards have evaluations structures other than the one previously described. They stipulate to their licensees that the board, not the licensees, pays for and "owns" the report (the board then charges the licensees for it as part of the legal costs they assess the licensee), and they stipulate that the licensees have no access to the report at all. In this model, the evaluator functions as a consultant to the board. The appropriate analysis of the dilemma in this context would have been very different. My currently preferred structure, one that would have prevented the dilemma described here, is that the licensee be required to produce an evaluation report by an evaluator chosen by the board, with accompanying releases, by a certain date. The licensee still contracts with the evaluator, pays for the report, and fully retains the right to rescind. But if the report, predicated on the releases being operationalized, is not produced, the licensee's license is indefinitely suspended. The professional being evaluated can truly give informed consent and make decisions about confidentiality, the board retains a powerful mechanism to protect the public, and the forensic evaluator remains independent, yet is not caught in the middle should the release be rescinded. That solution eventually occurred in this case, but with extra steps and much Sturm und Drang. After the experience of this case, I began suggesting this recommended structure to licensing boards. In truth, few listened.

In an adversarial legal system, however, no solution remains forever viable. Legal counsel has an ethical duty to operate in the client's best interests, and that means creating advantage. As a result, forensic psychologists will be called upon to respond to novel ethical dilemmas created by attorneys discharging their ethical duties by creating the dilemma. I am not being facetious or covertly critical of attorneys here. That is simply how the adversarial system works, and forensic psychologists must find ways to respond that are consistent with our ethical requirements because it is we who have elected to practice psychology within the constraints of their legal system.

When I later discussed this case with colleagues, some wondered whether I might have bypassed the angst and multiple consultations. A few opined to simply respect the rescinded release and forget about the board. Others suggested that getting any opinion that supported releasing it against the professional's wishes was an adequate discharge of my obligations, and it was sufficient for me to do so. The former seemed insufficient; the latter, frankly suicidal. The point, however, is that optimal solutions to ethical dilemmas are not merely plausible but facile rationalizations that address only part of the competing demands, but instead a considered course of action that attempts to prioritize and satisfy all of them. This is not always possible, but if the resolution ends up as mere compromise, it should not be because of a lack of trying, but because the dilemma is not currently known to be solvable.

I have also noticed geographical variation in colleagues' reactions. Those in my home state generally come to the same analysis previously outlined, but colleagues in some other states perceive this analysis as an excessively rigid construction of data privacy and confidentiality requirements. The reason for this is state-to-state variation in licensing board regulations, data privacy laws, and how these are typically interpreted. The optimal solution will have a distinctly local flavor shaped by the particular jurisdiction's requirements; yet, the broader issues involved and the processes of analyzing such a case remain fairly consistent across jurisdictions.

Most importantly in this case, I came away feeling like a true psychologist: one who not only did what was legally required, but who also attempted to treat all with beneficence, responsibility, integrity, justice, and respects for rights and dignity. I remain idealistic enough to think that this is the best ethical stance and risk management of all.

Key ethical principles and standards

APA (2002): Principle D (Justice), Principle E (Respect for People's Rights and Dignity), Standard 3.04 (Avoiding Harm), Standard 3.07 (Third Party Requests for Service), Standard 3.10 (Informed Consent), Standard 4.01 (Maintaining Confidentiality), Standard 4.02 (Discussing Limits of Confidentiality), Standard 4.05 (Disclosures), Standard 9.01 (Bases for Assessments), Standard 9.03 (Informed Consent in Assessments).

REFERENCES AND FURTHER READING

Bronstein, D. A. (2007). *Law for the expert witness* (3rd ed.). Boca Raton, FL: CRC Press.

Donner, M. B., VandeCreek, L., Gonsiorek, J., & Fisher, C. (2008). Unbalancing confidentiality: Protecting privacy and protecting the public. *Professional Psychology: Research and Practice, 39,* 369–376.

Gonsiorek, J. C. (Ed.). (1995). *Breach of trust: Sexual exploitation by health care professionals and clergy.* Newbury Park, CA: Sage Publications.

13

The Siren Song of Silence: Ensuring a Basis for Professional Judgments

Robert Kinscherff

Some years ago, I found myself appointed as a guardian ad litem in a high-conflict divorce case in which allegations of sexual abuse had arisen in the context of a prolonged and very bitter child custody dispute. The allegations involved sexualized touching and fondling of the genitals of the six-year-old daughter during overnight visitations, perhaps in the guise of caretaking activities such as bathing. The allegation followed the sudden onset of anxious and compulsive genital self-touching by the child that the primary custodial parent and some (but not all) school staff interpreted as troubling "sexualized" behavior.

While in psychotherapy initiated three months earlier to help her cope with anxiety arising from the separation of her parents and their ongoing conflict, the child had also become electively mute. She had stopped speaking two months before the allegations of sexual abuse during a period of time when her mother and father had each apparently begun relentlessly interrogating her to get information about the other parent. As a result, the child had made no statements to her therapist regarding either the potential sexual abuse or her self-touching. As often happens in these matters, a pediatric examination revealed no conclusive physical findings of abuse.

The scope of my appointment as guardian ad litem was strictly limited to the investigation of the alleged sexual abuse.

The parent against whom the allegations had been made expressed considerable urgency because the court had suspended visitations pending a report and recommendations. I interviewed both parents and relevant collaterals, but the child remained mute during two efforts to interview her. I also conducted personality testing with both parents. Although assessment approaches and professional practices in the assessment of alleged child sexual abuse have been refined in the years since this case, the core issues raised by the circumstances of my involvement as a psychologist remain relevant today.

The information that I obtained was, in my opinion, insufficient to confidently "rule in" or "rule out" sexual touching of the child. The accused parent flatly denied any inappropriate or even questionable touching during the course of child care activities or otherwise. The parent making the accusations strongly rejected any potential alternative hypotheses, such as the possibility that the genital self-touching had emerged as an effort at self-soothing, given the child's high level of anxiety in the context of very strong and persisting parental conflict. Personality testing was not particularly helpful in clarifying this specific issue. The allegation and denial essentially boiled down to a determination of credibility that the psychological assessment could not particularly enlighten and certainly could not resolve.

During the investigation, however, I had formed strong impressions of the toll taken on this child by the ongoing parental conflict. I had some opinions about some potentially helpful clinical interventions for the child and parents, steps the court might take to more effectively shield the child from the parental conflict and a visitation structure that would be more developmentally appropriate for the child (should the court decide to allow the parents to resume shared physical custody and visitation).

One problem involved the fact that these impressions and opinions fell beyond the narrow scope of my appointment as guardian ad litem. Furthermore, although I had interviewed both parents and a range of collaterals, the focus of the inquiry had been on the emergence of the girl's "sexualized" behaviors and the possibility of her victimization during visitations. I had not conducted a broader assessment of parenting skills and capacities.

Additionally, although she had been unwilling to talk with me during our sessions, during one session she had willingly drawn some pictures and engaged in some doll play. The play and drawing reflected themes of rescue by a powerful outside force from circumstances of danger and fear arising from feeling trapped between opposing evil forces. I had also felt utterly taken with the stricken, sad gaze that she fixed upon me as she drew and played with me during that session, almost as though she were attempting to signal to me directly what she wanted, although she was literally "without a voice" because of her mutism.

Finally, I had to acknowledge that I personally found one parent seemingly more credible than the other during interviews, although I admittedly had no compelling objective data to either substantiate sexual abuse of the child or to dismiss the allegation.

While writing the report for the court, I found myself repeatedly recalling the look on the child's face during the two sessions and considering whether or how to craft the report in a manner that would let me act as an "advocate for the child" and to "give voice" to this literally silent child. On the one hand, it seemed clear that the child was paying a terrible price for the persisting and intense parental conflict, even before the allegations of sexual abuse came up and the visitation was suspended. On the other hand, if I were to pose myself as the "advocate for the child," for what would I advocate, and on what basis?

If the child were being victimized, then the anger and the staunch refusal to permit unsupervised visitation by the parent with primary custody would be well justified, even if it occurred in the context of broader conflict. The protection of the child might be a collateral consequence of that parent's broader hostility towards the other, but it would constitute a protective stance nevertheless. If the child were not being victimized, then the anger and staunch insistence that visitation with the child resume promptly would be understandable, and no clear indication existed that before the suspension of visitation the child had feared or resented the visits. As with the parent with primary custody, the insistence of the other parent for visitation might be an almost collateral consequence of anger and hostility that predated the allegations of abuse, but from the child's perspective, the visits might maintain a parent-child relationship that she valued.

And, she could not or would not tell me directly herself in her own words about her experiences with one or both parents. The drawing and play reflected more a sense of being trapped between her parents than a particular fear or other negative reaction to one parent rather than the other. The more I struggled with the notion of acting as an "advocate for the child," I realized that in her silence I had become particularly vulnerable to intruding, bringing my own personal and very subjective perceptions, experiences, and judgments into that void.

Discussion

Key ethical issues

Standard 2.04 of the APA *Ethics Code* holds that the work of psychologists "is based upon scientific and professional knowledge of the discipline." Although it would have made my decision-making process easier, I simply did not have reliable scientific or professional basis upon which to render an opinion as to whether or not the child had been sexually abused during visits with the noncustodial parent. There was simply no compelling information that settled the question.

I had a visceral and strong intuition of what I *wanted* to believe and did believe subjectively, but I did not have any scientific or professional basis for confidently making a judgment of relative credibility. To implicitly or explicitly allow my personal perspectives or judgments to masquerade as science-based or professional judgments would not only violate Standard 2.04 but would also put me into conflict with Standard 9.01. This standard holds that psychologists "base the opinions contained in their recommendations, reports, and diagnostic or evaluative statements, including forensic testimony, on information and techniques sufficient to substantiate their findings."

I simply did not have information or techniques sufficient to confirm or dismiss the allegation of sexual abuse or to hold one parent as more credible than the other. Additionally, Standard 3.04 imposes upon psychologists the duty to "take reasonable steps to avoid harming their clients/patients, students, supervisees, research participants, organizational clients, and others with whom they work, and to minimize harm where it is foreseeable and unavoidable." Although because I was a guardian ad litem working under court appointment the court itself was my client, the members of this disintegrating family were certainly "others with whom" I was working.

I was strongly tempted to propose a process of supervised visitation for consideration by the court but did not include this in the report. Standard 2.01f holds that when psychologists stand in forensic roles, they "are or become reasonably familiar with the judicial or administrative rules governing their roles." The narrow scope of my court appointment instructed me to investigate and report upon the allegations of sexual abuse. I had no authorization to make broader recommendations regarding custody or visitation. I understood that the court expected any guidance I could offer in making a determination of whether or not the sexual abuse had occurred, and in how to proceed once the court made that specific decision either way.

Work setting

Situations like the one in this case occur commonly in divorce, child custody proceedings, and other legal proceedings in which psychologists may be appointed by courts or retained by attorneys to investigate allegations of domestic violence or other various forms of child maltreatment or neglect before a court has made a legal "finding of fact." Indeed, psychologists often find themselves in situations fraught with ambiguous or disputed facts when the court or others anticipate that their training and experience may generate information that will make it easier for the court to make determinations of what has or has not occurred. Whereas here, I had no scientific or professional basis upon which to render a confident professional opinion of what probably occurred or not, I felt as though I had to refrain from offering an opinion one way or the other "substantiating" or "not substantiating" the allegation of sexual abuse.

Legal proceedings are typically structured to yield determinations and decisions that are both clear and final. Criminal courts find verdicts of "guilty" or "not guilty," family courts assign rights and responsibilities such as "sole" or "joint" legal custody for children, and other courts determine whether a respondent is—or is not—going to be involuntarily civilly committed. Legal proceedings are not structured to incorporate ambiguity, and courts rarely ask psychologists to conduct assessments or render opinions in unambiguous circumstances.

As a result, psychologists often grapple with ambiguity in aiding courts to make decisions that reflect a clear choice made somewhere along a continuum of ambiguity. This ambiguity may arise from disputed facts, as in this case illustration, or from attempting to apply clinical approaches to the interpretation of a legal standard. For example, a criminal defendant's competence to stand trial is ultimately a matter of "fundamental fairness," and some defendants show relative strengths in some areas of trial competence but relative weaknesses in others. How fair is "fair enough" is essentially a social and moral decision rather than a clinical one, but courts often want psychologists to weigh in on whether a specific defendant may be competent or incompetent to stand trial. Sometimes, the ambiguity arises from the current limits of our science and practice, such as when we are asked to opine whether a specific juvenile delinquent may be "amenable to rehabilitation." Forecasting the future of an individual, particularly an adolescent who is still developing, commonly requires weighing multiple factors and prognostication that may well stretch beyond our science. Many of the common ethical dilemmas for psychologists in family court or other forensic settings have, at their base, ambiguity that may lure a psychologist into making personal credibility determinations, covertly usurping the role of the finder of fact by confusing clinical with legal constructs or pushing beyond the limits of current science or professional practice, often in an effort to be helpful or to aid the court in making difficult decisions.

Reflection

I had a strong intuition about the relative credibility of the parents. Yet, in the absence of information that would allow me to demonstrate that the account of one parent should weigh in more favorably than that of the other, I felt that if I did so that I would actually be relying more on my own *personal* reactions and attitudes than any specific *scientific* or *professional* expertise. As I wrote up the information gathered in individual interviews with the parents, I noticed the differences in tone created by slight differences in language. For example, differences in tone exist among "this parent indicated... reported... asserted... claimed."

As I considered my reaction to my experience of the relative credibility of parents during interview, I appreciated that I could insert myself in a powerful but subtle way into the role of the judge in making credibility determinations by how I phrased language in the report, or even go so far as implicitly or explicitly endorsing the perspective of one parent. For example, I could submit a report that signaled my endorsement of one parent over the other by providing recommendations that presumed or rejected precisely the matter at issue: whether or not a parent had sexually abused this girl. I recognized that, as I imagine occurs with most people, others have successfully misled me on occasion by willful deception in my personal life, and that to assume that I could reliably divine (in the absence of concrete information) who might deceive me in my professional life would constitute a particularly toxic form of hubris.

To avoid usurping the role of the judge in fact finding and making credibility determinations, and to avoid the harms that would likely arise to one or more members of this family if I inserted my personal judgments in the guise of psychological science or professional judgment, I wrote up the report in as objective and balanced a manner as possible. I had a colleague review a copy without identifying information for bias and tone before submitting it to the court. I reported that I lacked sufficient information to render a reliable or confident determination as to whether or not the sexual abuse occurred, and I drafted sets of recommendations for the court to consider should it decide that the maltreatment did or did not occur. I noted for the court the tension between the child's safety and the importance of parent-child contacts if the relationship with the noncustodial parent were to be sustained over time.

I recommended that the court consider appointment of a guardian ad litem to assist in any formal assessment of parenting capacities once the allegations of sexual abuse were resolved, and perhaps to assist in creating a process to minimize the impact of parental conflict upon the child. I felt that I had the data to support that recommendation and felt as though I owed at least that much to this child, even if it was a step beyond the narrow scope of my court appointment.

When the court eventually decided to appoint a guardian ad litem for those purposes and asked me to accept the appointment, I declined to do so for the following reasons: Although I lacked a scientific basis or data to transform my personal intuitions and beliefs into a responsible professional judgment, I did react strongly when the court ultimately made its determination about the alleged sexual abuse; I felt that the court had "got it wrong," although I also had to admit that I could not articulate any particular reason why the court's determination of parental credibility was more or less warranted than my own. At least the court bears the awesome moral authority and responsibility for making those kinds of determinations when required to do so, guided by rules of evidence if not by the kinds of science and professional practices that are intended to guide psychologists. I realized that my own reactions during the investigation and then to the court's decision had likely substantially compromised my ability to be professionally objective or perhaps even professionally effective, given that neither parent felt validated by my initial report. I realized in making the decision to decline the new appointment that my impulse was to take the appointment so as to give "voice" to this still-silent child, but after considerable reflection, I had to acknowledge to myself that I could not be sure whether the substitute "voice" I would bring would genuinely be hers and not mine. Years later, I still think of her when in situations in which I perceive children "without voice" and caught in the conflicts and cross fire of the adults around them.

Key ethical principles and standards

APA (2002): Principle A (Beneficence and Nonmaleficence), Principle D (Justice), Standard 2.01 (Boundaries of Competence), Standard 2.04 (Bases for Scientific and Professional Judgments), Standard 3.04 (Avoiding Harm), Standard 3.06 (Conflicts of Interest), Standard 9.01 (Bases for Assessments).

REFERENCES AND FURTHER READING

Committee on Ethical Guidelines for Forensic Psychologists. (1997). Speciality guidelines for forensic psychologists. *Law and Human Behavior, 15,* 655–665.

Koocher, G. P. (2006). Ethical issues in forensic assessment of children and adolescents, In S. N. Sparta & G. P. Koocher (Eds.), *Forensic mental health assessment of children and adolescents* (pp. 46–63). New York: Oxford University Press.

Pope, K., & Vasquez, M. (2007). *Ethics in psychotherapy and counseling: A practical guide* (3rd Ed.). San Francisco: Jossey-Bass.

Smith, S. R. (2006). Working with courts, judges and lawyers: What forensic mental health professionals should know about being expert witnesses. In S. N. Sparta & G. P. Koocher (Eds.), *Forensic mental health assessment of children and adolescents* (pp. 88–96). New York: Oxford University Press.

14

"Thera-mail" for a Quarter Century: Managing Complex Boundaries With a Former Client

Frederic G. Reamer

My weekly group meeting with the prison inmates ended on schedule. As I gathered my materials, I headed out of the maximum security penitentiary's "education" building and entered the prison yard. One of the group members—an inmate serving two consecutive life sentences with no parole option, plus an additional 50 years—walked beside me and handed me a small brown paper bag. "I made this for you," he said quietly, and then he walked away.

I felt caught off guard and stunned by Dale's gesture. I didn't know what to make of it, and the event transpired so quickly that I hardly had time to process how best to respond. I simply said, "Thanks!" and wended my way through the mazelike prison corridors to the front gate. As I headed to my car, I opened the bag and discovered that Dale had handcrafted a leather wallet for me carved with my initials. The design wasn't my style, but that didn't matter. What mattered was that this inmate—a member of the prison group I had facilitated for nearly two years—clearly cared about me and had taken the time to convey his feelings nonverbally. What made this gift especially meaningful—and surprising—is that during the two years or so that Dale had been attending my group, he had uttered only a handful of words. Dale remained silent nearly all the time, yet he came faithfully. I often wondered about Dale and his reasons for coming to the group. Obviously it mattered to him, yet we had never really engaged in sustained conversation.

Dale gave me his gift in 1983. At the time, I was a young assistant professor of social work and worked part-time at the nearby penitentiary. I have worked in prisons most of my professional career. When Dale handed me his gift, I accepted it without hesitation. At the time, it didn't dawn on me that I might have put my foot on the proverbial slippery boundary slope. In the early 1980s, very few professionals thought or wrote about complex and subtle boundary issues. The topic hadn't come up in my professional education, with the exception of the usual admonitions about sexual relationships with clients.

Instinctively, I wrote Dale a short thank-you note and handed it to him the next time I met with him at the prison:

> Dale: It was very kind of you to make me the wallet. I'm touched that you took so much time to make it. I'm very impressed with your skill, especially the way you carved my initials.
>
> I can't help but wonder what's been going on inside of you. You've attended nearly every one of our group meetings during the past couple of years, yet you're silent almost all the time. Feel free to let me know if there's something you'd like to talk about.

One week later, Dale handed me an envelope with his reply. He began his letter with some mundane comments about quitting his leather craft business. He then responded to my comments:

> You are correct in your observation. I have thoughts I would not share with others in the group. I have thoughts I would voice only to one or two others around here. I have thoughts I would share with no one.

For several months, Dale and I continued to exchange letters. He began to open up to me about the horrible murders he had committed while under the influence of drugs and about his deep, seemingly sincere remorse. I marveled at the fact that I had connected in an intense way with an inmate who regularly attended group sessions that I facilitated, during which he stayed virtually silent. I once joked with my wife that I seem to have stumbled onto a new form of professional-client relationship: *thera-mail*.

Several months later, this fairly benign way of connecting with Dale became more complex. My wife, also a social work professor, and I had accepted new faculty positions at a graduate school hundreds of miles away. I told Dale and the other group members that I would soon relocate to a new job. We processed the termination as best we could. Before I left the prison for the last time, Dale handed me a note letting me know how important my letters had become to him and that he would miss me terribly. He explained that for the first time since the murders, he had begun to open up. Dale wrote that he was finally able to express his feelings, but that he couldn't imagine doing so verbally when meeting with me, or anyone else, face to face.

Shortly before my wife and I packed up and moved, I wrote Dale and mailed the letter to the prison. I wished him well. Several weeks later he replied. That was 25 years ago. During the past 25 years, Dale and I have exchanged letters approximately every other month, without interruption. Dale's letters to me include a complex mix of soul-searching reflections about the murders he committed and relatively mundane details about his life in prison. A typical letter includes Dale's insights about what was going on in his life when he committed the murders and details about his prison job, prison gossip, and current events (e.g., national politics, major sporting events). My letters to Dale usually include follow-up questions about issues that Dale broached in his most recent letter. Often, I include follow-up queries that respond to points Dale made about the murders, his remorse, prison visits with his relatives, and the quality of his prison life. My comments and questions resemble those one would hear if I were talking with Dale in person. Occasionally, my letters include relatively mundane details about current events. Our letters always seem like a therapeutic exchange in slow motion.

Discussion

Key ethical issues

Ethical issues often seem clearer in hindsight. Twenty-five years after our relationship began, I have a reasonably good understanding of the boundary issues involved in my contact with Dale. Back then, however, I didn't have the same level of awareness—partly because I had less experience and partly because the ethical norms in my profession (social work) did not address these boundary issues in that era.

For example, today I understand that a client's gift giving and a practitioner's decision about whether to accept a gift can carry significant meaning. Twenty-five years ago, I simply did not grasp the issue well enough.

Furthermore, it took me some time to understand that my decision many years ago to embark on an exchange of letters with Dale introduced, over time, complex ethical issues about the appropriateness of maintaining contact with a former client. Only now do I think I have a full grasp of the ethical issues this relationship evokes. The primary ethical issues include boundaries, confidentiality, client self-determination, and the termination of services. Of course, when I helped to set this trajectory in motion 25 years ago, I could not possibly have forecast that the two of us would sustain our contact for decades. Ideally, however, I might have considered these possibilities.

During the past 25 years, I have also struggled with issues related to personal self-disclosure. I have found it hard to correspond with Dale all these years with only one-way disclosures, from Dale to me. The one-sided nature of the correspondence initially seemed awkward, artificial, and a bit condescending on my part. At various times over the years, I have made a conscious decision to share some very limited, innocuous personal information—for example, where my family and I traveled for a summer vacation or details about an interesting public event in my home state that I attended. I have never disclosed sensitive information.

Work setting

I now understand that ethical challenges vary from work setting to work setting. Context matters. For example, when I conduct ethics workshops for staffers in drug and alcohol treatment programs, I feel struck by the ways in which norms surrounding boundaries and multiple relationships differ from those in many other mental health treatment and social service settings. I have found that many staffers in substance abuse treatment centers feel more comfortable with self-disclosure (particularly in relation to their own experiences with substance abuse and recovery) than do staffers in other mental health treatment and social service settings (family service agencies, mental health centers, and private practice). It is quite common for staffers in substance abuse treatment programs to be in recovery and to share this fact with clients. Staffers and clients in recovery may encounter each other in 12-step meetings; for many people in recovery, the unique norms in 12-step culture (especially those related to confidentiality) help them navigate these boundary issues in ways that would be more challenging in other settings.

Similarly, clinicians in a remote wilderness therapy program for struggling adolescents may feel comfortable sleeping near clients and eating with clients (in fact, they may not have much choice), whereas clinicians in most other treatment settings would never consider crossing these boundaries. In other words, boundary challenges and norms vary from work setting to work setting. It is hard to generalize across all of them.

Having spent most of my career working in prisons, I know that this unique setting requires remarkable skill and vigilance regarding boundaries. Disclosing personal information to inmates or accepting gifts from them can violate institutional policies or prove disastrous in other ways. Most prison staffers do not display in their offices photographs of their family members, although this commonly occurs in other clinical settings. Although many prison inmates I have known are reasonably trustworthy and would never seek to sabotage a professional's career for self-serving purposes, some inmates do, in fact, grab any opportunity to exploit a staffer's naïveté or vulnerability. I've encountered the occasional inmate who gleefully discloses that a staffer accepted a gift or disclosed personal information in order to retaliate against the staffer, who, the inmate believes, behaved in an uncooperative or "difficult" manner. Sadly, prisons can become like petri dishes for adversarial relationships, conflict, cynicism, and mistrust. The boundary issues in this setting are in stark contrast to the boundary issues in less threatening, albeit complex, settings, such as grade schools, hospice programs, and private psychotherapy practices.

When I work in prisons, I remain especially cognizant of the distinction between ethical impropriety and the *appearance* of impropriety pertaining to boundaries. In my experience, prison staffers and inmates become hypersensitive to appearances. If inmates see a staffer and another inmate standing and talking in very close proximity in the prison yard, suspicions arise instantly. Has the inmate "ratted out" another inmate? Is there something "going on" between the staffer and inmate? Put simply, in prisons the threshold that defines appropriate and inappropriate boundaries sits much lower than in nearly any other social service setting. Letting down one's guard in a prison in relation to boundaries can have dire consequences.

Ethical norms in prison also prove challenging in other respects. Mental health professionals in prison must operate under unique rules concerning client (inmate) privacy and confidentiality. Typically, prison-based mental health professionals must remain mindful of security and safety risks that do not arise in other clinical settings (e.g., inmates who disclose that they have homemade knives or "shivs" in their cells to potentially stab a staffer or another inmate). Conscientious mental health professionals who work in prisons provide inmates with a different "exceptions to confidentiality" speech than do professionals in other settings.

Also, I have always needed to stay mindful of the fact that my correspondence with Dale lacks confidentiality. Prisons typically screen mail for contraband and have the right to read correspondence for any evidence of threats or security risks.

Similarly, informed consent guidelines and norms in prisons also pose unique ethical challenges. For example, the protection-of-human-participants-in-research protocols standard in hospital settings, for patients who agree to participate in randomized clinical trials involving high-risk drugs, may not pass muster among prison inmates with similar medical diagnoses and prognoses because of concern about possible inmate exploitation by the research sponsors.

Reflection

My experience with Dale has had a humbling effect. Twenty-five years after the fact, I view my relationship with Dale through a very different lens than I did when our relationship began. Ideally, when our relationship began, I would have recognized and thought about what it means when a client offers a professional a gift and the implications of the professional's decision to accept the gift. It turns out that my decision to accept Dale's gift set a 25-year relationship in motion. In truth, I'm not sure the outcome would have been different had I fully grasped these boundary issues. In retrospect, I think accepting Dale's handmade gift constituted an appropriate decision. To not accept the gift would have wounded him, I'm certain. Although I think accepting gifts from clients is risky, in this instance I believe that accepting Dale's unsolicited, handmade gift was the right choice.

The more ethically complex issues involve my decision to continue contact with Dale through our letter writing. Generally speaking, I would not advise a mental health professional to maintain a long-lasting relationship with a former client. Sustaining such a relationship can create counterproductive dependency, trigger problematic transference and countertransference, and undermine former clients' efforts to engage with another professional to help them address whatever challenges they face in life.

But, as with so many ethical challenges, one must factor in the unique circumstances of each case. It has seemed clear to me all along that Dale had no interest in speaking with another professional. Indeed, Dale has written to me repeatedly that he cannot imagine *talking* to anyone—even me—about the murders he committed. Dale has made it quite evident that he will communicate on these issues only with written words.

I sensed then, 25 years ago, and continue to believe that our exchange of letters provides Dale with an emotional lifeline; I do not consider our communication as therapy per se, but I do regard it as having a powerful therapeutic effect.

I also realize that my offer to exchange letters provides Dale with a safe emotional outlet and a relatively nonthreatening way for him to acknowledge his remorse and vulnerabilities. In prison settings, inmates usually are loath to publicize remorse or any form of weakness because of the possibility that others in the prison environment (both inmates and staffers) will exploit them. Through his letters, Dale is able to communicate with me privately. The fact that I live hundreds of miles away may add a further layer of emotional safety and therapeutic benefit.

This case raises one more critically important ethical issue: how mental health professionals respond to the morality or immorality of their clients' behavior. Many professionals provide services to people who have become genuine victims of life's toxic circumstances: children who have suffered physical or sexual abuse, women beaten by their partners, patients with terminal illnesses, and newborns with serious congenital impairment. Professionals' hearts instinctively go out to people who suffer through no "fault" of their own, people whose life circumstances seem horribly tragic.

Some of us, however, work with perpetrators, the people who abuse others physically, sexually, and emotionally. Although many, if not most, perpetrators have themselves suffered horrific abuse, many practitioners working with them struggle with the heinous nature of their clients' behavior. I know I do when I sit in a prison talking to inmates convicted of murder, rape, arson, armed robbery, embezzlement, and causing a death while driving under the influence. On an intellectual level, I understand that Dale murdered three people, one of them a four-year-old girl, while in the midst of a drug-induced psychosis. He had ingested so many potent drugs just before the murders, and his mind had undergone such alteration, that he lost complete control of his senses. The forensic evidence and courtroom testimony in his case make that abundantly clear. Interestingly, Dale had never committed an act of violence in his life before that fateful night. During my 25-year relationship with Dale, I have seen only one side of this man: a remarkably kind, sensitive, compassionate human being. I find it difficult to reconcile the goodwill I feel toward Dale with what I know about his disturbing crimes. Indeed, this has become the most challenging ethical issue for me in my relationship with Dale.

This particular ethical issue forces me to wrestle with the moral implications of the ancient debate regarding free will versus determinism and the concept of moral desert. Mental health professionals often make assumptions about the determinants of clients' behavior. For instance, some argue that poverty stems from structural problems in a capitalist economy and institutional racism (a form of determinism), whereas others believe that poverty results from individual laziness and sloth (a form of free will). Similarly, some professionals believe that criminal conduct results from determinants such as mental illness and cognitive impairment, whereas others believe that criminals choose, of their own free will, to violate laws and harm others. How we respond to these and other social problems—whether we focus our attention on environmental and other determinants or on individuals' moral flaws—frequently depends on assumptions we make about the extent to which people's problems flow from factors over which they have control.

My relationship with Dale has taught me a great deal about ethics. I've learned that one's work setting and context matter, and that ethical issues that loom large in one setting, such as a prison, may seem relatively minor in other mental health settings. I've learned that ethical norms evolve in the helping professions. Contemporary thinking about boundaries and dual relationships has become much more refined and mature as the human service professions have evolved.

Furthermore, I've learned that my own ethical instincts and insights have evolved and matured over time. My grasp of ethical issues today feels more nuanced than much earlier in my career. I can only wonder what I will understand more fully years from now than I do in this moment.

Finally, I've learned that ethical issues sometimes involve much more than our intellectual wrestling with matters related to privacy, confidentiality, informed consent, boundaries, conflicts of interest, paternalism, and so on. Ethical dilemmas involving professionals' response to their own sense of clients' morality are especially complex.

Key ethical principles and standards

NASW (1999): Standard 1.01 (Commitment to Clients), Standard 1.02 (Self-Determination), Standard 1.06 (Conflicts of Interest), Standard 1.07 (Privacy and Confidentiality), Standard 1.16 (Termination of Services).

REFERENCES AND FURTHER READING

Corey, G., Corey, M. S., & Callanan, P. (2006). *Issues and ethics in the helping professions* (7th ed.). Pacific Grove, CA: Brooks/Cole.

Reamer, F. G. (2003). *Tangled relationships: Managing boundary issues in the human services*. New York: Columbia University Press.

Reamer, F. G. (2006). *Ethical standards in social work: A review of the NASW Code of Ethics* (2nd ed.). Washington DC: NASW Press.

Reamer, F. G. (2006). *Social work values and ethics* (3rd ed.). New York: Columbia University Press.

Zur, O. (2007). *Boundaries in psychotherapy: Ethical and clinical explorations*. Washington DC: American Psychological Association.

15

Jonas and His Protective, Delusional, or Alienating Mother: Advocacy, Forensics, and Boundaries With Battered Women

Lenore E. Walker

Michelle sat in my office looking quite frightened. She had missed her appointment the previous day, but I agreed to see her when I had a cancellation. "I'm sorry, I forgot," was all she could say. A colleague, who had supervised her for two years in a hospital-based program where she worked, had referred her to me. "She's a quiet and competent professional," said the colleague, "but she is in trouble with the courts taking away her child. That's all we know, but we think she was in a domestic violence relationship."

I had left two hours for the initial interview, knowing that it would take at least that much time for Michelle to tell her story without my asking too many distracting questions. A "quiet" battered woman, as the initial referral suggested, probably would have some hesitation to give too much information at first, needing to gain support and assurance that I would understand and not judge her unfairly. But, the story that Michelle told that day took me by surprise.

Michelle had met and married Josef six years earlier, and together they had one child, a boy, Jonas, who was five years old at the time I first saw Michelle. Jonas was a difficult baby who often seemed inconsolable when he began crying. Although Michelle had planned to stay home with Jonas for three months, she ended up staying home for almost the entire first two years because no one else except for her mother could put up with Jonas' crying. All the doctors she consulted said Jonas seemed healthy, but he rarely smiled or played with others. Michelle's relationship with Josef, which had not gotten off to a great start, began to deteriorate as she became more preoccupied with finding out why Jonas seemed so unhappy. As he got older, Jonas began to play by himself, and his crying gave way to screaming and tantrums when he didn't get what he wanted. Exhausted at night from caring for Jonas during the days, Michelle let Josef put Jonas to bed while she would lie down in bed trying to ignore Jonas' screams. Her major relief became visits to her parents' large home by the beach, where they all could relax and play in the pool or ocean.

Occasionally, Michelle would accept work as a consultant for a day or two, and her mother would babysit with Jonas while Josef went to work. Michelle found herself beginning to pull away from Josef, and he became more controlling and demanding, often criticizing her for failing to fill the role expected of a traditional wife and mother. He actually physically hurt her on two different occasions during an argument over his demands. Their lovemaking became more "rough" and abusive to Michelle, and she tried to avoid him by going to sleep before he came to bed at night. Several times she awoke to his having sex with her even though she had fallen asleep. Although horrified and disgusted by this, she did not stop him because he became less verbally abusive afterward.

One night, after a particularly difficult day with Jonas, Michelle lay down in her bed while Josef gave Jonas a bath. She thought she had fallen asleep, but she awoke hearing Jonas pleading with his father. "Put it in slowly, daddy. Please don't hurt me like before. It hurts, daddy. Please. Please. Please. No more, daddy. No more, daddy." "Ok, Jonas. I'll be careful. Don't worry. I won't hurt you. It will be okay. You will feel good, just like daddy."

The words and tone of his pleading reminded Michelle of what she said when Josef tried to insert his penis into her anus. She sat up in bed, horrified. She thought for a minute and then reached for the telephone. But, she didn't know whom to call. She put down the telephone. She became frightened as she heard the door to the bathroom open and Jonas came running out, with no pajama pants on and dripping from his bottom. He ran into bed with Michelle and started to cuddle with her. A few minutes later Josef came in, took the child from Michelle's arms, put on his pajama bottom, and carried him into his own bed. By the time Josef finished putting Jonas to bed, Michelle had fallen back to sleep.

When Michelle awoke the next morning, she had a vague memory that something terrible had happened, but she could not remember the details. Life went on as it had before, but Michelle became more and more depressed and anxious. It bothered her that she couldn't remember what horrible thing had happened, but she didn't know what to do about it. At one point, she even went to see a hypnotist, but all that happened was that she remembered something bad had happened to Jonas. Josef yelled more and began cursing at her more often. When Jonas turned three years old, he seemed more compliant, so they placed him in a preschool program. He would do well for awhile and then, without warning, would become aggressive with other children and, when reprimanded, would scream for long periods of time.

After another episode of domestic violence, Michelle took Jonas to her parents' home and told Josef that she planned to end their marriage. Josef begged and pleaded with her not to leave him, so she and her parents invited him to live with them. When I asked her why she let him come into their home, she said she felt safer at her parents' house and she didn't really want to break up their marriage; she just wanted the abuse to stop.

Josef came to live with her parents for several days, and Michelle, who was feeling protected by her parents, began to remember the incident that had occurred six months earlier in the bathroom that she had forgotten. Jonas, who was three and a half years old by then, began to scream every time Josef tried to give him a bath in the grandparents' home. He demanded that his grandmother bathe him and would sleep only in his grandma's bed with her. Josef became angry, accused Michelle and her mother of alienating him from his son, and after a major fight packed his things and left the house. Jonas told his grandmother that he was happy his daddy had gone because daddy had hurt him. When she asked how he hurt him, Jonas said, "Daddy puts a toothbrush in my butt and wiggles it around like I do when I brush my teeth." He repeated it for his mother, whom his grandmother called into the room. As he said the words, Michelle flashed back to the night when she heard Jonas telling Josef not to hurt him, to do it slowly. After Jonas had gone to sleep, Michelle told her mother what she had heard. Together, they called the social services hotline and reported the child's sexual abuse.

Michelle started sobbing as she got to this part in her story. "I really thought they were going to help me protect my child. Instead, it became a nightmare for all of us."

She reported that during a physical examination, when the pediatrician turned Jonas over on his tummy, the boy pleaded with the doctor not to put "it" in his butt too hard and go slowly so it wouldn't hurt. When the doctor asked if anyone else put anything in his butt, Jonas said, "Yes, a toothbrush." When asked who did it, he closed up and wouldn't say. The doctor didn't even put the comments in his notes. In the taped psychological interview, the examiner asked Jonas if anyone hurt him. He said, "Yes, daddy hurt my butt." When asked further questions, he became agitated and began throwing things around the room and screaming. He never said anything further. No follow-up occurred. Child protective services closed the case as "unfounded" with a note stating that the child was too young to give adequate disclosures.

Josef did not have contact with Michelle or Jonas for four months after the accusation of child sexual abuse. He told the evaluators that it was a lie, that Michelle and her mother were conspiring against him to alienate him from his child. During this time, Jonas's behavior in school dramatically improved. He paid better attention and seemed more like a normal four-year-old child. Michelle's depression and anxiety became less debilitating. She filed for divorce from Josef and began to apply for jobs so she could earn her own money. When Josef got the divorce papers, he demanded visitation with Jonas. Michelle refused, stating it was not good for Jonas, especially since he had shown so much improvement. She attempted to have Jonas's teachers document the changes in the child. But the court ordered a visitation schedule despite the evidence Michelle presented. The judge warned Michelle that if she continued to alienate Jonas from his father, she would lose custody.

Within several weeks after visits with his father began, Jonas began fighting with other children in school. He took another boy in the bathroom, pulled down his pants, and attempted to put his penis in the boy's butt. The teacher walked in and found the children. She separated them, made them get dressed, reported what she had seen to the principal, and called Michelle to come in. They suspended Jonas from school and made a child abuse report to child protective services. They performed a second interview with Jonas, who again refused to tell them anything except he didn't want to see his father. Again they closed the case, calling it "unfounded."

During the next year, Michelle reported that both she and Josef went to see several different mental health professionals. Josef went to Dr. Nonotes, who wrote a short report stating that he thought Josef might have a sexual addiction problem. But Dr. Nonotes couldn't remember much about his few visits with Josef, nor could he find his notes or the test data from two years earlier when I asked for it later with a court order. Of course, this was a violation of the ethical principle that requires professionals to maintain records and the state licensing board rules mandating (in this particular state) preserving such records for seven years.

A family court hearing followed, and that judge ordered a custody evaluation to be performed by Dr. Toomany Roles. He appointed Ms. Child as guardian ad litem to represent Jonas's best interests. Even before completion of the evaluation, Dr. Roles testified at a hearing that Michelle seemed delusional and in a folie-à-deux relationship with her mother as they both believed that abuse had occurred when no evidence existed to show that it had. He asked the court to remove Jonas from the mother's care immediately and give custody to Josef, who hadn't seen his child for several months because Michelle appeared engaged in parental alienation syndrome. He seemed unaware that the ethical guidelines prohibit the use of diagnoses not based on empirical data. Not only did the judge listen to Dr. Roles, but he also ordered Michelle into therapy with a psychiatrist and ordered the psychiatrist to prescribe antipsychotic medication to cure her delusions and alienating behavior, and he ordered Dr. Roles to conduct supervised visitation between Michelle and Jonas.

That night, before Michelle or her mother could prepare Jonas for the court-ordered switch in custody, and before Michelle's lawyer could file for a stay pending an appeal, Dr. Roles and the guardian ad litem, Ms. Child, went to Michelle's parents' home, took the screaming child out of the house, and brought him to his father's house. The only times Michelle could see Jonas would be under Dr. Roles' supervision and at a fee of $400 per hour. Furthermore, Dr. Roles had received sole authority from the court to determine when Michelle might prove ready to have unsupervised visitation with Jonas, which would, of course, end his $400-an-hour supervisory job. At the same time, Michelle had to continue the custody evaluation with him. Although the ethics code does not expressly forbid multiple roles, the roles approved by the court in this case could potentially exploit the client and cause a loss of objectivity on the part of the mental health professional.

Michelle went back to work to pay for all her legal bills despite the emotional devastation that her family had experienced. She couldn't afford to pay for more than one to two hours of visitation with her son per week. She refused to take the antipsychotic medication prescribed by the psychiatrist, whom she did not trust. Just as her lawyer prepared to petition for a rehearing, the judge left the court for personal reasons, and everything stopped until the court had a new judge appointed. Six months later, as she still awaited a court date with the new judge, she was in my office.

Michelle's case presented a host of ethical quandaries. Following my intake session with her, I began to focus on several salient ethical issues. First, I wondered whether multiple roles and relationships in this case had harmed Michelle and Jonas because of decreased objectivity or exploitation. Although I criticized Dr. Roles and Ms. Child for their multiple roles in the case, I initially choose to play multiple roles myself. Second, I was concerned about issues of confidentiality; requesting the mother's data from prior professionals who also had data from the father required either the father's permission or a court order. The same was true for data regarding Jonas. Third, I was concerned that other mental health professionals involved in the case practiced outside their areas of competence. Although I was well positioned to evaluate the competence of these professionals by reviewing the case records, I wondered if this was an appropriate role for me. Finally, I felt constrained not to bring the unethical behavior of these professionals to the attention of regulatory boards because of the legal admonition not to attempt to tamper with a witness in a legal case.

Discussion

Key ethical issues

CLARIFYING MY ROLE. My first consideration was whom I owed a client duty and what role I would perform. Did Michelle seek me out as a therapist, consultant to her lawyer, coach, advocate, or forensic evaluator? She appeared to need some parts of all of these roles. She felt emotionally distraught and needed psychological support to continue her attempt to protect her child, if he really remained in danger of being sexually abused. Her story included many factors consistent with child sexual abuse, including Jonas's spontaneous admissions and behavior changes when his father was not present. However, his age and mental state made precise realities hard to assess. I would need more data to evaluate the strength of the complaint. I would also need to perform an evaluation to determine if Michelle did indeed have delusions, as Josef's asserted. In order to help support Michelle, I would need to understand her lawyer's legal strategy, if he had one. This would call for consultation. If Michelle did not follow her lawyer's advice, I would need to coach her appropriately. If the advice seemed inappropriate, I would need to advocate to help protect her and the child. She would also need a parental fitness examination, which would involve the role of forensic evaluator, and if my findings proved different from those of the other psychologists, expert witness testimony might also be necessary.

Admittedly, these roles also involve multiple relationships, but in the ethics code, these do not pose a conflict unless they create bias or pose harm to the client. Although the American Psychology and Law Society forensic guidelines suggest that forensic evaluations and psychotherapy should not typically be performed by the same person, in this case, to help Michelle, I might have to perform a little of each of the roles previously discussed. For example, I would have to assess her reality testing in order to work effectively in treating her and giving consultation to her counsel.

JUDGING COMPETENCE OF PRIOR MENTAL HEALTH PROFESSIONALS. The second area that I had to consider involved what, if anything, my role might entail in assessing the competence of Dr. Roles, Dr. Nonotes, and Ms. Child. Ethical principles enjoin psychologists to pursue justice and prevent harm wherever possible, and ethical standards impose an obligation to report clear ethical violations when they cannot be resolved informally and when reporting will not compromise client confidentiality. Did the multiple roles already in play actually harm Michelle? Dr. Roles seemed to think that because the court ordered him to perform all these roles, he was not exploiting the client or harming her. Rather, he believed he had a duty to protect the best interests of the child as a court-appointed custody evaluator. He believed he could objectively evaluate when Michelle no longer required supervision based on the child's needs and did not regard his own need for the $400 per hour he gained by keeping her supervised as a biasing factor. He claimed he had simply done his duty by taking the child out of Michelle's home, as he believed she would not follow the court order and turn Jonas over to Josef. If a mental health professional truly believes that a child is suffering harm, does he or she have the right to go beyond normal boundaries and enter a parent's home, without consent, to transfer the child to the other parent? Even if he had such a moral right, given the court's order that the child must be turned over to Josef, did he handle it in a harmful manner? Why not allow the custody change to flow from court personnel?

And what of Dr. Roles' relationship with Ms. Child and the judge? Did they hold biases against mothers, who find themselves accused of alienation more often than fathers? Did other undisclosed personal or professional relationships come into play? How could I separate out the gossip from the known facts? Did it seem reasonable to believe that a continued relationship existed between the judge and the professionals he regularly appointed that gave those professionals an advantage in having their recommendations followed, in contrast to others who rarely worked in that court? All these questions floated in my mind as I tried to decide how to proceed in the case.

Finally, I decided to ask Michelle's lawyer to obtain any available records from the other mental health professionals, and I would go through them carefully to determine if the data seemed properly obtained and interpreted. This would also help me determine what further assessment would prove necessary to evaluate Michelle's parental fitness. I also asked for the videotapes of the child protective services interviews and doctor's notes to assist me in assessing the competence of their evaluations of Jonas. Because Michelle did not have custody of Jonas, I could observe him on a supervised visit only if the supervisor, Dr. Roles, permitted it. Because he would not give the data to a lawyer, according to Florida licensing board rules that require raw data to be turned over to another psychologist, I obtained Michelle's written permission to call and talk with him and request copies of the data, which he provided voluntarily. Nothing in the data indicated that Michelle had a delusional disorder. Furthermore, if Jonas really had suffered abuse by Josef, then his refusal to spend time with his dad could indeed follow as a consequence of the abuse and not any alienation by Michelle. Later, with a court order, I obtained his data for Josef and Dr. Nonotes' report stating his opinion that Josef might have a sexual addiction problem. Although not dispositive, these data supported Jonas's allegations and Michelle's belief that Josef had harmed Jonas. However, it did not suffice in persuading the court to change custody back to Michelle.

Do I have a duty to report Dr. Roles and Ms. Child to the ethics committee or state licensing board if I believe they violated any rules? This raises interesting questions. My own experience with licensing boards suggests that although they can protect the public from unscrupulous mental health professionals, like ethics committees, they often have limited investigative abilities, and committee members may or may not have expertise relative to domestic violence and child abuse. Instead, I decided I would encourage the client to file a grievance or complaint and would even go so far as to help her word it, if she wished, but I would not file the complaint on my own. So, in this case, I explained the grievance process to Michelle and asked her if she wanted to file a complaint against Dr. Roles and Ms. Child. Although no decision about whether I would testify or not in this case had been made, filing a complaint against them and then testifying on behalf of Michelle might be considered witness tampering. Therefore, my filing a complaint before settling the case might preclude my entrance as an expert witness. However, some ethics committees and licensing boards enforce a time limit on how long one has to file a complaint after the problem behavior has occurred.

Did Dr. Nonotes violate state rules and the ethics code by not having notes from his treatment after two years? Did he actually have data that supported a finding of Josef's sexual difficulties, which he later destroyed? Could his motivation have involved protecting himself from not having reported the danger to child protective services? If so, then Michelle might also have a cause of action against him for malpractice. However, absent some sort of legal finding that Josef actually sexually abused Jonas, it would be difficult to prove such damage.

I decided that my primary role must focus on supporting Michelle by continuing to evaluate the data provided to me and performing a parental fitness examination for her. This put me more clearly in a forensic evaluator role than in any of the other roles, which seemed appropriate because the information continued to support the view that Jonas had told the truth about the abuse.

Work setting

I saw Michelle in my private practice office, where three other psychologists worked at the time. However, I also worked as a professor at a nearby university, a fact well known in the forensic community in that town. Furthermore, one of the major reasons my colleagues referred Michelle to me relates to my national reputation as an advocate for battered women.

Reflection

I chose this case because it represents a common type of referral that I see in my forensic practice. Many battered women file for divorce from their abusive partners, thinking they will soon feel safer than when they lived with the batterer. However, upon separation, once the children feel safer, they often disclose child abuse. Statistics indicate that approximately 60% of men who batter women partners also abuse children. A high percentage of such child abuse has a sexual component. Batterers, who often seek to tightly control their partners and create a traditional marital home where the woman has most of the control over the children, rarely have much alone time with the children. However, once the family court becomes involved, they invoke shared parental responsibilities and time sharing, so that the mother becomes less able to protect her children.

The result, as in Michelle's case, is that the children feel safer without the father around to abuse and frighten them and subsequently disclose the abuse, usually to the mother. Often, professionals and the court invalidate the allegations of the mother and children, and then the children are forced into more time alone with the abuser. Because the children must learn to accommodate to the parent and the abuse, they stop disclosing and try to make the best of the situation. The mother feels rendered powerless to do anything to protect the children, and as in this case, if she protests too much, she will find herself accused of causing parental alienation syndrome (if the children protest and do not want to spend time with the father) or psychological Munchausen syndrome by proxy (if the children develop psychological problems), or she may simply be labeled as mentally ill herself (like Michelle, who was diagnosed as having a delusional disorder).

Unfortunately, many professionals think that their role in a child custody evaluation involves determining whether or not domestic violence or child abuse has actually occurred. However, the forensic standard does not require such proof, and furthermore, most custody evaluators do not have the expertise to make a determination about what constitutes abuse. Rather, there are two standards applicable here. The first standard mandates the mental health professional to report suspicions of abuse, and child protective services performs the evaluation. The second and more relevant standard focuses on the *best interests of the child*. If it appears that the child's best interests require removal from the offending parent for a period of time, it is not necessary to prove that abuse occurred. Furthermore, it is important for the psychologist to offer that opinion to the court despite any personal beliefs, such as that children need both parents, and let the court make the final decision. Dr. Role's belief that Michelle would not follow the court's decision and turn the child over to the father was not sufficient to justify his violation of her civil and legal rights and may be considered unethical and perhaps even illegal.

Mental health professionals sometimes think that their role involves determining if abuse can be proved. If they find no sign of recognizable abuse, they may accuse the mother of alienation. Interestingly, of the hundreds of cases that I have reviewed, the parent accused of alienation is almost always the mother, who has accused the father of abuse. Why professionals so readily believe that the father did not contribute to the child's dislike of him seems curious. No empirical data support the belief that children must have a relationship with both parents all of the time, especially if the father behaves in a controlling and abusive manner. Furthermore, no empirical data support that changing custody from a mother who has acted as the child's primary parent to the father is in the child's best interests, even if some alienating behaviors on the part of the mother have occurred.

Key ethical principles and standards

APA (2002): Principle A (Beneficence and Nonmaleficence), Principle B (Fidelity and Responsibility), Principle D (Justice), Principle E (Respect for People's Rights and Dignity), Standard 1.04 (Informal Resolution of Ethical Violations), Standard 1.05 (Reporting Ethical Violations), Standard 2.01 (Boundaries of Competence), Standard 2.04 (Bases for Scientific and Professional Judgments), Standard 3.04 (Avoiding Harm), Standard 3.05 (Multiple Relationships), Standard 3.07 (Third Party Requests For Services), And Standard 3.08 (Exploitative Relationships).

REFERENCES AND FURTHER READING

Bancroft, L., & Silverman, J. G. (2002). *The batterer as parent: Addressing the impact of domestic violence on family dynamics.* Thousand Oaks, CA: Sage.

Campbell, J. C. (1995). *Assessing dangerousness: Violence by sex offenders, batterers, and child abusers.* Thousand Oaks, CA: Sage.

Shapiro, D. L., Walker, M., Manosevitz, M., Peterson, M., & Williams, M. (2008). *Surviving a licensing board complaint: What to do, what not to do.* Phoenix, AZ: Zeig, Tucker, & Theisen.

Walker, L. E. A. (2009). *Battered woman syndrome* (3rd ed.). New York: Springer.

PART III

In Medical Center Corridors

16

Determining a Patient's Capacity to Refuse Dialysis and Die: When Professional Competence and Credentials Do Not Overlap

James DuBois

During an ethics committee meeting at a local hospital, I listened to a report of an ongoing case involving a 52-year old man with end-stage renal disease (ESRD), recently admitted via the emergency department. He had undergone dialysis treatments for many years to manage his chronic kidney disease, a complication of diabetes. He was not listed for a kidney transplant. We had no information about whether this resulted from a failure of the system, personal preferences, or medical contraindications.

The patient had previously presented to our emergency department on multiple occasions. In this episode, his brother brought him to the hospital because he noticed that he was bruised and itchy and seemed very weak. As it turned out, he had stopped going to his dialysis appointments. After admission to the hospital, the treating physician explained that he urgently needed dialysis or else would die. The patient refused.

In and of itself, this is not shocking. There are many reasons why a patient may want to discontinue dialysis. As ESRD progresses, a patient may need to sit connected to a machine several times per week for many hours. The travel, the clinic environment, and the persistent symptoms of ESRD can all weigh heavily on a patient. Nephrologists estimate that approximately 20% of dialysis patients discontinue treatment, even though they know they will die without it.

However, in this case the patient said he did not want to die. He said he would accept dialysis when he felt sick, but right now he felt fine (despite his symptoms at presentation). The physician explained again to the patient that he was in fact very sick and would die within a week or so without dialysis. He explained that his symptoms—the bruising, itching, and fatigue—were all related to his kidney disease. Nonetheless, the patient continued to insist that he felt fine and did not want dialysis until he felt sick.

The physician sought an ethics consult. He recognized that ordinarily a patient has the right to refuse treatments, even life-sustaining treatments. But he felt unconvinced that this patient had intact decisional capacity. The physician wondered: should the staff accept the patient's informed refusal? Should they seek surrogate consent to force the patient to resume dialysis? What should they do?

The ethics committee requested a psychiatric evaluation to determine whether the patient had adequate decisional capacity. The psychiatrist wrote in the patient's chart that he did have decisional capacity and should be allowed to make his own decisions. Apparently, the psychiatrist reached this conclusion on the basis of the patient's Mini-Mental State Examination (MMSE) score, which was appropriate for his age and level of education (high school graduate), and the fact that the patient could paraphrase key information that the physician communicated to him.

Although I had no inclination to force the patient to undergo dialysis (which probably would have involved the use of some physical and chemical restraints), I also felt very uncomfortable with the psychiatrist's judgment that the patient had adequate decisional capacity. I feared that his life-or-death decision might not be a competent decision, and I also feared that family members might object to honoring his wishes. His brother, who had ongoing involvement in his care, really wanted to see him continue dialysis.

In my opinion, although the MMSE did assess basic cognitive functioning (e.g., orientation to time and place, list recall, and basic calculation), it did not qualify as an appropriate test of capacity to consent to medical treatments. Based on legal reviews and years of clinical trials with different patient populations, Grisso and Appelbaum (1998) have offered the most broadly used set of criteria. To have decisional capacity, they note, patients must understand consent information, appreciate how the information pertains to their life, reason with the information (e.g., evaluate risks in the light of probable benefits), and articulate a clear choice. One commonly recognized component of "appreciating" information involves *believing* the information. This patient appeared to disbelieve that he was sick and dying unless he felt subjectively sick at the moment. He appeared to understand what he was told and could paraphrase it, but he did not accept that the information was true and would gravely affect his life.

In determining decisional capacity, it is appropriate to focus on manifested abilities rather than on etiology or underlying psychopathologies. In fact, my concerns arose precisely from his failure to appreciate the information shared with him. Nevertheless, I thought it also relevant to consider that patients who have undergone dialysis for long periods of time become susceptible to chronic dialysis–dependant encephalopathy and other cognitive disorders that may involve impaired intellectual capability and depression. Although the patient's nephrologist had not diagnosed encephalopathy, it certainly seemed reasonable to assume that—even with other mental health diagnoses excluded—an organic explanation existed for the patient's confused pattern of reasoning.

Finally, I expressed to the ethics committee the view that decisional capacity is not an all-or-nothing phenomenon. One always possesses degrees of understanding and appreciation. In setting a threshold or determining "how much" capacity constitutes enough, it seems most appropriate to consider the consequences of a decision. In this case, I thought the level of capacity should rank higher than, say, capacity to consent to survey research: the man's life was at stake.

Fortunately, the chair of the ethics committee fully understood and shared the concerns I expressed. Furthermore, he was a physician with a wonderfully nonthreatening manner of engaging other physicians in dialogues about their practice of medicine. He suggested that the psychiatrists we used for consultation might not fully understand what the ethics committee wanted to know about a patient. We then began a process of developing a decisional capacity assessment form that we would provide to our psychiatric consultants. We decided not to use any of the existing objective decisional capacity assessment forms because such forms are often controversial among psychiatrists and because most do not provide clear cutoff points that are appropriate to a variety of clinical settings. Rather, we decided to provide the consultant with six open-ended items that addressed the ethical criteria for decisional capacity detailed by Grisso and Appelbaum, such as the following: "Describe how well the patient appreciates how his/her medical decision will affect him/her (e.g., the permanence of the decision, anticipated quality of life, etc.)." We concluded the form by asking, "If the patient does not adequately demonstrate any of the above capacities, do you think the capacities in question might be restored in the short term (e.g., by waiting, through further explanation of information, by providing a less threatening environment, or other means)?" This last question struck me as pertinent to our case at hand because in the initial ethics consultation, no one considered encouraging the patient to continue dialysis for, say, just two weeks while an attempt was made to ensure that his decision was ethically and legally valid. Dialysis, perhaps combined with the use of antidepressants and further discussion, might have enabled him to make a competent decision—which might very well become a decision to discontinue dialysis.

After the ethics committee achieved unanimous support for the new decisional capacity assessment form, the chair of the committee circulated it among the department of psychiatry. The entire department, including the original psychiatric consultant, received the form very favorably—suggesting no modifications (a rare feat for a hospital policy). In fact, they expressed gratitude because they said they did not enjoy a consensus among themselves regarding how best to assess decisional capacity, and they often wondered what precisely the ethics committee wanted to know when it requested a consult. However, in the process of developing the form, we also realized that the treating physicians—even internists with little background in psychiatry—often stood poised in the best position to assess decisional capacity because they know best the patient's history, prognosis, and treatment options. They have the best grasp of the information that a patient should understand, appreciate, and reason with. Thus, we made our decisional capacity assessment form available to all physicians, and in future cases, we often asked the primary care or attending physician to complete the form rather than call for a psychiatric consultation.

Returning to the case that prompted our committee to revise its process for assessing decisional capacity, within 48 hours the patient gave into pressure from his brother and resumed dialysis. However, this lasted only a few months before the brother and the patient both decided that further dialysis was simply too burdensome. However, when this decision was made, no one felt concerned about the quality of the informed consent because both the patient and the patient's surrogate were in agreement, and at least one of them appeared to fully understand and appreciate what was at stake.

Discussion

Key ethical issues

From the perspective of patient care, the key ethical issue in this case involved a decision of whether to accept a patient's refusal of dialysis. As a general rule, a patient's right to demand treatment is fairly limited, but a patient's right to refuse treatment is nearly absolute—assuming the patient is an adult with decisional capacity. When a patient lacks decisional capacity, we inquire into whether the patient has a designated attorney or legal proxy for health care decision making. If not, Missouri allows the next of kin (not defined) to serve as a surrogate decision maker. When no surrogate can be found, we seek a guardian ad litem appointed by the courts. In this case, we felt fortunate because we had a local surrogate decision maker available, a brother who was involved in the patient's care.

However, from my own personal perspective, the case gave rise to a second ethical issue, a question of professional ethics: *What should I do when I possess knowledge relevant to improving patient care but lack the professional credentials to provide patient care?* Nearly every code of ethics discusses the need to provide only those services that one is competent to provide. But credentialing is another matter altogether. In an ideal world, competence and credentials would always overlap nicely. But in this particular case, I possessed some relevant expertise without the relevant credentials. I had recently developed materials—a Web site, DVD, and textbook—for a National Institutes of Health–funded training program on mental health research ethics. In the process, I had researched decisional capacity in great depth—competing theories, concrete assessment approaches and tools, difficult cases, and a fair amount of recent data from studies of decisional capacity. Nevertheless, my education and training lie in experimental psychology and philosophy. I held no clinical license, yet I had a basis to contradict the opinion of a licensed psychiatrist with staff privileges.

Work setting

Apparently, nurses and some other allied health professionals face this kind of dilemma rather frequently. When confronted with an incompetent physician or a physician with unusual convictions, nurses may well know what is best for a patient, yet they may lack the authority to provide referrals or to write treatment orders. Thus, they may observe physicians who consistently undertreat pain, ignore advanced directives, fail to communicate with families, or simply have consistently worse outcomes than those of other physicians on staff. This can lead to a phenomenon known as moral distress, which in turn contributes to higher rates of job-related burnout. Nevertheless, those who lack formal credentials, regardless of their expertise, may feel silenced or marginalized in the process of deciding upon patient care. Although there are very good reasons for this, it can create ethical dilemmas when those without formal credentials have something valuable to offer to patient care.

Moreover, even when individuals hold appropriate credentials, hospitals, especially academic medical centers, operate in a very hierarchical manner, and informal understandings pervade physician relationships. Physicians often feel reluctant to challenge the practice of other physicians, especially those outside their own specialty.

These factors may affect the behavior of ethics committee members. Membership typically crosses professional discipline lines, yet members do not come to the table as equals—at least not in all respects. Furthermore, one typically serves on an ethics committee at the pleasure of hospital administrators. One's consulting relationship may be terminated at any time. I know ethics consultants who behave in a very reserved manner out of fear that if they say too much they may find their services are no longer needed.

Reflection

Whereas many ethical dilemmas end in an unfortunate manner, I believe the dilemma described here had a generally happy ending in terms of quality of patient care and policy development. Several factors contributed to this. First, the psychiatrist involved was not incompetent. He simply had an understanding of decisional capacity different from that of the ethics committee members (or some of us, at least). He proved open to dialogue and willing to serve our needs. Second, I had the audacity to speak up when others seemed more inclined to accept the expert's opinion. Third, the chair of the ethics committee was a physician with an understanding and diplomatic nature. This enabled us to elicit support from other physicians on staff to develop a policy that would better meet our needs. Finally, the typical process of developing a policy within a hospital, which involves circulation through relevant clinical departments and patient care committees, provides a peer review process that often allows for policy improvement even while achieving buy-in from key stakeholders. That is to say, our happily negotiated ethical solution, like so many others, involved a mixture of patience, courage, critical thinking, teamwork, and simple good fortune.

Key ethical principles and standards

APA (2002): Principle A (Beneficence and Nonmaleficence), Principle E (Respect for People's Rights and Dignity), Standard 2.01 (Boundaries of Competence), Standard 3.09 (Cooperation with Other professionals), and Standard 3.10 (Informed Consent).

REFERENCES AND FURTHER READING

Arieff, A. I. (2007). Nervous system manifestations of renal failure. In R. W. Schrier (Ed.), *Diseases of the kidney and urinary tract* (8th ed., vol. III, pp. 2460–2481). Philadelphia: Lippincott Williams & Wilkins.

DuBois, J. M. (2008). *Ethics in mental health research. Principles, guidance, and cases.* New York: Oxford University Press.

Faden, R. R., & Beauchamp, T. L. (1986). *A history and theory of informed consent.* New York: Oxford University Press.

Galla, J. H. (2000). Clinical practice guideline on shared decision-making in the appropriate initiation of and withdrawal from dialysis. *Journal of the American Society of Nephrology, 11*(7), 1340–1342.

Grisso, T., & Appelbaum, P. S. (1998). *Assessing competence to consent to treatment: A guide for physicians and other health professionals.* New York: Oxford University Press.

17

When Boundaries Intersect in Cyberspace: Facebook, Multiple Relationships, and Confidentiality in a Hospital

Nabil Hassan El-Ghoury

The advent of social networking is changing the way people interact in a virtual world. With the initial use of the Internet, information generally flowed in one direction, from the creator to readers. New tools in social networking now allow information to move in both directions; they also allow user-defined options and interactions, now called Web 2.0, for the second generation of the World Wide Web.

One of the largest and most important social networking sites is Facebook. As of April 2008, Facebook had more than 200 million users worldwide, with 100 million logging in daily (retrieved April 19, 2009, from www.facebook.com/press/info.php?statistics). Originally used exclusively within universities, Facebook is now open to any user older than 13 years of age. Users may connect to friends and acquaintances from school, work, and the community. To connect to someone, a user makes a "friend request"; upon receipt of the friend request, the requested user may choose to accept or decline the connection. Clicking on another user's name can reveal mutual friends of the two users. A key function in Facebook is the status update, in which people may post a brief message about what they are doing; this update automatically passes to all the friends in their social network. Conversations may occur when people comment on status updates. A feature called *the wall* allows users to post publically viewable messages to anyone with access to that profile. By providing particular e-mail addresses, one may join networks based on a workplace or universities attended.

I joined Facebook in January 2008 after hearing about it from my relatives and some friends. Initially, I felt somewhat reluctant to join and become active. But I soon realized that Facebook had become the primary means of communication for many of my younger relatives. Rather than send e-mails to friends, my cousins would update their status and passively send their news to everyone they knew. Through Facebook, I learned of one cousin's diagnosis of a significant chronic illness, and that a second cousin might soon qualify for the Olympics. As I became more comfortable with Facebook, I started using the status update to share different things, such as "Nabil is traveling to DC for a weekend of meetings" or "Nabil really enjoyed last night's American Idol!"

Reconnecting with friends from elementary school, high school, and college proved another positive experience. I had moved across the country for graduate school before most people had e-mail, so I had lost contact with many old friends. Many located me on Facebook, and we started having conversations and catching up on our lives. I have found this experience one of the greatest benefits of belonging to Facebook.

However, along with all these great connections and reconnections have come more difficult ones. As a clinical psychologist working with children and families in a department of pediatrics at a public hospital, I became concerned that adolescent patients might find me online. From my clinical interviews, I learned that most of my patients participated in MySpace, a different social networking site, so I thought I would encounter fewer problems. I never joined MySpace because I knew that many of my patients participated in it.

One day, I received a friend request from a person whose name and profile photo I did not immediately recognize. After ignoring this request for a while, I took a closer glance at the profile of the user requesting this connection. I soon recognized the individual as the parent of a former patient of mine, who was using a name different from the one I had known during the course of psychotherapy. For the purposes of this chapter, I will call this parent John. He had brought his teenage son to counseling sessions for help with academic concerns, attention problems, and depression. Over the course of various counseling sessions, I learned that John and I were of approximately the same age, had a number of interests in common, and shared political views and favorite movies. We worked at the same hospital, although I rarely if ever saw him because of different work schedules and departments. I enjoyed working with John's son, who was very smart and always interesting as a patient.

I consulted with this family over the course of about a year and a half. My work with John and his son began about one year before I joined Facebook. By the time this friend request had come, I had not seen the family for about six months.

The friend request raised issues that worried me as a clinician and as a Facebook user. How would John react to either decision, to accept or to decline the friend request? How much of my profile could John see? Because John worked in the same hospital, he fell in my workplace network category. Further complicating this situation, John and his son were no longer actively in treatment. I therefore had no ability to adequately discuss and process this interaction in a therapeutic setting. How might a process discussion be interpreted (or misinterpreted) over e-mail?

Because we were listed in the same network through our work setting, I began exploring whether my profile was visible to those in my network. Although I thought I had limited my profile to "Friends Only," I learned that those in my work network could see all aspects of my profile. Although I had not disclosed anything embarrassing, I immediately changed my privacy settings to ensure that my full profile was visible only to friends I had accepted, and I limited the view accessible to general searchers on Facebook.

I recognized the transference and countertransference issues inherent in this situation. Based on the friend request and our interactions in psychotherapy sessions, it seemed likely that John liked me and enjoyed our conversations. Had I met John in a nontherapeutic context, I likely would have developed a genuine friendship with him. Our similar backgrounds, interests, and experiences could have contributed to a pleasant friendship. However, given the nature of our meeting through a patient-psychologist interaction, a friendship would have represented a potentially inappropriate boundary crossing. Many of my patients cease psychotherapy when they have accomplished their initial goals but return at a later time when the same or new issues emerge. Developing such a friendship with John would have precluded or complicated the opportunity for his son to return for counseling. I consulted with a few colleagues who also had profiles on Facebook. We agreed on the appropriateness of declining the friend request. The more important question became whether or not to discuss this with John, and how. If John and his son were current patients, this would have become an additional topic for discussion in the counseling relationship, and we both would have had the opportunity to appreciate the rationale behind declining the friend request. However, their status as former patients made this conversation more difficult.

Ultimately, I declined the friend request. I chose to not send a message out of concern that the discussion about the rationale would prove too difficult for an e-mail message. I never saw John or his son again, so we never had a chance to verbally discuss this process. Since then, I have left the hospital setting and moved out of state, so it seems very unlikely that I will ever see them in a professional context again.

Discussion

Key ethical issues

The primary clinical and ethical issue in this situation involves multiple relationships. A multiple relationship exists when a psychologist or other mental health professional has a professional relationship with an individual, then develops a second type of relationship, such as a personal relationship (American Psychological Association, 2002). Multiple relationships are not inherently unethical; for example, casual interactions such as belonging to the same health club as a patient or seeing a patient in public are not necessarily considered inappropriate.

In the case of John, however, the nature of the nontherapeutic interaction would possibly have created inappropriate multiple relationships. Although not disclosing inappropriate information, I certainly shared much more information about myself on Facebook via status updates than I would with a patient or family in a therapeutic setting. I regularly share details about my current or upcoming social plans (e.g., "Nabil is going to the Pride parade") that I would prefer to keep private and so reduce the likelihood of encountering patients in public. I occasionally share more personal details (e.g., "Nabil is missing his mother") that may prompt my closer friends to contact me in real life; these statements are typically less appropriate to share with patients. Because the purpose of psychotherapy focuses on helping a patient or family, it seemed appropriate for me to avoid sharing my particular feelings and activities at any given time.

A second ethical issue relevant to this situation involves confidentiality. Social networking creates and maintains connections between different individuals; one's list of friends becomes available for other friends and potentially strangers to see. I have asked my Facebook friends about how they knew a mutual colleague. If I listed a parent of a former patient as a friend on Facebook, it might invite questions about how I met this parent. Because of ethical principles and legal requirements about confidentiality, I would not be able to disclose the nature of the origin of our relationship. Rather than having to provide vague answers to such inquiries about mutual friends, I would rather limit such connections and eliminate those types of questions.

Work setting

As an outpatient psychologist in a public county hospital, I treated a large number of patients. At any given time, my open caseload of patients seen in the last month or so ranged from 60 to 80 families; this could result in a circle of up to 200 individuals if parents, grandparents, and siblings were included. Former patients (over six years) could increase that number to more than 1,000 individuals.

With such patient volume, it seemed inevitable that a multiple relationship would occur on Facebook. More and more users are joining Facebook and other social networking sites, and eventually one would certainly find me there and request me as a friend. Even without my being directly requested as a friend, overlapping social networks increased the likelihood that I would eventually have a patient who connected as a friend of one of my Facebook connections.

Providing psychological services to a fellow employee at my hospital increased concerns about confidentiality and multiple relationships, as it became possible to run into patients (or parents of patients) throughout the hospital. The group network options on Facebook simply provided additional means for employee/patients to locate me in cyberspace. A patient/employee who used Facebook would have multiple means of finding me on Facebook: by my name, e-mail address, work-related group network, and any mutual or shared friends on Facebook. Each search option has potentially different security options that users must change if they wish to minimize contacts through such means.

Reflection

In hindsight, this encounter offered an excellent opportunity to think about the nature of social networking and its relationship to psychotherapy. How could this situation have been prevented?

At the beginning of each therapeutic relationship, I always have a discussion about confidentiality and its limitations. That conversation includes how everything we talk about in counseling sessions is confidential, with some limitations, such as child abuse or risk for harm to self or others. Another aspect of the confidentiality discussion includes my promise to keep the person's status as a patient private if I encounter him or her in public; patients have the right to choose to acknowledge me or ignore me if they want to, without concern for my reaction. I follow their lead on how they wanted to interact with me in public.

We should consider social networking sites such as Facebook another extension of that confidentiality discussion. Similar to respecting a patient's confidentiality in person, I could discuss with patients and families how I would ignore any requests to connect to them on any social networking site (e.g., Facebook, LinkedIn, Twitter) for confidentiality reasons. By preemptively discussing the possibility of social networking connections, patients and parents would be informed of my likely response. If someone wanted to test that limit and request a connection afterward, I could ignore that request, knowing that I had already discussed this outcome with him or her, and discuss it in a therapeutic context afterward, if possible. Such preemptive discussions have been suggested for other ethical concerns as well.

When working with adolescents, adding the social networking clause to the confidentiality discussion may prove advantageous. It would communicate to the teenager that I had familiarity with social networking sites and could have reasonable discussions about the issues that develop on such sites, without need for education about the site. Having this discussion could provide me with credibility to a teenager as someone who understands the unique needs and socializing strategies of adolescents. If I were going to view an adolescent's profile, which might be appropriate in a therapeutic context given the amount of cyberbullying and difficulties adolescents may be subjected to while online, I would discuss this with the patient before doing so, and ideally review it with him or her.

Because I met John and his son before I ever joined Facebook, I did not think of having that type of discussion with them. Since then, I have added this as part of my confidentiality discussion with patients. Furthermore, I have changed my privacy settings to make it more difficult for individuals to find me on Facebook, and I have raised the restrictions on who can view my profile. I have also introduced both of these topics to graduate student supervisees, who relished the opportunity to have frank discussions about how to safely and appropriately use Facebook as graduate students.

Key ethical principles and standards

APA (2002): Principle B (Fidelity and Responsibility), Principle E (Respect for People's Rights and Dignity), Standard 3.05 (Multiple Relationships), and Standard 4.01 (Maintaining Confidentiality).

REFERENCES AND FURTHER READING

American Psychological Association. (2002). Ethical principles of psychologists and code of conduct. *American Psychologist, 57*, 1060–1073.

Gutheil, T G., & Gabbard, G. O. (1993). The concept of boundaries in clinical practice: Theoretical and risk-management dimensions. *American Journal of Psychiatry, 150*, 188–196.

Koocher, G. P., & Keith-Spiegel, P. (1998). *Ethics in psychology: Professional standards and cases* (2nd ed.). New York: Oxford University Press.

Zur, O. (2007). *Boundaries in psychotherapy: Ethical and clinical explorations*. Washington DC: American Psychological Association.

Zur, O., Williams, M. H., Lehavot, K., & Knapp, S. (2009). Therapist self-disclosure and transparency in the internet age. *Professional Psychology: Research and Practice, 40*, 22–30.

18

Second Chances: Decision Making in Pediatric Transplantation

Lisa M. Farley

When I first met Grace, I had the feeling of meeting an old soul. Although my job focused on helping and supporting her, I sensed that *she* would be the one teaching me. Grace had a way about her that seemed sweet and engaging, but also fiercely courageous, with a strength that belied her tiny frame. She was insightful beyond her years. There are some people you never forget, and Grace is one of them.

Grace was 13 years old and contending with end-stage cystic fibrosis (CF). If she didn't receive a lung transplant, she would likely die within the year. I met her because the medical team had asked me to conduct a psychological assessment as part of her pre-transplant evaluation. Before children can qualify for the lung transplant list, they must undergo a series of evaluations (medical, physical therapy, psychological, social work) to ensure that they present as good candidates for transplant and can manage the lifelong post-surgical medical regimen.

As part of a pre-transplant evaluation, I typically meet with the child, the child's parents or caretakers, and the medical team. My goal involves assessing the child's psychological functioning and identifying symptoms (i.e., depression, anxiety) that could affect the child's adjustment to the transplant process and/or that might benefit from treatment. Inclusion of the family also becomes important in the assessment process, particularly in the case of a child. Parents or caretakers often take charge of medications and scheduling, as well as providing the child's primary support as he or she navigates the illness. The medical team often provides a history of the patient's management of the illness to date, including difficulties with adherence to prescribed treatments or medical recommendations.

I decided to meet with Grace first. She was an absolute delight—warm, funny, and insightful. Grace evidenced no signs of psychopathology; she was not depressed, exceedingly anxious, or behaviorally dysregulated. She was a good student who loved spending time with her peers. Grace impressed me with her knowledge of CF and her understanding of what a lung transplant really entailed. She had grown up around other kids with CF and had watched some go through the transplant process. Grace knew kids who had done well after surgery and kids who had suffered multiple complications, even death. She understood the full implications of her decision to pursue a transplant, and she felt confident that she wanted to take that course. Grace had battled CF her whole life, and she knew that she had started to lose the fight. She wanted to receive a transplant so that she would have more time with her family. Grace described so many things she still wanted to do, including graduating, going to the prom, and becoming a nurse. She said to me, "I'm just too young to die."

Upon meeting with Grace's family, I discovered that they were very loving and kind, but that they were having difficulty helping Grace meet the many demands of her illness. The family had limited financial resources and four other children in addition to Grace. They described their life as both chaotic and stressful. Grace's mother had a history of anxiety and depression. Grace's parents often worried about losing their jobs and how they would provide for the family. Grace's illness required adherence to a strict medication schedule, regular clinic visits, physical therapy, and overnight feedings delivered through a G tube. The family found it extremely difficult to supervise and monitor this regimen, and Grace found it challenging to manage it on her own. As a result, Grace did not receive the full "dosage" or benefits of her treatment, and she often became sicker than necessary.

The medical team expressed significant concerns about Grace and her family's difficulty with adhering to her medical regimen. These issues had existed for many years, and Grace's already precarious health status had deteriorated further because of inconsistent treatment. Although the team acknowledged how challenging maintaining a demanding medication and treatment schedule over the long course of a child's chronic illness can become for families, they had to look ahead to how this pattern of nonadherence might affect the outcome of Grace's transplant.

Although issues of adherence have relevance to the care of any illness, they become absolutely critical to consider when a patient is evaluated for transplant. A lung transplant does not provide a "cure" for CF; in fact, I have frequently heard transplant teams describe the process as "trading one illness for another." Post-transplant care is complex, the side effects of the required immunosuppressants are unpleasant, and the necessity of regular medical appointments becomes a lifelong commitment. Additionally, the demand for transplantable organs far exceeds the availability. The medical team must evaluate whether a patient and her family can undertake this commitment. Although medical adherence does not guarantee a positive outcome, it offers the best way to increase the odds of a successful post-transplant course. Nonadherence ensures failure.

These issues present the pediatric psychologist with the challenge of assessing the emotional health of both the child and the family and whether or not they are ready for transplant. If barriers to adherence exist, as in Grace's case, where does the decision point lie in terms of recommending transplant as a prudent course of action? The stakes of this decision are very high, not only for the child receiving the transplant, but also for the unknown child in some other hospital who *will not* receive that particular organ.

If Grace did not receive new lungs, she likely had very little time left to live. However, the question of whether she would receive a transplant had little to do with her, and more to do with her family's difficulty caring for her complex medical needs. The team, including me, felt torn over this dilemma. At age 13, Grace could not fully care for all of her medical needs, but in developmental and psychological terms, she was as happy and well adjusted as we could expect of any teenager. Should Grace, in a sense, receive life-threatening "punishment" for the difficulties and challenges posed by her parents? If we recommended transplant, would we set Grace up for a failed post-transplant course and possibly further pain and suffering? Furthermore, if Grace received a transplant and the family was not medically adherent, would that waste the chance of another child who might qualify as a good candidate for a transplant?

In the end, after much discussion and consideration, the team came up with a solution we thought would address the importance of adherence and provide the support to Grace and her family that would maximize the chances of success. The medical team, including me, recommended that Grace receive a lung transplant. In addition, we secured approval for at-home nursing that would help Grace with her post-transplant care. We hoped that the nursing services might also assist with teaching Grace's parents how to administer her medications on a consistent schedule and follow other medical recommendations.

The team had a formal meeting with Grace's parents to discuss their concerns about post-transplant adherence and the proposed solution of home nursing care. It involved a good deal of discussion about how the nursing services might affect their family life, as well as the pros and cons of at-home care in helping Grace recover from her transplant procedure. Both Grace and her parents decided to try this arrangement.

After the decision to place her on the active transplant list, Grace received new lungs only a few weeks later. She recovered beautifully in the hospital and went home with the nursing plan in place. Despite the need for some initial adjustments, the family came to really appreciate the expertise and help of Grace's at-home nurses. The nursing team helped her parents become more involved than ever before in Grace's care. Grace came to her outpatient appointments regularly, and she rarely became sick enough to warrant admission to the inpatient unit. I continued to follow Grace supportively throughout the next several years. She continued to amaze me with her insight, her strength, and her appreciation of life. Sadly, Grace died of complications of her illness unrelated to nonadherence at the age of 18. The transplant afforded her five extra years of life—a chance to be a teenager. She even went to the prom.

Discussion

Key ethical issues

The primary ethical issues addressed in this vignette involve beneficence/nonmaleficence and respect for people's rights and dignity. In mental health treatment, psychologists seek to help others and to avoid harm. Specifically, the principle states that psychologists "safeguard the welfare and rights of those with whom they interact professionally and other affected persons." During a pediatric transplant evaluation, the duty of the psychologist focuses on assessing the patient and the patient's family to determine if any mental health difficulties might serve as barriers to transplant adjustment and adherence to post-transplant care. Thus, a primary consideration lies in addressing the needs of the patient and the patient's family.

The principle of beneficence guides psychologists to ask the following questions: How can I best help my patient? What are the wishes of the patient? Is the patient willing and able to manage the transplant process? In pediatric transplantation, this necessitates evaluating not only the child for mental health symptoms, but also the parents/guardians. If there are psychological symptoms that interfere with daily functioning and/or the ability to manage the demands of the medical illness, mental health treatment is often recommended. Because the family is so crucial to the care of a pediatric patient, supportive intervention for parents can often be quite helpful.

Benefitting others and doing no harm in transplantation means thinking beyond the needs of the patient. Transplant teams must also remain aware of the larger context of the transplant process. This involves consideration of those patients whom you *do not* see in your care, the other potential transplant recipients who wait as competitors for the same organ. I have heard physicians comment that "saying yes to one patient means saying no to another." The limited supply of available organs creates a situation in which decisions must be made that benefit the transplant community as a whole. Thus, the team seeks to provide organs to those patients who will "take care" of the organ by adhering to the medical regimen and maximizing the odds of success. Additionally, the maxim of doing no harm is considered in the evaluation of a patient who may not be willing or able to manage the post-transplant process. If patients do not take their medications or attend follow-up appointments, the likelihood of organ rejection, illness, and death is greatly increased.

The principle of respect for people's rights and dignity also applies to Grace's case. Although pediatric patients are legal minors and their parents have ultimate decision-making authority, it is important to deeply consider the wishes of the child with regard to a transplant. The decision to pursue a transplant affects children at the most basic level—they experience the surgery, bear the scars, take the medications, and endure the discomfort and pain. We have an ethical duty to attend to children's experience and understanding of their illness, and to fully explain the transplant process and post-transplant care at a developmentally appropriate level.

This principle is also evident in the informed consent process. The goal of informed consent before a psychological evaluation is to provide patients with information on the assessment process and how the information they provide will be used. This respects patients' rights and allows them to determine if they would like to proceed. In the case of a transplant evaluation, patients are told that the team is attempting to determine if they are appropriate transplant candidates at that point in time. Generally, I provide patients and their families with a rationale as to why the evaluation is important—namely, the team wants to avoid potentially dangerous complications and optimize the chance of success.

As a psychologist on the team, I saw my role as that of identifying psychological symptoms that might negatively affect post-transplant adjustment. If the evaluation did yield significant psychological symptoms, such as depression, I would recommend appropriate services to help address these difficulties. It is conceivable that patients might be denied immediate placement on the transplant list because of psychological concerns (i.e., depressive symptoms that are negatively influencing adherence behaviors). These symptoms would then require attention before the patient was placed on the transplant list.

The standard highlighting boundaries of competence also has relevance to this case. In order to provide competent psychological services in a pediatric medical setting, one must receive training in child development and the assessment and treatment of childhood psychiatric disorders. In addition, it is important to garner supervised experience working with medically ill patients, specifically the transplant population. In order for psychologists to make appropriate and clinically indicated recommendations to the pediatric patient, they must have knowledge of the symptoms and sequelae of the medical illness and its associated treatments. Adequate training helps to ensure that a psychologist is competent to assess and treat a specific medical population. Without this experience, it would be challenging for a psychologist to fully appreciate the psychological toll of chronic illness on patients' quality of life and/or provide comprehensive assessments of patients in this specialized population.

Finally, it was important for me to consider the ethical standard regarding the bases for my professional judgments in this case. In making recommendations to the team about a transplant, it is important to carefully consider the information relevant to the case and to make determinations based on objective data. However, objectivity can be challenging when one becomes attached to the patient and witnesses him or her struggling with a life-threatening illness.

In Grace's case, I assessed her for transplant and then followed her supportively while she was an inpatient before, during, and after her transplant. Would I have been able to do this had the team not found her to be a candidate for transplant? My best answer is, "It depends." In most cases, I have found that I can continue to work with the child and the family to provide assistance with coping and adjustment while they are admitted to the inpatient unit (they may also have an outpatient therapist in the community). Often, the decision by the team to delay transplant is not a permanent judgment, but an opportunity to address factors, such as nonadherence, that might be impeding a transplant at that point in time. The spirit of the evaluation is one of teamwork and of collaboration between the medical team and the patient, which lends itself to an ongoing therapeutic alliance.

In a related vein, would it be possible to assess patients for transplant if the psychologist had already met them in a clinical capacity through his or her work with the medical team? Often, a psychologist works for a particular service (i.e., the pulmonary service for CF patients), and he or she follows inpatients from this service at various points in time. Therefore, it may be possible for a psychologist to have met the transplant candidate for supportive inpatient work before being asked to evaluate him or her for transplant.

In these cases, close clinical supervision and the team approach can prove quite helpful. Supervision or peer consultation can help the psychologist assess and evaluate the factors most relevant to proceeding with transplant. Supervision can also help the psychologist process the complex feelings that arise when participating in such a weighty decision-making process. Furthermore, it is important to keep in mind that psychologists do not make the ultimate decision about transplant; rather, they provide consultation to the transplant team about psychological issues that have the potential to negatively affect post-transplant adjustment. Medical teams make decisions about transplant through consideration of a multitude of medical, psychological, and psychosocial factors. Ideally, the team works closely together to integrate these various areas to provide the best care for patients.

Work setting

Consulting as a psychologist on a transplant team involves working closely with other medical professionals in a hospital setting. The approach taken is one of collaboration and sharing the information and insights of one's specialty area to inform patient care. Transplant evaluations usually occur in an inpatient unit or in an outpatient office in the hospital. Ongoing supportive treatment most often takes place while the child is hospitalized. This overall approach differs from traditional outpatient therapeutic intervention, which tends to be a more solitary endeavor.

A psychologist working as part of a transplant team must also become knowledgeable about the nature and course of the illnesses that can lead to transplant, as well as with the transplant process itself. It is important to be aware of the types of medications patients take, as well as common side effects. For instance, transplant patients often take steroids to help the body accept the transplanted organ. Steroid medications can affect mood; this should be taken into account when post-transplant adjustment is assessed.

In general, working within the context of a busy medical setting challenges psychologists to be flexible, team-oriented, and both clear and efficient when expressing their clinical opinions to other medical professionals. The hospital environment also requires a certain comfort level with the signs and symptoms of medical illness; for instance, I have been in the middle of meeting with a patient when a staff member needs to draw blood or quickly examine the surgical site. My training opportunities prepared me for these moments, and regular supervision/consultation helps me process the emotions that often arise when I am working with a seriously ill child.

Reflection

I consider myself very fortunate to have had the opportunity to work with children and families contending with life-threatening illness and the experience of transplant. My interactions with these children have been a gift, and I often feel as if I am learning unexpected life lessons. At times, however, I have felt overwhelmed—nervous about the gravity of the process and my ability to help patients through it. I felt all of these things in my work with Grace.

The evaluation process required for a pediatric transplant is multilayered and complex. In adult transplant evaluations, patients who do not adhere to their medical regimen will most likely not get a favorable recommendation for transplant. Adults are considered independent agents able to make their own decisions regarding their health-related behavior. With children, so much of their adherence is influenced by their parents. In Grace's case, I really struggled with the idea that she seemed potentially at risk for not receiving a transplant because of the challenges of her family situation. It didn't seem fair. I think most of the team members felt this way, which led to the solution of providing extra nursing help for the family.

I have often wondered what would have happened had we not received approval for the additional nursing care or if Grace's parents had rejected the idea. In similar situations, we have worked closely with the family to pursue every available option for support, from engaging the help of extended family members to providing further education regarding medication management to teaching various strategies designed to improve adherence. Often, it is important to listen closely to the family's concerns about possible interventions (i.e., home nursing) and solve the problem of how to address both the family and the team's concerns. My observation is that the intention and goal of the pediatric transplant evaluation focus on identifying those factors that might create particular vulnerability under the stress and strain of transplant, and then providing interventions to meet those needs.

Key ethical principles and standards

APA (2002): Principle A (Beneficence and Nonmaleficence), Principle E (Respect for People's Rights and Dignity), Standard 2.01 (Boundaries of Competence), Standard 2.04 (Bases for Scientific and Professional Judgments), Standard 3.10 (Informed Consent), and Standard 3.04 (Avoiding Harm).

REFERENCES AND FURTHER READING

Levenson, J. E., & Olbrisch, M. E. (1993). Psychosocial evaluation of organ transplant candidates. A comparative survey of process, criteria, and outcomes in heart, liver, and kidney transplantation. *Psychosomatics, 34*, 314–323.

Rapoff, M. A. (1999). *Adherence to pediatric medical regimens.* New York: Plenum Publishers.

Shaw, R. J., & DeMaso, D. R. (2006). *Clinical manual of pediatric psychosomatic medicine: Mental health consultation with physically ill children and adolescents.* Arlington, VA: American Psychiatric Publishing.

19

On Being There: Boundaries in Emotionally Intense Contexts

Gerald P. Koocher

I admit it. I once spent what was supposed to be a psychotherapy hour holding hands with a 26-year-old female client, sitting alone in her room. Actually, the appointment ran over—closer to two hours. We spent most of the time looking into each other's eyes, exchanging hushed words every few minutes. I struggled internally and uncomfortably for part of the time, wondering if this interaction constituted appropriate behavior in a professional relationship. Finally, I stopped fretting and decided that being there just felt right.

Karen had cystic fibrosis (CF), with severe pulmonary disease. The self-referral surprised me. I'd consulted to the CF treatment team for almost a decade and knew about her through case review presentations at clinic rounds, but she'd never wanted to chat with the "psych consultant" before. When I knocked at the door of her private hospital room, she sat propped up in bed with the ceiling lights dimmed and window shades drawn. I introduced myself while pulling a chair up to her bedside and asked, "How can I help?"

As I sat down, she gripped my left hand tightly and tensely blurted out, "Don't let go!"

Karen's 5-foot 6-inch frame had shrunk to 85 pounds, a consequence of the gastrointestinal malabsorption that accompanied her condition. A transparent mask held against her face by a thin green strap provided the maximum permissible flow of oxygen to her severely damaged lungs but could not fully satisfy her body's urgent need. Every 15 to 20 minutes, she broke into a bout of raspy coughing that usually ended with hemoptysis, spitting a few teaspoons of bright red blood into a bedside basin. She needed several breaths of oxygen amid the frequent coughing spasms to give voice to each sentence. The high levels of carbon dioxide in her blood created a frightening sense of air hunger and anxiety bordering on panic.

No evidence-based treatment manuals could have prepared me for that encounter. Karen had no psychopathology. Relaxation training, hypnosis, cognitive-behavioral therapy, EMDR (eye movement desensitization and reprocessing), forget about it! Lonely and terrified by the symptoms modern medicine could no longer keep at bay, Karen wanted human contact. In a moment of intense emotional intimacy, she asked me, a relative stranger, how she could tell her parents that she no longer had the will to keep fighting for her life.

Solid advances in psychological science have given us powerful tools to treat all manner of psychopathology and human distress. Considerable professional debate has focused on the importance of investigating, teaching, and applying evidence-based techniques. Such debate has directed us to rely chiefly on well-validated evidence as we assess and intervene professionally with our clients. I agree these are worthy activities and important aspirations. At the same time, I often find myself considering the distinction between performing psychotherapy and engaging in behaviors that seem likely to have psychologically beneficial effects. Many studies have taught us that empathy, the ability to form an emotional connection, and forging an alliance with the client will create a far stronger foundation for change and improved quality of life than any treatment manual validated by a plethora of randomized clinical trials.

Karen and I passed the time talking about how she could best communicate several important things she wanted to say to her parents about the 26 years they'd shared together—the love and support she'd felt from them, her sadness at the times when frustrations about her illness led her to direct anger at them, and her decision not to seek a lung transplant. She had an intravenous line in place and told me that she planned to ask her pulmonologist to start a "morphine drip," knowing that it would both reduce her discomfort and suppress her respirations, quietly ending her life in the course of a few hours. She hoped her parents would understand. I held her hand until her parents arrived. She died later that evening.

I had shared a few intensely emotional hours with a young woman I hardly knew, seeking to provide comfort at the very end of her life. Focusing on the laws and rules that guide our professional lives, one can find many flaws in my behavior. I failed to inform her of the limits of confidentiality and HIPAA

(Health Insurance Portability and Accountability Act) regulations. I did not take a careful history or perform a mental status examination. I did not seek her consent or formulate a treatment plan. Although I had reviewed her medical record, my brief closing session note in her chart would provide little guidance for future care providers. I assigned no diagnosis and never turned in a billing slip.

Some therapists might find fault with the fact that I also went to her funeral. Having spent many years treating children and families affected by life-threatening illness, I have decided that attending a funeral can serve two useful purposes. One important function focuses on the survivors mourning the loss. I have no pretense that my presence at such times constitutes a professional service. Rather, I seek to convey a message of respect and caring that I hope may bring some measure of comfort. The second important function of attending a funeral feels purely selfish. I need to feel a degree of closure and come to terms with the loss of a person about whom I too had intense feelings. I cannot appropriately express my personal distress to the family, but it lurks in need of self-care nonetheless.

At her funeral a few days later, Karen's parents handed me a note she had written on a strip of cardboard she had torn from a bedside tissue box after I'd left her room. It read simply, "Thank you for being there."

Discussion

Key ethical issues

Many aspects of this narrative reflect decisions to override standard operating procedures in psychotherapeutic practice. We teach psychotherapy students that any physical contact with patients, even at their request, must involve careful understanding of the meaning, purpose, and appropriateness of the act. One might typically address such a patient request by asking, "How will that help you." In the context of this case, a degree of beneficent exigency seemed to dictate a spontaneous gesture of emotional support. At the same time, the physical response, prolonging the session, and emotional intensity raise the ethical question of boundary crossing: how does a psychotherapist understand and decide to take action in a nontraditional manner for the well-being of a patient?

The key issues to consider involve whether the boundary crossing will likely enhance the therapeutic intervention without posing a risk for harm to the patient. What chance exists that the therapist's behaviors will prove incorrect, insensitive, or harmful to the client? To what extent will the therapist's behavior lead to a loss of professionalism that may compromise the relationship? Does the boundary crossing benefit the patient, or does it meet some inappropriate need of the therapist? These critical questions lie at the heart of the intervention but sometimes require an instinctive response.

Knowing the background of the referral from having read the medical chart and consulted with the patient's pulmonologist, I understood the seriousness of the young woman's circumstances. I made the decision to respond empathically in the moment. I understood that this was not the time to provide an HIPAA briefing on the limits of confidentiality or to ask, "Why do you think holding your hand will help?"

Another important ethical issue involves practitioner competence in terms of content knowledge, interdisciplinary practice, and personal attributes. In such situations psychotherapists must work hard to deal with their own intense emotional reactions to their patients' situations. Working as part of a treatment team, having supportive colleagues to review cases with, and understanding one's own limits become important for preserving the emotional competence to persist in such work. It also helps if one can tolerate talking with people who occasionally cough up blood, vomit, or become incontinent during psychotherapy sessions. Many practitioners have expertise and a degree of personal comfort in acute medical or palliative care settings, but a generalist psychotherapist would do well to avoid such situations without solid preparation. Understanding one's own reactions to loss, managing one's private grief reactions, and preventing personal issues from compromising patient care constitute essential professional competencies. Recognizing what might make us feel too uncomfortable to function effectively as psychotherapists for particular subsets of patients helps us to uphold the principle of *nonmaleficence* and the standard of *avoiding harm* most effectively.

Work setting

Working in an acute care medical setting requires psychotherapists to adopt a number of nonstandard practices; the absence of a typical office setting, scheduling around acute medical needs, atypical working hours, and involvement with a team of medical professionals of varying psychological and empathic sensitivities become the rule. Scheduling psychotherapy will often necessarily take a backseat to patients' symptoms, medical treatment, lab tests, and institutional routines such as scheduled meal times and privacy issues. Not all patients have private rooms or can be moved to accommodate therapy sessions. In an acute care setting, one must expect to hold bed-side sessions at odd hours, followed by the need to put immediate notes the medical record. All of these conditions focus on meeting the needs of the patient while challenging the psychotherapist to maintain the most appropriate degrees of privacy, respect, and professionalism possible.

Working in such settings requires some very specific competencies, as alluded to previously. Some of the skills needed involve the recognition of and ability to cope with emotional reactions evoked by the experience. An aptitude for teamwork and ability to support or motivate other members of the medical team also require some professional dexterity that extends beyond the usual realm of psychotherapeutic practice. At times, one must offer therapy-like interventions to modify the behaviors of medical team members in the interests of one's patient.

Practicing psychotherapy in medical acute care contexts also demands that one acquire a degree of knowledge-based competence about diseases and treatment protocols. Knowing the natural history or typical course of a particular chronic illness, understanding the purpose of various medical therapies and their side effects, and grasping the consequences of decisions at various choice points in the life trajectories of one's patients become critically important. Attending medical rounds and case conferences and asking one's medical colleagues for readings and candid appraisals of patients' conditions involve a degree of flexibility and effort not usually required in traditional office-based psychotherapy practices.

Reflection

I seldom tell casual acquaintances or even professional colleagues that I treat children and young adults with life-threatening illnesses. Such disclosures tend to stop conversations or evoke a response of "I could never do that." In some ways, the work offers exceptional rewards. Patients and families in acute distress, who are highly motivated to use my help, allow me into their lives at particularly intimate moments. Beneficial change occurs far more rapidly than one finds when trying to intervene in cases involving entrenched psychopathological or character-disordered conditions.

In another aspect of my clinical practice, I work with divorcing couples to resolve child custody disputes and improve post-divorce co-parenting. At moments when I find myself sitting between two hostile adults, squabbling over a few disputed vacation hours in a visitation agreement, I feel an urge to jolt them into perspective. I want to say, "Feel grateful that you're not facing the loss of your child from a devastating illness. Stop feuding, and focus on helping the other parent effectively without animus." Of course, I do not say such things because they do not share my experience across these different patient populations and can focus in the moment only on their own realities. I must bring myself into their present context and push the critically ill patient from my consciousness, so as to help them with their own issues.

Still, the nature of the work spills into my life in other ways. My spouse of 35 years, a clinical social worker, has no difficulty recognizing when I come home from work following a session of the sort I have described. Based on her silent appraisal of my mental status, she will often ask, "One of your patients is very sick?" My typical response is a hug, followed by a need to turn on an escapist video of some sort, typically involving gratuitous violence, alien invaders from another galaxy, and lots of explosions.

I keep a personal journal of my work as a psychotherapist, sarcastically titled, "Great Moments in Psychotherapy." I do not have "great moments" every week or even every month, but I do consider the anecdote recounted in this chapter among them. I feel as though I used my knowledge of the patient's illness and basic needs and a measure of empathic understanding to consciously reach across a traditional boundary to offer comfort at a critical point in time—a care point. Although I lack objective pre- and post-test measures, I believe I made an important positive difference in the life of another person. When I find myself in the midst of frustrating experiences that comprise life's speed bumps, I find myself reflecting on such care points, drawing patience and comfort.

Key ethical principles and standards

APA (2002): Principle A (Beneficence and Nonmaleficence), Principle E (Respect for People's Rights and Dignity), Standard 2.01 (Boundaries of Competence), Standard 2.06 (Personal Problems and Conflicts), Standard 3.04 (Avoiding Harm), Standard 4.06 (consultations).

REFERENCES AND FURTHER READING

Emanuel, E. J. (1991). *The ends of human life: Medical ethics in a liberal polity.* Cambridge, MA: Harvard University Press.

Koocher, G. P. (1986). Memorable patients: A contrast effect. *The Psychotherapy Patient, 2,* 39–44.

Meyer, E. C., DeMaso, D. R., & Koocher, G. P. (1996). Mental health consultation in the pediatric intensive care unit. *Professional Psychology: Research and Practice, 27,* 130–136.

Randall, F., & Downie, R. S. (1999). *Palliative care ethics* (2nd ed.). Oxford, UK: Oxford University Press.

Williams, J., & Koocher, G. P. (1999). Medical crisis counseling on a pediatric intensive care unit: Case examples and clinical utility. *Journal of Clinical Psychology in Medical Settings, 6,* 249–258.

PART IV

In National Security Settings

20

"I've Got This Friend": Multiple Roles, Informed Consent, and Friendship in the Military

W. Brad Johnson

Tony was a 30-year-old US Navy pilot serving in Hawaii. I was a US Navy psychologist and an officer—of equivalent rank to Tony—stationed at a mental health clinic on the island's naval base. Tony and his wife, Angie, lived just down the street from us in navy housing. Because we had children of approximately the same age, my wife quickly became friends with Angie. Families living in military quarters often become quite close, especially during periods when the service members are away from their families. In addition to spending time together as couples, we often shared child-care duties, and Tony and I went running together at least twice each week.

Nine months into our friendship, Tony was promoted to squadron intelligence officer, a position with responsibility for all classified material. A high volume of sensitive material that required very exacting protocols for transmission, storage, and disposal regularly came to his attention. Finishing a tour of duty as an intelligence officer without security mishaps almost always served as a career boon and ensured subsequent promotion. Any slipup, however—something not uncommon given the volume of classified material transmitted each day and the myriad challenges involved in effectively managing it—could just as easily become a "career stopper."

After a brief whirlwind training period, Tony assumed the mantel of chief intelligence officer. Immediately inundated with protocols, requests, and a backlog of work courtesy of the outgoing officer, his stress level skyrocketed. Terrified of violating a security protocol and aware of the zero-defect expectation from his superiors, Tony began spending long hours on intelligence duties at work, in addition to maintaining normal flight hours. He quickly began to feel overwhelmed.

In military settings, spouses often become better informed of families' emotional stresses than the military members themselves. I did not know the full extent of my friend's distress until my wife asked me to "take Tony out for coffee." Perplexed, I asked, "Why?" and learned that Angie was "very upset" about Tony's increasing insomnia and anxiety. In light of his reported sleeping problems, I decided not to invite Tony for coffee and instead asked him to lunch the following day. When we sat down, I confessed up front the reason for my invitation and asked how he was doing. True to Angie's report, Tony admitted a stress level "beyond anything I've ever known." Given the volume of classified material coming across his desk each day and the elaborate protocols for keeping it secure, he believed it was simply a matter of time until an error occurred.

Tony appeared haggard with circles under his eyes. He admitted to rather severe insomnia, stomach upset, and pervasive rumination about his job. As a friend and a psychologist, I felt immediate concern for Tony and began to consider a range of cognitive-behavioral strategies that might prove useful in helping to ameliorate his distress. I shared with Tony that his symptoms seemed consistent with insomnia and adjustment disorder; both were quite common in situations such as his and highly treatable. I suggested that he owed it to himself to let me refer him to a colleague at the mental health clinic.

Without hesitating, Tony said, "No way in hell." He reminded me that any whisper of a mental disorder or of a mental health consultation would trigger a swift evaluation by the flight surgeon and a near-certain grounding period with potential suspension of his security clearance. Failing to log flight hours due to an emotional problem would certainly be seen negatively when the next promotion board reviewed his record, a risk Tony—like most other military pilots—would not accept. Although being grounded and losing his security clearance would mean Tony could not function as the intelligence officer, he was staunchly opposed to even discussing the possibility of seeing my colleague. When Tony suggested that he and I meet "off the record" for therapy, I explained that, short of an emergency, our friendship precluded me from beginning a professional relationship with him. I also explained my ethical concerns about carrying on an undocumented therapy relationship. Frustrated, I cautioned Tony about the dangers of ignoring his symptoms and recommended a few self-help books related to insomnia and stress management. I appreciated my friend's predicament and understood his reticence to engage in mental health treatment. Military personnel with high-level clearances and those serving in submarines and other sensitive communities often show similar resistance to documentation in their health record of a mental health visit.

Tony and I continued to go running together twice a week. During our next run, he spontaneously offered, "I've got this friend who's really stressing out." A sideways glance revealed a sheepish smile. He continued, "It's not like the guy's going to go postal, he's just wrapped around the axle all the time and not sleeping very much." Playing along, I inquired whether his "friend" had read any books on sleep recently. He had. For the remainder of that run, we spoke in general terms about sleep hygiene, disputing catastrophic thinking, and actively practicing self-relaxation. At the conclusion of the run, I reiterated the benefits of professional assistance and offered to find the right practitioner for Tony's "friend" anytime. I also inquired whether this friend would tell someone if his symptoms worsened or if he ever began to feel desperate or contemplate suicide. Startled, Tony was quick to respond, "Of course! I know this guy. He'd never let it get to that point; he's got a family." Finally, I explained the potential problems involved in providing services to friends, as well as the circumstances that might lead me to report my concerns to a flight surgeon (e.g., if a pilot were so impaired that crew members or others might be in danger).

Back at the clinic that afternoon, I pondered my predicament. It was clear I had embarked on a trial of thinly veiled intervention for my friend. I worried about the blurring of friendship and provider roles, about what might happen if my friend's condition worsened, about the inability to formalize the new role and provide detailed consent, and about how much worse things might get for my friend if I proved unresponsive to his need. During a quiet moment, I consulted with another psychologist and outlined the essential elements of my dilemma. We agreed that the cleanest solution would be to cease all discussion of Tony's distress and insist that he seek professional help. We both understood, however, that no promotion-conscious aviator would do so unless so ordered to by his or her commanding officer.

On one hand, I worried about providing informal therapy to a friend—even if for nothing more than situational stress. On the other, I knew that a distressed service member would receive no help unless I continued to do what I could informally. In the end, I decided to proceed with a regimen of "friendly therapeutic runs" focused on stress management, sleep hygiene, and the disputation of negative self-talk. My colleague agreed with this approach but also cautioned me to remain alert to signs of deterioration that might necessitate a different course of action.

During the next three months, I spent roughly two hours per week running with Tony. A portion of each run was spent discussing his job, his irrational thinking, and various strategies he might employ to reduce his stress, make his job more manageable, and achieve a reasonable level of sleep each night. Although Tony's symptoms seemed to ebb and flow, he evidenced steady improvement in mood and a decline in overall distress. A single bump in the road occurred when the squadron prepared for a major inspection. During this time, Tony's anxiety and sleeplessness hit such a level that he admitted to struggling to stay awake and attend to tasks in the cockpit. Although he was successful in staying awake, and although his aircraft always had three pilots in the cockpit, the incident left me wondering if at some point I would feel ethically obligated to report Tony's condition to the flight surgeon to protect other crew members.

Nearly four months into his intelligence officer duties, Tony's distress evaporated entirely when he won promotion to department head within the squadron. With the intelligence officer duty delegated to another junior officer, Tony's burden dissipated, and he entered a period of nearly euphoric relief. He expressed genuine gratitude for my friendship and assistance during what he began describing as his "dark age." He also described a renewed commitment to making the navy a career. Although my friendship with him continued for another nine months, until he transferred to a new duty station, we socialized less often and our spouses arranged fewer get-togethers—perhaps sensing the need for greater personal distance. In the end, I observed that Tony—or his "friend"—had become more self-aware and better able to cope effectively with stress. He appeared to have benefitted from developing better control of his cognitive life and from greater sensitivity to his stress responses.

Discussion

Key ethical issues

The most salient ethical issue present in this case is that of multiple relationships. When a practitioner is in a professional role with someone and at the same time is in another—often personal—role with the same person, a multiple relationship exists. These relationships are risky in that the professional's judgment and performance may be compromised by the blurring of roles, with the outcome being that the client is exploited or otherwise harmed. Of course, multiple relationships that would not reasonably be expected to cause impairment or risk exploitation or harm are not unethical.

Other ethical issues germane to this case include informed consent and documentation of professional work. Mental health professionals are careful to obtain informed consent for their services before proceeding. This practice is especially important when embarking on any form of psychological treatment. Practitioners are also careful to create an adequate record of their work, a record that might facilitate subsequent care by other professionals.

Finally, the ethical principles of beneficence and respect are quite relevant to Tony's case. Mental health professionals should strive to benefit others, and when conflicts occur among competing obligations, they should try to resolve the conflict in a way that minimizes harm. Professionals also respect the rights of individuals to privacy, confidentiality, and self-determination.

Work setting

Military psychologists are often deployed or *embedded* within military units. As such, they are members of the military force, legally obligated to place the mission first and even housed among the very personnel they must serve. In this work environment, close personal contact and multiple roles with several clients are not uncommon. Further, as lone mental health practitioners in many geographic locations, military psychologists often have no choice about commencing clinical relationships with friends or coworkers and may have little capacity to predict when multiple relationships will arise. Although many members of any military unit will appreciate the psychologist's varied roles within the community, others may be less inclined to respond positively. Another complicating factor is the military psychologist's dual identity as mental health provider and officer. Active duty psychologists are legally obligated to hold subordinates accountable, to promote order and discipline, and to place the mission above the interests of individual service members. These demands mean that the military psychologist is always an officer—even when exercising, attending a social function, or talking with a friend.

For these reasons, military psychologists are often encouraged to recognize that every member of the military community is a potential client and to increase tolerance for routine boundary crossings. *Boundary crossings* are departures from commonly accepted clinical practice regarding professional boundaries, but they do not necessarily imply boundary violations or predict harmful outcomes for clients. To the extent that military psychologists are both prudent and comfortable with day-to-day extratherapy contact with clients, they will be more effective as both officers and clinicians.

Finally, it is important to note that military personnel are often justifiably reticent about seeking mental health care. Military physicians and psychologists wield profound power over all aspects of a service member's life and career. Psychologists are often directed to make critical go/no-go decisions or provide key input in determining fitness for duty, ability to deploy, security clearances, flight status, and other career-impacting matters. Military mental health practitioners understand that personnel in certain work settings are unlikely ever to initiate treatment voluntarily.

Reflection

As a military psychologist embedded within the navy community, I occasionally offered supportive and psychoeducational assistance to colleagues, supervisors, and friends without formalizing the relationship or opening a client record. In some respects, this approach allowed me both to earn the trust of military members and to further the preeminent mission of keeping the fighting force healthy and ready for the next mission. As military mental health jobs become more and more operational or embedded, practitioners will need to become increasingly comfortable with such informal consultation. But this situation raises an important ethical question: At what point along the continuum of helping does supportive advice to a friend or colleague become a professional relationship? Tony suffered from acute situational distress, something any supportive friendship would undoubtedly help to ameliorate. So where is the threshold between support and psychotherapy? Factors such as symptom severity—including evidence of serious mental illness, signs of impairment, and level of intervention required—may all be relevant in deciding when a professional must insist that a relationship be formalized.

Tony's case exemplifies a more extreme and unusual example in that his initial distress might have been most appropriately managed in a clinic setting. I wrestled with several ethical concerns in this case, not the least of which was the decision to provide some measure of psychoeducation, consultation, and support outside of a documented therapeutic relationship. In light of Tony's flat refusal to seek professional help in a mental health clinic, I reasoned that the navy would be well-served by any informal effort to keep a good pilot and officer functional. But I experienced some tension about the potential risk associated with enabling Tony to evade more formal care, and I worried that if his distress actually worsened, he could put others and himself at risk.

I also struggled to balance my multiple roles with Tony. Although it is not at all unusual for military practitioners to find that good friends or coworkers suddenly require clinical care, and although I attempted to offer Tony an explanation about why our multiple roles could at some point feel uncomfortable or problematic for one or both of us, it is doubtful that I would have been willing to offer so much informal professional support had Tony not been a friend first. In the end, my professional role made our friendship—both as individuals and as couples—less comfortable; as our "consultative runs" continued, I found it necessary to become more attentive to boundaries in our personal lives.

In retrospect, I believe that ethical standards enjoining professionals to work actively to resolve conflicts between ethics and either laws or organizational demands should have compelled me to become more vocal about the apparent conflict between the best interests of service members (e.g., fully confidential access to basic mental health care) and federal regulations and military policies that clearly inhibited distressed service members from seeking professional assistance. Mental health professionals have an abiding obligation to make conflicts between ethics and organizational policies known to the organization. When focused at the level of an individual client, the clinician can easily lose sight of this ethical requirement.

Throughout my decision-making process, it was imperative for me to seek consultation from another military psychologist. This consultation helped me normalize the boundary crossing and multiple roles and make decisions in light of military policy and our overarching mission. My colleague also helped me to think carefully about those signs, symptoms, or events that would trigger a different course of action (e.g., contact with the flight surgeon). In the end, I hope that my imperfect solution benefited both the military and an excellent naval aviator—in whom much had been invested. But I am mindful that there are genuine risks involved when any service is rendered outside the umbrella of formal documentation and organizational recognition.

Key ethical principles and standards

APA (2002): Principle A (Beneficence and Nonmaleficience), Principle E (Respect for People's Rights and Dignity), Standard 1.02 (Conflicts Between Ethics and Law, Regulations, or other Governing Legal Authority), Standard 3.04 (Avoiding Harm), Standard 3.05 (Multiple Relationships), Standard 3.10 (Informed Consent), Standard 4.06 (Consultations), and 6.01 (Documentation of Professional and Scientific Work and Maintenance of Records).

REFERENCES AND FURTHER READING

Barnett, J. E., Lazarus, A. A., Vasquez, M. J . T., Moorehead-Slaughter, O., & Johnson, W. B. (2007). Boundary issues and multiple relationships: Fantasy and reality. *Professional Psychology: Research and Practice, 38*, 401–410.

Gutheil, T. G., & Gabbard, G. O. (1993). The concept of boundaries in clinical practice. Theoretical and risk-management dimensions. *American Journal of Psychiatry, 150*, 188–196.

Johnson, W. B. (2008). Top ethical challenges for military clinical psychologists. *Military Psychology, 20*, 49–62.

Johnson, W. B., Ralph, J., & Johnson, S. J. (2005). Managing multiple roles in embedded environments: The case of aircraft carrier psychology. *Professional Psychology: Research and Practice, 36*, 73–81.

Kennedy, C., & Zilmer, E. A. (2006). *Military psychology: Clinical and operational applications.* New York: Guilford.

21

Establishing Rapport With an "Enemy Combatant": Cultural Competency in Guantanamo Bay

Carrie H. Kennedy[1]

Mohammad, a detainee from Afghanistan, estimated his age to be somewhere in his late 30s or early 40s. He was held in Guantanamo Bay (GTMO), Cuba, for reasons unknown to me. I was a military psychologist and an American woman deployed to provide mental health care in the detention camp. Mohammad was Muslim, with only a few years of formal education. He had multiple wives, and his children numbered in the double digits.

I met Mohammed on a hot, muggy day while I was out on his block seeing another detainee. This block was in one of the outdoor camps and held about 40 men in individual cells. After meeting with my intended patient, I began my walk back out through the block. As often happened, the linguist who had accompanied me was requested by several other detainees, one who had a cold and needed a corpsman, one who wanted a copy of the Koran in a language different from the one he had, one who

---

[1] *Disclaimer*: The views in this manuscript are those of the author and do not represent the official policy or position of the United States Navy, the Department of Defense, or the United States Government. Please note that this case represents a conglomeration of cases in order to protect the identity of the patients in Guantanamo Bay.

strongly recommended in colorful language that the linguist stop working for the Americans, and finally Mohammad, who requested an appointment. Getting new business while out seeing patients was common, and it was not unheard of to arrive on a block with the intention of seeing one detainee and then leave having spoken to as many as five to eight.

Mohammad's request made him a new patient, one not already on the panel of the Behavioral Health Services. After I conducted a brief screening to assess for acute symptoms, the staff provided him the next available routine appointment at the Behavioral Health Unit for an outpatient diagnostic interview. During this assessment, it became apparent that Mohammad had no mental health disorder. He felt bored, frustrated, and homesick in GTMO, feelings which were exacerbated by the uncertainty of the length of his detention. His central concern focused on missing his wives and his children. Apparently, none of his wives had been writing, effectively cutting him off from all news of his family, as well as the social and emotional support other detainees received via letters from home.

Providing mental health treatment, especially psychotherapy, proved a bit tricky in GTMO. The nature of the work environment was unprecedented and the cultural variability inordinately wide. In order to do any work there, a psychologist had to get exposure to a variety of diverse materials: readings from the Koran, the professional psychology literature, and even the Manchester Document (i.e., a purported terrorist training manual found in Manchester, England, which among many things discusses hunger striking and the importance of insisting one has been abused while in captivity). A psychologist also had to learn the therapeutic approaches most acceptable to the population and learn the history of the relationships between different religious and cultural groups, such as Sunnis and Shiites, Arabs and non-Arabs, and infidels and the devout.

Mohammad and I began a fairly traditional supportive therapeutic relationship, meeting weekly for sessions for several months. As had become typical in my experience, it took several sessions to establish sufficient rapport before any more meaningful discussions could successfully ensue. Consequently, the first several sessions involved him testing my boundaries and getting to know me, while I tried to understand his points of view, given his geographic region of origin, life experience, and educational level.

As one might expect of an American, woman, and a military officer, my views and feelings about individuals and societies that do not provide equal rights to women run fairly strong. While certainly not my first GTMO therapy patient, Mohammad was my first patient who focused on experiencing problems related to women in his life as a primary issue. Just how effective could I be? I hold strong views that do not align with his, and I felt concerned about my ability to provide the empathy needed to help a man I might have difficulty relating to, particularly when his family played a pivotal role in his presenting problem. Since I constituted his only option for supportive therapy given the absence of referral sources, I clearly had to work it out.

My first task was to further my understanding of the cultural issue of multiple wives. The Internet and available professional literature proved only mildly helpful. So as with many of our other cultural issues, I turned to the linguists for help. The linguists were from a wide variety of countries, and many came from the same geographic areas as the majority of the detainees. These men, in general, did not hesitate to explain some of these cultural concepts in straightforward ways. These informative sessions were often accomplished over dinner, where the linguists and clinical providers took turns providing ethnic meals, or during the language lessons that some of the linguists provided informally for the clinicians so we might more easily establish rapport with the detainees and, secondarily, recognize if we had entered a hostile environment. We also learned about the background and current state of polygamy in various Muslim countries.

So with a little knowledge under my belt and, probably more importantly, some practice in comfortably discussing the issue, as he tested my boundaries, subtly questioned me on my values, and tried to get a measure of me, I did the same with him. Over the course of his therapy, he educated me on his background, his life circumstances that resulted in his large family, and the finer points of managing more than one wife. My obvious interest in his life, willingness to listen openly to his different views, and subsequent ability to form a strong working relationship with him resulted in his willingness to adopt some of the strategies I taught him to better manage his boredom, frustration, and longing for home.

Discussion

Key ethical issues

The most salient ethical issue present in this case is that of competency, in particular cultural competency. The detainees presented multiple challenges in GTMO with regards to cultural issues, as they came from many different countries, had a wide range of education and experience, spoke many different languages, and held a range of non-Western or anti-Western views of men and women.

Other ethical issues germane to this case included mixed agency and confidentiality. By the term "mixed agency," I refer to the perpetual balancing act required of the military psychologist, whose primary client is always the military. This requires constant consideration of the best interests of both the military and the patient and proactive measures to ensure that the needs of both are met. For instance, the mixed-agency dilemma was present in a related case of a detainee who provided information of intelligence value during a therapy session. In that instance, the psychologist worked to preserve the confidentiality of the detainee/patient while still ensuring the information was received by appropriate personnel. Balancing dual obligations to the military and to detainee-patients in GTMO required constant ethical analysis.

Preserving the confidentiality of patients is also always of the utmost concern for psychologists. This was compounded in GTMO given the patient's status as subordinated to military rules and procedures and the presence of the guards as mandated for the safety of the staff and detainees. Ensuring privacy always presented a challenge and was largely accomplished by not having sensitive conversations on the cell blocks, where your presence was often announced loudly down the tier and neighbors and guards were able to easily listen. Depending on a detainee's specific neighbors, at times some additional commentary was volunteered to both myself and the detainee-patient. Consequently, with the exception of one urgent visit, all of Mohammad's psychotherapeutic care took place in the recreation area of the Behavioral Health Unit. This prevented other detainees from becoming aware that he was getting mental health treatment, as well as allowing for safe visual-only monitoring by the guards.

Finally, the ethical principle of respect for people's rights and dignity was quite relevant to Mohammad's case. In many ways, the two of us seemed about as diametrically opposite as two people can get in terms of background and life experience. However, by finding some common ground and remaining open to understanding his beliefs, I was able to establish rapport fairly easily, which paved the way for effective psychotherapy. Striving to reduce or eliminate personal biases about patients' backgrounds and choices, and becoming a culturally competent provider, became exceptionally important in GTMO.

Work setting

From a clinical perspective, the work environment in GTMO seemed largely comparable to a criminal forensic or penal facility, though with the added dimension of intense public scrutiny. Strong public perceptions of the current wartime detention facilities and human rights concerns for those held within generated constant external evaluation. Additional professional complications included limited access to mentorship and supervision given the isolated nature of the job, issues related to classified information further reducing the pool of potential consultants, and a lack of professional resources directly addressing the unique challenges that arose in the course of the work.

The physical environment added unique challenges in terms of heat and humidity. The need to dress in long sleeves, long pants, boots, and antistab vests made routine interactions incredibly uncomfortable. Endangered species of iguanas also roamed everywhere at GTMO. These animals assumed the role of pets for both staff and detainees alike. In the context of mental health, they provided a readily available topic of discussion that often served as the common ground needed to begin building rapport.

Reflection

Mental health providers have to take significant initiative in GTMO to address issues related to cultural competence, mixed agency, and confidentiality, not to mention issues related to situational awareness and appropriate self-care. Working in GTMO also provided another unique environmental element in that most patients recognized a kind of truce when one arrived to provide care, despite the fact that some detainee-patients had made clear their desire to kill Americans, including you, if presented with the opportunity. Fortunately, among the mental health patients, these were exceptions and not the rule. However, compartmentalization of this understanding when providing assessment or care became key to efficacy in GTMO, while still requiring the mental health personnel to remain constantly on guard for our own personal protection, as is the case in many forensic settings.

At times, media scrutiny proved even more trying than the openly hostile motives of some of the detainees. Mental health providers found themselves called upon to provide media interviews 1–2 days per week, every week, necessitating the cessation of all mental health care in the vicinity of such tours to avoid putting our patients on display. In addition, prior to taking on the job in GTMO, I did not realize the frequency with which the media inaccurately portray things or engages in selective reporting because the truth seems simply too boring.

Such stress profoundly affected the professionals working at GTMO and had the capacity to significantly impact efficacy on the job. Fortunately, during my tenure there, all of the mental health providers were females of the same rank and so we lived together. Nightly debriefings occurred in our house without interruption, and this served to assist us in maintaining objectivity, problem solving, and taking care of each other. In the context of war and stressful deployments, one cannot overemphasize the importance of mental health providers addressing their own stressors and seeking mutual support.

With constant problem solving and examination of our own decisions and options for the detainee-patients, we had significant opportunities to make a difference as mental health providers in GTMO. Another special irony of GTMO was that the patients routinely thanked medical and mental health staff for our care of them, usually when they thought no one else could hear.

Key ethical principles and standards

APA (2002): Principle E (Respect for People's Rights and Dignity), Standard 1.03 (Conflicts Between Ethics and Organizational Demands), Standard 2.01 (Boundaries of Competence), Standard 2.06 (Personal Problems and Conflicts), Standard 4.01 (Maintaining Confidentiality) and Standard 4.02 (Discussing the Limits of Confidentiality).

REFERENCES AND FURTHER READING

Howe, E. G. (2003). Dilemmas in military medical ethics since 9/11. *Kennedy Institute of Ethics Journal, 13*, 175–188.

Kennedy, C. H., & Johnson, W. B. (2009). Mixed agency in military psychology: Applying the American Psychological Association's ethics code. *Psychological Services, 6*, 22–31.

Kennedy, C. H., Jones, D. E., & Arita, A. A. (2007). Multicultural experiences of U.S. military psychologists: Current trends and training target areas. *Psychological Services, 4*, 158–167.

Kennedy, C. H., Malone, R. C., & Franks, MM. J. (in press). Provision of mental health services at the detention hospital in Guantanamo Bay. *Psychological Services*.

McCauley, M., Hughes, J. H., & Liebling-Kalifani, H. (2008). Ethical considerations for military clinical psychologists: A review of selected literature. *Military Psychology, 20*, 7–20.

22

Psychotic, Homicidal, and Armed: The Delicate Balance Between Personal Safety and Effectiveness in a Combat Environment

Heidi S. Kraft

It was over 130 degrees outside that afternoon. As I traversed the light brown dirt between my barracks and our surgical company's tiny combat stress platoon office, my feet actually baked inside my tan suede combat boots.

By the time I met PFC Johnson, US Marine Corps, on that stifling desert afternoon in western Iraq, I had already seen ten patients. My psychiatrist colleague, our two talented psychiatric technicians, and I stayed very busy out there. We worked seven days a week most of the time, taking turns covering the duty radios and nighttime emergency watch. As some of the only mental health providers in Iraq, we took seriously the charge to care for the many marines and sailors serving there.

PFC Johnson was escorted that afternoon by a gunnery sergeant in his chain of command. The gunny told us the junior marine had recently started acting "strangely" in his shop. The young private had reportedly picked up his Ka-Bar, a Marine Corps–issued knife, and yelled at it while others watched with a combination of amusement and concern—after which he threw it at the wall in a dramatic display.

When he arrived in our tiny office, PFC Johnson was obviously uncomfortable. Of course, in 130-degree heat, it is difficult to assess whether profuse diaphoresis is actually a symptom of anything psychiatric in a new patient. But he also shifted constantly in his seat, looking around often, and nervously transferred his M-16 automatic rifle from one side to the other on his lap.

We were deployed to a hostile area of a chaotic combat zone, during a time when casualties ran high. We all carried weapons and ammunition. My own 9mm pistol hung from the holster around my shoulders, with a loaded clip inserted. For that reason, I did not give much thought at the time to the fact that the Marine sitting in front of me had a loaded firearm resting across his thighs.

Our conversation started reasonably enough. I explained the limits of confidentiality and began to ask questions to attain basic demographic information and history. He answered my questions in a terse but respectful manner. He made it clear that he had not chosen to come to mental health of his own accord, and that he disagreed with his gunny's assessment that he needed help. I validated his uneasiness and explained that sometimes misunderstandings could be cleared up with my assistance. That seemed to appease him temporarily.

Then the questioning got more personal. I asked about his family history, to which he replied they were "all nuts." I asked if he had ever been hospitalized on a psychiatric ward. The muscles around his jaw and eyes visibly tensed. He nodded yes but did not elaborate. I asked how many days. He shrugged.

"I don't know, three? Four?"

"What can you tell me about that?"

"Nothing." His eyes began to dart around the room, and he made progressively less eye contact with me. I reminded him that I couldn't help him without more information. He reminded me in no uncertain terms that he didn't want my help.

I told PFC Johnson that I needed to take care of something quickly. I left the room and crossed my fingers that my psychiatric technician—a navy petty officer—was on duty next door doing paperwork. He was. I asked him to do everything he could to get hold of the psychiatric ward at the naval hospital at the marine's duty station back home in the United States. Our phone lines worked inconsistently at very best. I knew it was a long shot.

I re-entered the room, thanked the marine for his patience, and sat down. PFC Johnson's eyes squinted at me, and his mouth twisted into an angry line. His boot tapped nervously on the deck, and his thumb and forefinger tapped on the handle of his rifle. He reiterated that he had no interest in my help.

"Fair enough. But let's figure out the Ka-Bar thing, so I can explain to your command for you. Okay?"

He seemed to calm appreciatively then. He told me, matter-of-factly, about throwing his Ka-Bar against the wall. He said "she" had angered him and that he'd lost his temper. But they made up, he explained, and now "she" understood that he didn't mean to hurt her. "It's not a good thing, you know?"

"What's not?"

"The sun. If it penetrates directly, it can derail a train."

I reminded him we were talking about his knife.

"I know that!" he shouted. "It's all a matter of timing." He quickly moved his head to stare at the corner of the ceiling. I asked if he saw something up there.

He looked directly at me for the first time and accused me of insinuating he never sang in his church choir. I realized the situation was quickly deteriorating, and that I'd sent my only backup to find a working phone and try to call the States. I quickly ran through the situation in my head, assessing options, while attempting not to *look* like I was assessing options. I realized that I was working to balance my patient's best interests with concern for my own safety. I was alone with a possibly psychotic and armed patient who was clearly agitated. My first priority had always been the safety of the patient, but I'd also never been in a situation in which my own safety could have been threatened to this extent. I knew I needed to keep the patient calm, and that this required distracting him from the truth of the treatment that was inevitable for him. My mind raced; I felt pressured to make the right decision. He tapped his boot furiously.

A knock came at the door. I stepped out and my petty officer informed me that he had reached the hospital. The marine had stayed twenty days on the inpatient ward, was discharged with a provisional diagnosis of schizophrenia, but then returned to duty when his symptoms cleared completely without medication. I knew there was a great deal of important psychiatric information bearing on this patient that I could not immediately access. I also knew that people with schizophrenia can behave erratically, especially when disorganized and paranoid, as my patient appeared to be. Despite my uncertainty about what waited for me behind that door, I knew the patient needed our help. I took a deep breath to steady the anxiety that accompanies such an uncontrollable situation. I asked the psychiatric technician to stay nearby, and again I entered the room.

Once again, I sat across from my patient, although I became acutely aware that the patient's seat was positioned between my own and the door. I decided to use his rank as often as possible from that point on; aware that his reality testing was compromised, I wanted to remind him that he was a US Marine, with the pride and self-discipline that implies. I began, "Private First Class Johnson—"

"I know you," he interrupted through clenched teeth. "You're trying to fillet me, like a hamster." I explained to him that we had contacted the hospital and that their story about his inpatient stay differed quite a bit from his. His tense look relaxed completely, and he grinned at me. The hair on the back of my neck stiffened.

"Doesn't your husband ever forget your birthday?" he asked sweetly.

"Excuse me?"

"It's not like that means I'm guilty."

Still using his rank in nearly every sentence, I told the marine I would like to have him come into the hospital. I went after the safety angle, trying to convince him that I could keep him safe.

He did not like this. He began to yell, telling me I was only here to fillet him, and that he wanted to leave. I spoke softly, assuring his safety and asking him again to let me help him.

And then, without saying a word, he slowly, deliberately moved his rifle around on his lap until it was pointed directly at me. His finger rested on the trigger. He told me again that he wanted to leave.

In that one moment, I mentally juggled the buzz words from myriad ethical concepts that had been emphasized and re-emphasized early in my training: do no harm; duty to warn; self-protection; and limits of confidentiality. There was a brief instant in which I felt nearly dizzy with the dilemma. I suppose instinct trumped all others.

I told him it was fine if he left.

He swaggered out the door, his rifle still in his hands. I made eye contact with the petty officer, who looked at me questioningly, and I shook my head slightly to indicate that he should let the patient go. The petty officer watched PFC Johnson exit the building, then entered the room and asked if I was okay. I asked him to help me track down the patient's executive officer (XO), as soon as possible. The petty officer decided not to rely on inconsistent phone lines and instead hitched a ride in one of our ambulances and spoke to the XO personally.

I knew when that conversation took place because the XO immediately came to the hospital looking for me. He asked me, not mincing words, what I thought I was doing, requiring the involuntary admission to the hospital of one of his most productive marines. I lowered the volume of my voice to counter the rising volume of his. I told him his industrious marine was psychotic and could be a danger to himself or others. He glared at me. I spoke nearly in a whisper as I let him know this was a psychiatric emergency and it was not open for discussion. He turned on his heel and stomped away. Four hours later, my patient was returned to the hospital, unarmed and cooperative. I let my partner handle his medical evacuation, so as not to further agitate the patient with my presence. This also gave me a chance to consult with my psychiatry colleague. He agreed we had no other appropriate course of action.

We had ineffective mechanisms at the time to track our mental health patients once they returned to the United States, but we ensured that hospital in the United States to which the PFC would return was alerted to his situation, waiting for him, and that the psychiatry staff there had sufficient information to make critical decisions about his treatment and disposition.

I stood in the sand alone and watched his helicopter take off. I hoped that the providers at each of his next steps would take care of him for me. I felt empty fatigue and more helpless than I had four hours before, when he had pointed his rifle at me.

Discussion

Key ethical issues

We are taught from day one to "do no harm." It transcends nearly everything we do as psychologists. And until the moment that my marine patient used his weapon to make his point, I proceeded with that principle in mind. He was a young man suffering an early psychotic break, and my duty to him was clear: he required treatment that we could not provide onsite, and he needed a transfer to a safe environment. Despite earnest attempts on our part to support the operational mission by keeping marines and sailors in the combat zone for treatment if at all possible, we did have to MEDEVAC the most severe cases.

And then, in one moment, legal responsibility trumped any ethical desire I had to protect the patient's fragile emotional state. At the instant he expressed (through his actions) homicidal intent, one word flew into my mind: *Tarasoff*. There was no specific identifiable victim (except me), but he was acutely dangerous to anyone in his path. I needed to keep myself and the petty officer safe. I also knew we did not have a mechanism in place to "take down" a violent patient carrying a loaded weapon. So, despite all ethical and legal responsibilities screaming to the contrary, I had to confront a situation in which my choices narrowed to one. I had to allow a psychotic patient, carrying a loaded weapon, to leave my office. I would have given anything to have stopped him. But I could not take that chance.

Work setting

Through the conflicts in Iraq and Afghanistan, operational psychology has evolved as a field. Based on continued, and increasing, requests by line commanders to station military psychologists as far "forward" as possible—to treat combat trauma and other outcomes of war where they occur—this evolution has been well-received by those we serve.

In combat zones, the proximity of a psychologist to his or her patients is not only helpful—it is vital. For psychologists embedded with units like marine infantry battalions, visibility and familiarity make the clinician "one of us" in the eyes of unit members, effectively breaking down the barrier of stigma and enhancing the psychologist's credibility. Psychologists at mobile hospitals or surgical companies live and work side-by-side with the majority of service members who might seek their services. Our combat stress platoon quickly developed a reputation for keeping our patients in Iraq for treatment or follow-up if at all possible, we had low numbers of psychiatric MEDEVACs, and we made a serious effort to work around operational schedules so patients were seen immediately. Marine commanders on the base appreciated this; they knew they could count on us to emphasize the importance of the mental health of their marines to mission readiness and do our part to keep them there, in the fight. Of course, this defines a long-standing ethical dilemma in military psychology, the balance between what is best for the individual patient and what is best for the mission or the organization. But in combat, it is even more acute. Each person is vital to the overall success of the campaign. If at all possible, we needed to keep them with their units.

In addition, of course, we also shared many experiences and concerns with the marines and sailors operating in our area; at the time, these included incoming artillery, inconsistency in the cooling systems and the fresh food supply, and heavy casualties. They knew we understood; they trusted us.

We wanted it this way. And it allowed us to be effective. But in retrospect, I now understand that the same trust we strove to maintain among our line counterparts led directly to the unsafe situation that developed in the case of PFC Johnson.

One hundred percent of my patients carried weapons and ammunition. I carried a pistol myself. We certainly could never ask them to check their weapons. Not a single marine would have come to see us if we had; weapons are ubiquitous in a combat zone. Carrying a functional personal weapon at the ready is considered an inalienable right and a fundamental responsibility for every combat theater service member. So despite this glaring potentially dangerous situation each time someone walked through our doors, we had no plan for anything resembling a "code green," a hospital term for a psychiatric emergency that requires the involvement of security. There were additional logistic challenges as well, given that communications were so archaic. But it didn't matter. Just as our patients trusted us, we trusted them.

Reflection

I have thought about this patient often since my return from Iraq. I wondered how his treatment progressed at the naval hospital, how quickly his medical board was processed, which medications and therapies were helpful for him, and what he is doing today. I hope we were able to provide the care he needed and deserved.

When I remember his case, I am certain that I took the right course of action; he required an immediate MEDEVAC from the combat zone. However, the manner in which that MEDEVAC eventually happened was anything but optimal and potentially put many people at serious risk.

The patient walked into my office armed. There was no reason, based on the referral question and background information from his command, to expect him to walk in otherwise. As it became obvious that I was dealing with psychotic symptoms, I attempted to convince him to accept treatment voluntarily, still never expecting the patient to actually threaten me. My past experience with young and newly psychotic patients taught me that the marine was afraid. So I spoke calmly and quietly to assure him of his safety, all the while attempting to help him with reality testing. I believed that my priority was to help him to *not* be afraid.

In the past, that strategy had worked. But my experience before I entered the combat zone had never included the possibility that the patient might be holding a loaded automatic weapon and be trained in how to use it. The moment he pointed the rifle at me and demanded to leave, my priority instantaneously changed, and it no longer involved making the patient feel unafraid. I let a psychotic and homicidal patient walk out the door, with no one to stop him. I was helpless to do anything else, and in that moment, I also felt completely incompetent.

Every reference I have ever studied with regard to the management of violent patients preaches safety, both for the clinician and potential victims, as paramount. I mismanaged my own safety in several different ways. But the part that still haunts me is that by allowing him to leave, I exposed my psych tech, and then any random number of the ten thousand people who shared our base, to great risk. People outside our office had no idea that this marine—who looked like everyone else—might open fire if agitated, hallucinating, or both.

And yet we did not have the resources or the ability to protect them. We followed the best possible course of action, and it took four hours for the command to track down, disarm, and deliver the patient. Four hours. He did not harm a soul. But those were the longest four hours of my life.

Obviously, the patient I've described in this chapter is the very rare case. In this case, trusting a patient caused an unsafe situation. But even knowing that today, I cannot say that I would have changed the way I practiced in Iraq. The mutual trust and respect that developed between our small team of mental health providers and the marines and sailors entrusted to our care allowed us to help many people we never would have reached without it. The risk was worth taking.

Key ethical principles and standards

APA (2002): Principle A (Beneficence and Nonmaleficence), Principle B (Fidelity and Responsibility), Standard 1.02 (Conflicts Between Ethics and Law, Regulations, or Other Governing Legal Authority), Standard 1.03 (Conflicts Between Ethics and Organizational Demands), Standard 3.04 (Avoiding Harm).

REFERENCES AND FURTHER READING

Dubin, W. R., & Lion, J. R. (Eds.) (1992). *Clinician safety: Task force report No. 33.* Washington, DC: American Psychiatric Press.

Kraft, H. S. (2007). *Rule number two: Lessons I learned in a combat hospital.* New York: Little, Brown and Company.

Lion, J. R. (2008). Psychotherapeutic interventions. In R. I. Simon & K. Tardiff (Eds.), *Textbook of violence assessment and management* (pp. 325–328). Washington, DC: American Psychiatric Press.

Theinhaus, O. J., & Piasecki, M. (1998). Emergency psychiatry: Assessment of psychiatric patients' risk of violence toward others. *Psychiatry Services, 49,* 1129–1147.

23

"What Do You know That Can Help Us?" Behavioral Science in National Security Settings

Susan E. Brandon[1]

I manage a behavioral science research program for the US Department of Defense (DoD). The goal of this research program is to enhance capabilities within DoD to collect and validate information from human sources. We award research contracts, primarily to academic institutions, to conduct this research. More than 95% of our research is unclassified.

Because my coworkers know I am a Ph.D. psychologist, they sometimes come to me with stories about what they have been taught about influencing or persuading others, collecting information from human sources, detecting deception, or enhancing cognition. Although I have no authority to determine what methods or tools are used by DoD personnel, I think they tell me their stories because they want to share their successes with me, to promote a particular tool or technique, or because they are uncertain whether to trust a particular method or tool and want my professional opinion. As an example, one such story is paraphrased below. The names and specific questions are fictional, as are any relationships among people, places, and groups.

---

[1] Department of Defense, Washington D.C. The views, information, and analysis presented are the author's and do not represent the U.S. Department of Defense.

Report of examination

> Summary: On April 4, 20XX, interrogator Bill requested a voice stress analysis test on Detainee X being held in Camp A. The examination was conducted to verify information provided by Detainee X. On April 5, 20XX, Detainee X was interviewed and consented to a computer-based voice stress analysis examination to verify the information or statements made by or pertaining to Detainee Y. Mr. Hamdon, a linguist expert in Modern Arabic, served as a translator during the conduct of the examination. (A list of 12 questions followed. The responses to the questions and the outcomes of the voice stress test are noted.)
>
> 1. Have you ever lied to interrogator Bill? No. (Deception indicated)
> 2. Are you a member of the Libyan Islamic Fighting Group? No. (Deception indicated)
> 3. Do you know anyone associated with the Libyan Islamic Fighting Group? No. (Deception indicated)
> 4. Do you know why Hassan was in the United States? No. (No deception indicated)
> 5. Do you know Hassan's real name? No. (No deception indicated)
> 6. Was Hassan training to be a suicide bomber? No. (No deception indicated)
> 7. Did you ever live in the same apartment building as Joseph in Bosnia? Yes. (No deception indicated)
> 8. Is your nephew in the United States? Yes. (No deception indicated)
> 9. Are you scared to go back to Algiers? No. (Deception indicated)
> 10. Did you pay for your travel to Iraq? Yes. (Deception indicated)
> 11. Did you complete training at the camp? No. (No deception indicated)
> 12. Is this a picture of Dubai? No. (No deception indicated)
>
> After analysis of the information collected during the voice stress analysis test, it was the opinion of the examiner that Detainee X responses resulted in a deception.

It should be noted here that current DoD policy is that the polygraph and the Preliminary Credibility Assessment Screening System (PCASS) are the only accepted technologies to be used for "credibility assessment" (DoD 5210.48). Voice stress–based technologies are prohibited by DoD. Users of credibility assessment instrumentation other than the polygraph are required to provide a "written assessment" to the undersecretary of defense "reflecting instrument type and numbers, how such instruments were used, overall utility, validating factors, lessons learned, limitations, and depictions of 'success' or 'failure' irrespective of circumstance of context" in order to "assist in the validation and approval of future technology" (DoD Memorandum, 2004).

Discussion and reflections

I hear many such stories about various technologies and methods that have no empirical basis: These include the use of "neurolinguistic programming" as a persuasion tool, the detection of deception via "microexpressions" analysis, and the use of "kinesics" to determine whether someone is telling the truth. To try to prevent the use of such tools does not pose an ethical challenge. In my view, to fail to try to prevent the use of such methods is a violation of scientific ethical standards. (On this note, those who argue that behavioral scientists should have no role in national security agencies are vulnerable to the charge that they are failing to address violations of scientific ethical standards, and in my view, such scientists are engaging in ethically risky behavior.) The ethical dilemma here is how much to protest about the use of methods and tools for which there is no empirical evidence of efficacy, or in some cases, for which there are numerous demonstrations of failure. I do not have the authority to decide what is used; the best I can do is speak out. Senior management has been willing to listen to my concerns about the use of technologies that have never been shown to be valid, and it is DoD policy that "research and improvements" on potential credibility assessment tools "continue to be a priority for DoD" (DoD Memorandum, 2007). However, I also have been asked to "not be so negative," "find something positive to say," and "suggest how we can improve the tool." Continual nay-saying risks making me someone who is avoided or characterized as not a member of the team, which will make me less effective in the work that I do.

My response to this dilemma has been to continue to speak out—but I do this as someone more towards the end of my professional career than towards the beginning. My motivation for working for the US Government, after twenty very happy years in academia, was to make a difference, and I will work where I work only for as long as I can convince myself that I do (however slight). For those more junior than me, whom I supervise, we "speak out" together by writing "review papers" that explain, using nontechnical terms, the science or lack of science behind particular methods and tools that are problematic. We do not publish these in scientific journals; they simply are shared with our coworkers as opportunity presents itself (after being reviewed and approved, of course, by the appropriate military channels). We coauthor all of these papers.

There are, of course, a variety of techniques currently available for use in the effective collection of information from human sources that have been shown to have efficacy in laboratory settings and, in some instances, marketing. For example, there are methods and tools that might be used to discern deception, persuade individuals to cooperate, and/or persuade individuals to provide information against their will or without their consent. Such methods include:

(1) Priming, where a category is either explicitly or implicitly activated or made salient to an individual, with behavioral consequences. For example, the presence of weapons in the room has been shown to produce aggressive behaviors (Anderson, Benjamin, & Bartholow, 1998).
(2) Demonstrations that one person shares values with another have been shown to reduce resistance and induce compliance (e.g., Brehm, 1966).
(3) Various persuasion techniques—"foot-in-door," "door-in-the-face," and "low-balling"—that work outside the person's awareness (Cialdini & Goldstein, 2004).
(4) The pique technique that disrupts cognitive scripts, or rules, that individuals have established in response to particular types of requests, with the ultimate outcome of piquing curiosity and increasing compliance (e.g., Burger, Hormisher, Martin, Newman, & Pringle, 2007).
(5) There now is abundant evidence that false memories can be created inside and outside the laboratory (Loftus, 2004).

I face three ethical dilemmas with respect to the promotion of these evidence-based methods. The first is that, although I have no experience with such, I cannot guarantee that these, or those developed within my research program, will not be used in places where international laws are violated or where users engage in unethical practices. The second dilemma is that I cannot guarantee that some of these methods—perhaps such as those listed above—do not violate the "inalienable rights" of individuals to privacy and self-efficacy. Should behavioral scientists create and develop methods of implicit or indirect behavior manipulation that violate an individual's right to self-determination? This issue is made more problematic by the fact that US Government distinguishes US citizens from non-US citizens in terms of their rights and privileges; while the use of implicit and indirect methods may be limited by state or federal laws for application to US citizens, there are likely to be fewer restrictions for "non-US persons." The third dilemma is that evidence-based methods and tools have been validated only in laboratory settings (most often, only with American study participants). These may not generalize for use with people from other cultures, held perhaps in harsh conditions and against their will. Related to this point, acceptable field validation may prove impossible.

My response to the first of these three ethical dilemmas is to assume that less harm will be done if effective methods are available for use, even though I cannot guarantee that these will not be used in contexts that violate national or international laws, standards, or codes. My reasoning here is the result of realizing, shortly after coming to work in Washington DC in August 2001, that if operational/military personnel perceive they need help to accomplish some task—for example, interrogation—they may ask scientists "What do you know that can help us?" If the answer is, "Not much; we need more research," these people do not wait until the research is done (in fact, of course, they cannot; doing nothing is unacceptable). Instead, they turn to industry or pseudoscience or to whomever will offer help. In addition, good science is public, and if as a behavioral scientist I want to help decide *how* methods and tools are used, I have to be on the inside, not on the outside—I have to be at the table if I want a voice.

By constructing research contracts with scientists who study implicit and indirect measures, and by offering descriptions of such methods to those who teach or conduct interrogations, I also accept the risk that the use of such methods invades the private domains of other people. However, my decision regarding this particular challenge is colored by my own scientific view that we are largely unaware of what determines our own behaviors anyway. For example, it is my view that reinforcement shapes behaviors in ways that go largely unnoticed and that setting up reinforcement contingencies to shape behavior is not fundamentally different from the application of the kinds of indirect or implicit methods described above.

The dilemma regarding the use of methods and tools without validation is highly problematic for me. If I decide that evidence-based methods should not be used until they are field validated, I cannot recommend any new methods or tools to interrogators or to those who teach interrogation. All I can do is manage a basic research program that the military eventually will regard as useless; if the research does not have some operational impact, it will not be supported for very long. Also, as described already, ineffective and perhaps unethical methods will be used—some actions will be taken.

As an example of the challenge here, field validation of the Preliminary Credibility Assessment Screening System (PCASS) has not yet occurred, although the device has been purchased for use by the military in Afghanistan (MSNBC, 2008). The challenges to such field validation are obvious. First, many decision-makers do not understand what validation is or how to evaluate the relevance of experimental studies to field-use conditions. Second, it is difficult to find independent information regarding an examinee's veracity in the field, and without such, validation testing cannot be conducted. Third, the military is understandably reluctant to deploy research scientists to combat areas (it is necessary to go to combat zones because this is where the device is being used). Those conducting the validation must have the appropriate research skills; however, researchers deployed to Iraq or Afghanistan at present would pose a security risk to themselves and to the service personnel around them—they would, as well, require additional security measures be taken on their behalf.

My response to the dilemma of inadequate field validation changes with time, so I worry that my scientific ethics are slipping: Two years ago, I would not have agreed to use any method or tool without sufficient field validation. Recently, I agreed to a single opportunity to do just this, with the understanding that "deployment" of the tool occured in partnership with the researchers so the field use can approximate field validation testing. The problem here is that I have no way to enforce this arrangement; feedback to the researchers will occur only by the good will of those involved and with the support of their senior management and security officers, both of which may wish to guard outcome data for various political and security-related reasons.

I have two sons whom, had their lives gone in different directions, might now be serving in Iraq or Afghanistan. They would be, as their cohorts now are, in need of the kind of help that behavioral science can provide. I would be highly motivated to discourage the use of invalid tools, support research on useful methods and tools, and try very hard to conduct appropriate field validation studies. If I would take the ethical risks described here for my own children, am I not obligated to take the same risks for the sons and daughters of others?

Key ethical principles and standards

APA (2002): Standard 1.01 (Misuse of Psychologists' Work), Standard 3.04 (Avoiding Harm), Standard 5.01 (Avoidance of False or Deceptive Statements), 8.10 (Reporting Research Results).

REFERENCES AND FURTHER READING

Anderson, C. A., Benjamin, A. J., & Bartholow, B. D. (1998). Does the gun pull the trigger? Automatic priming effects of weapon pictures and weapon names. *Psychological Science, 9*, 308–314.

Brehm, J. W. (1966). *A theory of psychological reactance.* San Diego, CA: Academic Press.

Burger, J. M., Hornisher, J., Martin, V. E., Newman, G., & Pringle, S. (2007). The pique technique: overcoming mindlessness or shifting heuristics? *Journal of Applied Social Psychology, 37*, 2086–2096.

Cialdini, R. B., & Goldstein, N. J. (2004). Social influence: Compliance and conformity. *Annual Review of Psychology, 55*, 591–621.

DoD Memorandum (2004) to Secretaries of the Military Departments, Combatant Commanders, Inspector General of the Department of Defense, Directors of the Defense Agencies, and Directors of DoD Field Activities, from Stephen A. Cambone, Undersecretary of Defense, June 8, 2004.

DoD Memorandum (2007) to Secretaries of the Military Departments, Combatant Commanders, Inspector General of the Department of Defense, Directors of the Defense Agencies, and Directors of DoD Field Activities, from James R. Clapper, Undersecretary of Defense, October 29, 2007.

Loftus, E. F. (2004). Memories of things unseen. *Current Directions in Psychological Science, 13*, 145–147.

MSNBC News (*April* 9, 2008). "New anti-terror weapon: Hand-held lie detector," by Bill Dedman. Retrieved from http://www.msnbc.msn.com/id/23926278.

PART V

In Organizations

24

A Disaster in a Suit and Tie: When Organizational Policies Undermine Ethical Obligations

Charles A. Morgan III

Up until that moment, the interview had gone well. Or to be more precise, up until that moment the candidate appeared composed, easy going, mature, talented, and well suited for employment within the special mission unit to which he had applied. He came from an intact family, the middle of three boys born to his parents. In elementary school and high school, he was known for his ability to excel in both academics and in athletics. Offered a college scholarship for football, he turned it down in favor of one in mathematics. His record clearly reflected his ability to balance scholastics and sports and excel in both. College completed, he accepted a commission as an officer in the US Army, and according to his report and his service records, the candidate seemed to have performed in an exemplary manner.

Indeed, in the interview process, to meet him was to like him. He was polite, displayed an appropriate sense of humor, and spoke directly when providing answers. He seemed, on the whole, reasonable and thorough in all his answers. As I interviewed him, I found myself wondering about the results of the psychological testing the candidate had completed one day prior to our meeting; this was a standard part of the special mission unit application process. Testing revealed an image management style, as well as elevations on indices of impulsivity, hostility, anger, and paranoia. In addition, he'd endorsed almost twice the number of traditionally endorsed items on his polygraph screening form. The polygraph form contains queries about specific instances of breaking the law, doing drugs, having affairs, stealing from the government, and many other behaviors that might suggest impaired judgment, impulsivity, illegal activity, or antisocial behaviors. In effect, on paper this candidate appeared to be a hostile, impulsive, paranoid, and antisocial person; in person, however, he appeared to be the personification of the ideal special mission unit candidate.

To resolve this discrepancy, I elected to pursue a line of inquiry that was gently provocative and designed to assess the competing hypotheses I entertained. First, I asked directly about the responses on testing that had contributed to the worrisome testing results; in response, he provided answers that were plausible and compatible with having spent a significant amount of time deployed in a war zone.

Then it happened: the candidate transformed from his mild mannered, jovial appearance into something quite different. The proximal cause was a directive I'd given him to tell me about a specific time when he disagreed significantly with a peer or superior and how that disagreement was resolved. I'd added the caveat that it should describe a time that he "knew that he took the right course of action even if it got him into trouble." He sat still for nearly a minute and then began to speak. As he relayed his story, his face reddened with anger. He relayed a situation that occurred when he served in a forward operating base and when, in midargument with a difficult peer, he drew a loaded weapon and held it to the peer's head; he saw this as the only way of "getting the point through his thick skull." When I asked about the intensity of the anger he was displaying about the incident, he stated that he had not forgiven his command for removing him from theatre for the incident. I asked if there had ever been other circumstances during which he felt physical aggression was the only way to "make his point" to someone who was "thick headed." He said, "YES—just last fall, I had to make a point with an idiot (a master sergeant) who couldn't get it that I needed time off for family. I had an argument with him in front of the 7-Eleven store. He thought he won the argument, but I got him back. I slashed his tires. All four of them." I mused aloud that I thought it was hard to puncture tires these days. He quickly corrected me, "Nope. It's easy, Doc, I've had practice, and I've never been caught."

As I made statements conveying my desire to understand his point of view, he calmed and began to disclose a number of important additional facts: he had a history of slashing the tires of cars belonging to people from work who annoyed him; a history of being so angry he had no memory of events that transpired during the argument or fight; he had a history of seeing a psychiatrist who'd prescribed a medication called Haldol (an antipsychotic) that he'd stopped taking; and a history of gambling that had resulted in a debt of $90,000 at the time of my evaluation.

After disclosing all of this, his more cheerful disposition returned, and he stated that he'd put that behind him and was looking forward to "life out of the military but working in a civilian position that was involved in the current fight." Based on the intensity of his affect and his apparent lack of insight as to how this all might bear on his application for employment, I considered thanking him for his time and wishing him well on his interview with the board the following day and exiting the room. However, I didn't. I felt I had an obligation to share my thoughts honestly with him, let him know that I would inform the board about these events, and that, from a mental health evaluation perspective, I thought these events were important and represented a degree of psychiatric risk. I stated this to him. He smiled and said, "Well, like you said, Doc, you're not the one making the hire/don't hire decision, but I appreciate you listening to me. If they ask, I will explain it to them, and they will see my side of things too." He shook my hand and left the evaluation room.

That night, I prepared my notes for the briefing I would give to the board. I shared my experience with the other psychologist doing selection, and he expressed alarm and said, "So this guy has admitted he's $90,000 in debt, has been so out of control he was removed from theater, is supposed to be on meds, and has slashed tires as recently as six months ago? He's a disaster! And you know what? They [the board] will probably want to hire him cause he looks good in a suit and tie!"

The next morning, as I sat waiting to brief the board I felt confident; I felt useful. After all, I had meaningful and relevant data to convey about a significant psychiatric risk associated with a candidate who, as far as I could tell, would likely charm the members of the board. As I began to speak and describe the developmental history, the director of the board interrupted me and stated, "Now you know, Doctor, you are not allowed to tell us anything about his age, a history of criminal behavior, drugs, his sex life, marital status, etc. These are all forbidden areas of information when we evaluate candidates. All I need you to tell us is whether or not he is smart enough from your IQ testing and whether or not there are any personality quirks we should be aware of."

"I'm sorry," I said, "are you telling me that I cannot say whether this person is a felon, is or has been actively violent with coworkers, is doing drugs, or whether he is on major psychiatric medication or deeply in debt from gambling?"

"Yes, that is what I am saying," responded the board director.

I then asked, "Is there someone else to whom I may convey what I have learned?"

"No, it is just me and this panel," stated the director.

"Well, I've got a serious problem," I said, "because this guy is smart and looks good in a suit and is a disaster, but I am not allowed to tell you why I think this is the case. If I am not allowed to put this material into my report, then I must say this man is high risk without any data to back it up in the record, or I must say that he is a low psychiatric risk to be consistent with the record. However, the truth of the matter is that he is a high risk candidate!"

At this point, the director raised his voice and said "WE CANNOT know any of this; it is not permitted. This is for a GS (government service) position, and you can tell us about his IQ but not information from the personality tests, which are not allowed for GS employees. They do not have to take the MMPI or the NEO tests that you guys give, so you cannot brief us on that information. We therefore [he now addressed the other members of the board] must disregard what the doctor has told us and only judge him on whether he can do the job he is applying for!"

I then said, "Well, this is very awkward in that I cannot see how a psychological assessment is helpful to your process of interviewing. If you are not allowed to hear what I have learned and there is no one else to whom I can express my concerns, then I am not sure how a psychological assessment is part of this process. I understand that you believe you are keeping to the government guidelines, but we should explore this issue further to protect the integrity of the unit." I excused myself from the room. Later that evening, I discussed these events and my feelings about these events with my colleague. I relayed to him that it felt unethical to be asked to perform a thorough psychological evaluation and then be prevented from divulging findings that were relevant to security and psychiatric risk issues.

It seemed to me that to behave in this way would give an appearance of meeting the screening requirements while not actually doing so, in that I would have to avoid the substantive and relevant elements of such an evaluation. In my opinion, it would be better to opt out of this process rather than to give it legitimacy by conducting evaluations from which most data could not be utilized.

My colleague and I have recommended that the command consider two possible solutions to this issue: the first is that we not evaluate the GS candidates; the second is that suitable candidates receive a provisional offer of employment that is contingent on successfully passing the security/threat assessment process. It would be during this process that individuals would be assessed by both security personnel and by psychologists in order to assess whether they present security risks. At the present time, the new command has not reached a decision.

Discussion

Key ethical issues

There are several ethical issues that are intertwined and relevant to this case: They are related to the principles of fidelity and responsibility, integrity, misuse of psychologists' work, and conflict between ethics and organizational demands.

Within the principle of fidelity and responsibility, psychologists strive, among other things, to clarify their professional roles and obligations. Nonpsychologists may not fully understand the ways in which our role and obligations differ from those of other professionals. In this situation—one in which the psychological assessment is meant to provide information about suitability and risk—it is incumbent upon the psychologist to provide all information that is relevant to the situation and that is the basis of their judgment. This provides customers who seek our opinions a picture of the purpose and scope of our activity and the ways in which it contributes to the larger context—in this case, the selection process.

The principle of integrity enjoins psychologists to strive to promote accuracy, honesty, and truthfulness in the science, teaching, and practice of psychology. In the case described here, it would be inaccurate and dishonest to withhold information that the clinician knows is relevant for two reasons: First, it would result in the psychologist providing a recommendation that is deliberately less than complete and misleading should the omission of the information lead to a positive recommendation rather than a negative one. Second, the omission of information that is relevant to one's official recommendation may result in the appearance of bias if our work is reviewed by colleagues or public entities.

With respect to the standard bearing on misuse of psychologists' work, psychologists strive to prevent misrepresentation of their work and take reasonable steps to correct the misuse of their work. In this case, the censoring or limiting of the information used to inform the conclusions of the psychological report to the selection board and the subsequence use of that report in making a decision to hire or not hire an individual would represent a misuse of the psychologist's work because it is used to an end that is contrary to the psychologist's professional opinion gained from the evaluation.

Finally, this case raises the ethical standard of conflicts between ethics and organizational demands, bases for scientific and professional judgments, third-party requests for services, psychological services delivered to or through organizations, and bases for assessments. In accordance with these standards, psychologists strive to make known (and resolve) identified conflicts of ethical standards when interacting with other professions or organizational bodies. In this case, the decision by the head of the selection board to limit what could be known from the psychological evaluation created a conflict between the ethical obligations for said professional and the operating procedures of the organization.

Work setting

The work setting is that of a relatively small special mission unit of the United States military. In this organization, all successful employees (military, contractor, GS) must function as subject-matter experts in their respective fields. As such, there is little oversight and supervision for each employee. This degree of autonomy when working with classified materials and when operating in sensitive work environments means that the potential damage inflicted by an individual with serious psychological problems or security risks could be very extensive before it was detected. The psychological component of the screening process was designed to permit the detection of problems in cognition, personality, and judgment that might impair the mission of the unit or present risk to others. All candidates are given information about this process and give consent to participate in psychological testing. The psychological interview is traditional in that one attempts to assess the degree to which a person's reported history gives evidence of normal development, cognition, judgment, and maturity or whether there are indications of illness or maladaptive behavior.

The restrictions on my ability to convey problematic disorders, behaviors, or thinking styles to the command thwarted this objective. Given the limitations that may be imposed upon psychologists who perform such evaluations, it may be useful to have a healthy debate on how one might best perform and report on a thorough evaluation. If one adopts the view that psychological assessments are performed, in part, to detect whether a candidate has specific vulnerabilities that would negatively impact the work setting, then it is reasonable to conclude that such information would be valid for the psychologist to report.

At the present time, many organizations tasked with national security issues have elected to give a provisional offer of employment to candidates;

the offer is withdrawn if that candidate does not successfully pass the security evaluation process of which psychological assessment is a part. It is possible that this solution may become standard practice for military programs that employ psychological evaluations in selection decisions; this solution, however, is not a perfect one and sets up the potential for situations in which individuals offered a job and found to exhibit significant psychopathology would then challenge the withdrawn offer of employment by claiming discrimination against individuals with psychological problems. The degree to which such claims will be found to be compelling is not known and likely related to whether or not one views working in national security positions as a right or a privilege.

Reflection

The director of the GS hiring board was correct on two main points: First, during the hiring process, board members are not allowed to ask the candidate questions pertaining to age, sexuality, marital status, mental health and criminal history, etc; second, during the process of candidate evaluation, tests such as the MMPI and the NEO are not permitted prior to a provisional offer of employment.

Given that a psychological testing battery and evaluation is not considered valid or within the standard of practice without an evaluation of a person's developmental, social, sexual, criminal, and mental health histories, in what manner can such evaluations contribute to the candidate selection process? To whom should the findings be given? Would psychological evaluations be best linked to security assessments so as to avoid the limitations imposed by the EEOC rules?

Key ethical principles and standards

APA (2002): Principle B (Fidelity and Responsibility), Principle C (Integrity), Standard 1.01 (Misuse of Psychologist's Work), Standard 1.03 (Conflicts Between Ethics and Organizational Demands), Standard 3.07 (Third Party Requests for Service), Standard 9.01 (Bases for Assessments), and Standard 9.03 (Informed Consent in Assessments).

REFERENCES AND FURTHER READING

Bronstein, D. A. (2007). *Law for the expert witness* (3rd ed). Boca Raton, FL: CRC Press.

Committee on Ethical Guidelines for Forensic Psychologists. (1991). Specialty guidelines for forensic psychologists. *Law and Human Behavior, 15,* 655–665.

Melton, G. B., Petrila, J., Poythress, N. G., & Slobogin, C. (2007). *Psychological evaluations for the courts: Mental health professionals and lawyers (3rd ed).* New York: The Guilford Press.

25

Risking Your Job: On Striving to be an Ethical Leader in Difficult Organizational Circumstances

Rodney L. Lowman

In a book intended for mental health professionals, this case may seem anomalous. Yet increasingly, mental health professionals—like it or not—will find themselves in managerial and leadership roles. This means they will have responsibility for others' behavior at work and if they rise through the ranks to any degree, they will have responsibility for overseeing larger and larger parts of an organization. How can mental health professionals who serve as managers retain their ethical integrity and their professional values while working in the "real world" of people with a variety of motives, not always benevolent? The case I present here is a combination of some of several managerial situations blended to make a single case. As an amalgam, this case touches on ethical quandaries from several of my personal organizational experiences.

I once served in an academic leadership role. Although my position was reasonably high up in the organization, I had both a boss and a boss's boss. After working in this role for a year or so, I hired a number two, a senior leader chosen as the "second in command" in my part of the organization. This hire was intended to fill a position that had been vacant due to an illness. The prior "second" had been well regarded, and I regretted that, for health reasons, he felt it necessary to take an early retirement.

As typically happens in academic settings, a search committee was formed and in this instance recommended three finalists to be brought to campus for interviews. One of the three dropped out of the search early for personal reasons. The second came for a campus visit and quickly decided he did not want to leave the comfort of his own institution for the uncertainties of this one and its somewhat isolated geographical area. The third candidate engendered mixed feelings among the search committee members, some of whom favored continuing the search while others found the candidate acceptable. The individual in question had a history of leadership in the corporate sector before returning to school to obtain the necessary terminal degree in her particular content area.

She pushed very hard for the job, and because I felt somewhat desperate to have someone in the position, I hired this candidate when the other two fell through. I worried a little at the time that the search committee, a broad and representative one, had not acted with more unanimity or even enthusiasm in its recommendation of this candidate and that she seemed to want the position a bit too much, but I decided other considerations outweighed these doubts.

For the first few months, things seemed to go well with this individual in her new role. She worked with considerable energy and apparent enthusiasm on her assignments, which involved tasks I could not closely supervise because of the demands of my own position and the diversity of areas in which she had to work. A few months into her tenure, however, a curious pattern of events began to emerge. A controversial decision had been made by a senior official at the institution (and assigned to me to implement) that would adversely affect students' fees. Because the institution found itself in trouble financially (I have generally been attracted to turnaround and start-up situations), it became necessary to generate more income. For fiscal reasons, we had to close that gap; I had to administer the directive by implementing a fee increase plan. Like many financially driven decisions in academia, this one proved necessary but unpopular, generating a lot of student and faculty angst. An implementation committee made up of students, faculty, and administrators chaired by the new number two began work.

Not long after this, I started to receive complaints from some of those in my supervisory line of reporting that criticisms about me, my leadership style, and my role in this particular implementation plan had begun to flow. Because this particular institution was located in a fairly small city in the South, word of these complaints had quickly reached into the community. One of the local trustees, the head of one of the locally large employers and a self-made businessman with a reputation for hot headedness, quickly raised concerns with certain officials at the university about complaints he had heard. In no case had anyone come to me directly about their concerns. I was apparently being castigated in ways that seemed very disproportionate to my role in the issue at hand. Over time, it became clear that the individual I had hired in the number two role had the apparent goal of ousting me so she could get my job, and she had begun subtly but systematically undermining me and my authority.

The style this individual employed was crafty and frankly sneaky. Despite meeting with me several times a week, she rarely brought up any issues related to the concerns that were being raised or her own role in fomenting them. Instead, I began to learn about these indirectly. I also discovered from confidential sources that she bitterly resented my efforts, which I regarded as mentoring, to guide her in a new position and that she wanted to be left totally alone to make her own decisions and, clearly in this case, to undermine me.

In time, I began to receive confidential calls from certain members of the university community identifying the senior manager as making disparaging remarks about me at every opportunity. Always, I was told, her remarks came framed in a manner more laden with innuendo than directness, but the intended meaning was quite clear. In time, subordinates started complaining that the conflict between the two of us made it difficult for them to get their work done.

Unfortunately, in this particular case, by the time I learned from a number of separate sources what was really going on, the problematic number two person had already done much damage. As information slowly started coming in about what was really going on (and as I struggled to address the concerns of some senior officials who suddenly began perceiving me as a problematic manager), I confronted the individual with what I had heard, my concerns about what she had said and done, and my concerns about the ethics of her behavior. She denied doing anything problematic and said that others had misunderstood her communications. Because she had complained about me in a way suggesting we did not get along well, I began to meet with her specifically on issues about which she had been quoted. I tried to make clear to her that it was essential that the two of us work out any differences we may have, and she continuously denied that any existed, that she reported liking the institution and working for me. It was only through the information obtained by "moles" (essentially spies who reported back to me on her behavior in sessions in which I was not present) that I obtained evidence of her continued efforts to undermine me. It became nearly impossible, however, to undo the reputational damage that she had caused.

Managing one's own emotions is a challenge in any situation like this. As a psychologist, I would like to think well of others and assume there always can be a common meeting ground even when there is conflict. I would also like to think that people deal with you directly and honestly. As a leader and as a human being, however, working with duplicitous, angry, deceptive people brings out other emotions. When a work environment like this has become overly polluted with fear, distrust, and divisiveness by behavior you consider unfathomable, paranoia can be a leader's natural reaction. Thoughts such as these were not infrequent: *I hired this person, how could she do this to me? How could anyone be so stupid as to take at face value the utterances of anyone as dumb, inexperienced, and disrespectful as this? How could people dislike me enough to take sides in issues as silly as these? How could I have made such a hiring mistake?* These are reactions a leader cannot afford to share with others or even to hold, at least not for very long. It is like receiving the sudden and unexpected diagnosis of a terrible disease: you have to get beyond "How could this happen to me?" to accept that it *is* happening and then formulate a plan to deal with those whose motives and actions are not benign. And if those to whom you report do not understand the dynamics of what is happening or support you in addressing them, there may be few options but to resign. That is what I ultimately chose to do in this situation. That said, I did not feel that I had to compromise my ethical values by stooping to the level of those who, in my opinion, were maliciously and vindictively fighting dirty. Then and now, I would rather not be in a job than behave in a way that is incongruent with my values, beliefs, and ideals.

Discussion

Key ethical issues

What is the appropriate and ethical thing to do in circumstances such as those described in this case? When dealing with another professional, one can almost always find a set of behavioral guidelines that say what one must (and must not) do. If any questions about their behavior come up, one can always find a rule book against which to evaluate their behavior. But as I have noted, managers do not hold any particular ethics code by virtue of their managerial profession. Nor is there any ethical tribunal to say that a manager or leader has screwed up or behaved unethically. At best, an organizational or institutional code of ethics or a set of values may exist, but these statements often prove to be lofty aspirations rather than enforceable standards. Particular industries may have laws and rules that constrain or mandate conduct, but these address mostly extreme behavior, not the petty conflicts that often constitute the realities of day-to-day organizational life. In my own case, I took inspiration from the APA Ethics Principles, especially Principle B: Fidelity and Responsibility, which states, "Psychologists establish relationships of trust with those with whom they work," and Principle C: Integrity, which states, "Psychologists do not steal, cheat, or engage in fraud, subterfuge, or intentional misrepresentation of fact. Psychologists strive to keep their promises and to avoid unwise or unclear commitments." Yet in both cases, these were broad general guidelines that really did not tell me precisely how to behave. I also kept in mind the APA ethical standard 3.04 Avoiding Harm, "Psychologists take reasonable steps to avoid harming their. . . supervisees. . . [and] organizational clients, and others with whom they work, and to minimize harm where it is foreseeable and unavoidable." In each case, however, these principles did not exactly apply to working with nonpsychologists, nor, it could be argued, was I functioning as a psychologist when acting as a university administrator. Such principles did keep me focused on what by nature I was inclined *not* to do (stoop to the low level of behavior of my subordinate) and reminded me there were higher principles at stake than my "winning" a fight.

In leadership roles, one must make many decisions, often affecting others' lives. When taking on responsibility for people in an organization, one must also take responsibility for setting the tone in terms of values, norms for acceptable or unacceptable behavior, and appropriate methods for addressing problematic behavior. Hopefully, your values remain consistent with those of the institution, or at least your part of it. Sometimes, however, that is not the case, and as a professional who finds him- or herself in leadership roles, you will have to decide what kind of ethical tone you wish to set and whether you can live with an institution that, in its actual behavior, practices values you find objectionable, sometimes abhorrent.

Work setting

Throughout my professional career, I've found myself in key administrative positions in which credentials as a psychologist were not an essential requirement for the job. I say "found myself" because I can't really say that I started out my career expecting to take on a leadership or management position, and my occupational interest patterns always looked more like those of a psychologist than those of the prototypical manager. Still, I have had more than my share of senior leadership positions, particularly in academia, and I have to say that every one of them has proved interesting but also presented its share of ethical challenges.

Among the professional roles I've served in over the years include serving as a department head, a dean, provost/vice president for academic affairs, acting university president, and a president in various academic institutions. I've also served as a senior leader in mental health settings and have run a private practice. For the most part, I've felt like I almost always stayed faithful to at least the spirit of my ethical standards as a psychologist even when not serving in a position that required (or even considered desirable) a professional background as a psychologist. But I have encountered a few situations while serving as an administrator in which I felt uniquely challenged and pressured to act in a manner not consistent with my principles, and I must occasionally deal with unethical behavior on the part of nonpsychologist subordinates or associates from the perspective of my own ethical standards.

I consider the essence of a manager's job to involve figuring out quickly and accurately what needs doing and then to help make that happen working through and with other people. Of course, strategy becomes involved in getting the goals right, but even when the goals appropriately target what the department or organization most needs, one must also enlist others to cooperate in getting the work successfully done. Depending on the level of the position, the job also usually involves the day-to-day oversight of others and making sure their work gets done properly, encouraging some and addressing the performance needs of others. And always, personnel matters will arise in addressing the needs or issues raised by employees—particularly the disgruntled or ineffective ones.

In thinking about ethics, one of the defining characteristics of a professional role involves adherence to a particular code of ethics. Although members of a profession usually receive careful training in the ethical expectations and required behaviors of their profession, a mechanism for enforcement where one can levy ethical complaints usually exists. For most professionals, behaving ethically is not simply an aspirational, "nice to do" thing. In contrast, as a manager or leader, one typically has no generally accepted professional codes of ethics and, other than through the courts when addressing extreme behavioral problems, no enforcement mechanisms when encountering ethically questionable behavior.

Reflection

I wish I could say that behind-the-scenes undermining and mischievous behavior by subordinates only rarely occurs. In fact, an organization is composed of individuals, each of whom has his/her own motives, network of allies and partisan groups, and a complex network of connections within the system that characterize any large organization. If mental health professionals have an obligation to follow consistent ethics and motives in their professional behavior, the same cannot always be said for organizational members.

I have to admit that by training and temperament I am not very well suited to deal with dishonest and undermining individuals. As a result, I am sure I miss cues that others, more sensitive to power dynamics, may quickly pick up and thwart. I generally expect people to behave honestly and directly and when, for whatever reasons (e.g., anger, greed, mischievousness), people pursue a negative, hostile, and undermining agenda, I often miss it until it is too late. I struggle with the ethical dilemma of whether to stoop to the level of my attackers, enlisting spies who report to me on problematic individuals' behavior, or whether I should rely on my natural instincts to assume integrity and honesty on the part of others until clear evidence to the contrary exists.

In my opinion, the best way to deal with this kind of conflict is not to get into it in the first place. By carefully choosing the organization or part of the organization in which you work, you will assess whether these are people and this is an organization to which you feel good about attaching your name.

Sometimes, however, such as in a bad economy or when the jobs dry up due to too many professionals chasing too few jobs, you take what you can get and feel lucky to have any job, particularly one that pays benefits. Alternatively, you may make a move because you want to progress upward or are looking for a new place to live for personal or professional reasons. Or the players may have changed and the people who hired you are replaced by those you don't respect. When, by circumstances or error, you find yourself in an organization in which behavior you consider unethical is tolerated, or when (as is often the case) the players change and the old rules become new ones that no longer work for you, it will be time to decide whether you stay or go and whether you confront what you consider objectionable or suffer in silence. Your job may be at risk if you object too strenuously or if you speak truth to power, but your integrity and sense of professional identity may be at risk if you don't. As a psychologist, I remain sensitive to my obligation under standard 1.03 of the APA Code: Conflicts Between Ethics and Organizational Demands. When, as an employee or as a consultant, an organization asks or requires me to behave in a way that would undermine the spirit—if not the letter—of my professional code of ethics, I am obligated to make this conflict known, try to resolve the conflict amicably, and in all cases, adhere to the APA Code of Ethics. In this case, I was compelled to cut ties with an organizational context likely to ultimately compromise my ethical integrity.

I would be remiss if I did not communicate just how strong the pressures can become to tolerate behavior in some institutional settings with which a professional may take exception. It is easy to behave ethically when working in an ethically supportive environment in which you feel you are valued for what you do well and for behaving ethically in complicated situations. It is much more difficult to maintain an ethical stance when you must fight for your values and ethics in an environment in which those values are not respected and in which the people with whom you work are behaving inappropriately. Few ethical codes for mental health professionals have yet considered that many of their members will serve as leaders and managers during some part of their career. Until there are clearly defined codes for practice as an ethical professional who is also a manager, you will to some degree be struggling in that ethical wilderness on your own.

Would I handle the situation differently in the future? I would certainly attempt to identify unprofessional colleague behavior early on, and I would be less concerned about trying to work through the issues if they were not amenable to early change efforts. I would try to act swiftly to protect my subordinates by terminating someone who was wreaking havoc in the organization no matter how long a contract she or he may have. And I would have better sources in the organization with whom to get an early warning of misbehavior by a direct report.

You may think that issues like these will not happen to you. Chances are, however, that sometime in your career you too will find yourself in a managerial or leadership role. There are many rewards in such roles, but don't ever forget that first and foremost you are a professional or ignore your code of ethics just because it does not explicitly address issues such as these.

Key ethical principles and standards

APA (2002): Principle A (Beneficence and Nonmaleficence), Principle B (Fidelity and Responsibility), Standard 1.03 (Conflicts Between Ethics and Organizational Demands), Standard 3.04 (Avoiding Harm).

REFERENCES AND FURTHER READING

Drucker, P. (1974, 2008). *Management* (Revised Edition). New York: HarperCollins.
Lowman, R. L. (2006). *The ethical practice of psychology in organizations* (2nd ed.).
   Washington, DC: American Psychological Association. *The Psychologist-Manager Journal.* Taylor & Francis.

26

When Bad Things Happen to People Who Try Really Hard: Ethical Quandaries in Test Validation

Nancy T. Tippins

Several years ago, I was asked to develop and validate a test battery for use in selecting people into a family of jobs that included a number of unique, hourly job titles. All the employees in this job family had strong labor union representation. The union did not participate in setting selection standards but had major concerns about the procedures for movement within and across job families, i.e., upgrades and transfers. The management team for these jobs had several objectives for the new test battery. First, they wanted to identify job candidates who would likely perform the job well and prove less likely to engage in counterproductive behaviors such as accidents and insubordinate behavior, as well as those who would leave the job prematurely. Second, the management team wanted a test that the test administrators in the staffing organization could administer without assistance from line managers. In other words, the use of department assessors or interviewers was not feasible. Third, the team also hoped that one battery might work well for all job titles so movement of employees within the department could occur without additional testing. Fourth, management wanted the selection procedure developed and validated in accordance with legal and professional guidelines so it would withstand legal or administrative challenges. Finally, the organization would own the selection procedures that were developed.

I wrote a proposal for the development and validation of the battery and made a presentation to the management team. Both the proposal and the presentation emphasized that I would conduct research with no guarantees of meeting the stated goals, although the research team would follow best practices that would enhance the probability of a successful outcome. I also participated in several union/management meetings in which I explained the test development and validation process and the protections the company provided those employees who participated in the project. After much deliberation, the union agreed it would do nothing to inhibit the test development and validation process, a result management considered very positive.

After establishing the client's goals for the project and its constraints, the next step involved forming a project team to guide the development and validation from the job analysis through the implementation. The project team consisted of representatives from my research team and the management team. Management did not include union representatives on the project team because the union customarily did not play a role in setting selection standards.

I began the project with a job analysis, following the *Standards for Educational and Psychological Testing* and the *Principles for the Use and Validation of Personnel Selection Procedures* as well as the *Uniform Guidelines for Employee Selection Procedures*. Because of obvious differences in the tasks performed by job incumbents in each job title, it became particularly important for the research team to determine if common knowledge, skills, abilities, and other characteristics (KSAOs) necessary for the performance of all jobs existed and could be measured via a single test battery. After the first stage of the job analysis, which included job analysis interviews, the research team developed a detailed list of tasks and KSAOs. At this point in the job analysis, the differences among jobs became clear, and one test battery that could serve as a good predictor for all jobs within the family increasingly seemed less probable. When informed of the differences across jobs, the management team expressed its concern and urged me to find the commonality across the jobs in the next stage of the job analysis.

The research team developed a job analysis questionnaire that included comprehensive lists of tasks and KSAOs that covered all of the jobs in the study. The project team discussed the pros and cons of using administrators from various organizations (e.g., the department, the research team, human resources department). Although using administrators from the department would have been the most cost effective, the project team had concerns about the resulting quality of data if inexperienced administrators were used. In the end, the research team collected the job analysis data.

Although a few people in the sample refused to participate, the job analysis data collection process proceeded without major incident; however, the results of the job analysis clearly indicated three groups of jobs existed within the job family. Some commonalities existed in KSAO requirements across the jobs, but significant differences also existed, particularly in the level of physical and mental abilities required. I met once again with the project team to explain the findings. Despite their disappointment with these findings, management recognized the need for three groups of jobs, each with separate selection standards, in light of both the level of prediction that would result from using one test battery for the three job families and the legal implications of using selection procedures that might prove irrelevant or inappropriate.

The labor union clearly knew of the job analysis data collection and clamored for the results, which we duly provided in a labor/management meeting. The labor union also expressed unhappiness with the results. In the past, the union had successfully moved injured workers from jobs with heavy lifting requirements to less strenuous jobs. If the three job groups had different selection criteria, this avenue of recourse would close unless the injured employee could meet the selection standards for the other job group. To ensure consistent administration of the selection program, the company had a policy of no exceptions to test standards, which it had strictly enforced for many years. Thus, the union knew it would not likely win a grievance or arbitration challenging this long-term practice.

Based on the results of the job analysis, the research team developed three experimental test batteries with some overlapping tests and scales and planned the validation study. Because of significant legal challenges to the selection programs in other parts of the company, the project team agreed that a criterion-oriented validation study based on concurrent data was the only acceptable approach. The research team developed a stratified random sample for each of the three job groups and presented the sampling plan to the project team. Although the research team explained that we would now conduct three separate validation studies, each requiring its own sample, the department management had concerns about the number of employees required in the validation effort. In addition, the management team became alarmed when they realized we had sampled a few employees known to create problems. The research team explained at length the importance of randomization in order to generalize the results. In the end, the representative from the legal department on the project team decided the issue, and the sampling plan stood as originally defined with a few exceptions of employees who actually did not perform the job because of their official union duties.

Once we established the sampling plan, the next major problem the project team faced focused on the extent of confidentiality afforded each employee who participated in the validation study. The research team argued for complete confidentiality; the department wanted test scores for all kinds of reasons, ranging from remedial training to performance management. In the end, the research team won this argument because everyone agreed we would not likely get enough cooperation without a promise of full confidentiality.

No one questioned the plan to collect the validation data, both predictor and criterion data, in face-to-face sessions using experienced test administrators. The research team assembled a team of test administrators and criterion data collectors, trained them, and started the data collection process, which began in an area of the country where the union was not particularly strong. A few employees chose not to participate, but overall the collection of experimental test data occurred without a problem. However, as we moved to other parts of the country and as word about the study got out, more and more employees chose not to participate. At first, people just didn't show up; later, they came but either appeared to put minimal effort into taking the tests or simply did not complete the tests. The department management was unhappy and wanted to require people to take the test. The research team insisted that participation must be voluntary if useful data were gathered and professional testing guidelines met; force would not work and would result in data that were not useful.

In one of the last data collection sessions, things blew up. We had scheduled approximately 100 employees to take the experimental batteries on a Saturday morning in the cafeteria of a work site. We scheduled their supervisors to provide criterion data in a session to begin an hour after the testing session. Once the session began, they peppered the lead administrator with questions obviously designed to amuse others and divert attention from the importance of the task. Once the first test began, things did not improve. Some employees talked loudly with each other, commenting on the questions, asking each other the answers, complaining about spending their Saturday mornings this way, etc.

After the first test was complete, the lead test administrator explained the importance of attending to the task at hand and allowing others to do their best. The employees were asked if anyone would like to leave; no one did. During the second test, a group of employees continued to talk throughout the test administration even when other employees asked them to be quiet. Test administrators stood by the employees and asked them to not speak out loud, yet this group continued its disruptive behavior. After the second test, the test administrators called an unplanned break. The test administrators conferred with the department's managers present and split those displaying disruptive behavior into separate rooms. A test administrator and a manager remained present in each room for the remaining tests, and no more disruptive behavior occurred.

After the administration of the experimental battery, we reviewed the answer sheets before entering the data. A large number of answer sheets had fewer than 10% of all items answered, even though we had set time limits so that 90% of test takers would finish 90% of the items. Many of the test takers had names such as "George Washington" or "Mickey Mouse." Approximately half the answer sheets were unusable.

The managers of the department were outraged over the behavior of their employees. They obviously knew who had acted disruptively, but they did not know who refused to participate fully or used false names. Because they had agreed to pay these employees and the assigned task involved taking the experimental test battery, they wanted the names of those who did not do their job. Because the research team had promised confidentiality, we refused to state who had provided few if any answers. In addition, although we suspected most of these people had behaved inappropriately, we could not know with certainty whether or not an employee had tried his or her best and simply could not answer many of the test items.

Once we eliminated the unusable answer sheets, the sample for each job group proved too small to yield sufficient statistical power, and we advised against analyzing the data until collecting more. The project team, however, saw no feasible way to collect additional data and insisted that we analyze the data "just to see what happened." Somewhat surprisingly, the results were positive, although several key analyses did not reach statistical significance. We spent several long meetings discussing what the lack of statistical significance meant for the achievement of the original goals: prediction of performance, counterproductive behavior, turnover, and legal defensibility in the event someone challenged any of the three selection procedures under federal EEO laws. We also tried to explain the limitations on the generalizability of any results due to the large number of people in the sample who provided unusable data. The attorney on the project team cautioned against implementation but stated he would not prevent it.

In the end, the project team emphasized how much money the project had cost to date, professed its trust in the research team, and decided to implement the three batteries anyway. We protested, but the management team explained that the organization owned the data and made the decisions about implementation of selection procedures—not consultants. We created a database for recording test scores and wrote a specific suggestion in the technical report that more research was needed.

Discussion

Key ethical issues

This study presented a number of ethical questions for the psychologists on the research team. Perhaps the two most important issues in the study involved 1) confidentiality and 2) interpretation of the validity evidence. Underlying both, however, one can see the inherent dual relationship industrial and organizational psychologists constantly face: serving the needs of the client, i.e., the organization, and protecting the individuals who participate in organizational research.

All of the psychologists involved were clear on the confidentiality commitment made to the employees participating in this study, and none advocated violating that promise. However, that promise did not alleviate the difficulties in dealing with a management team that believed strongly in its right to assign work to employees and its belief that the employees should perform their assigned duties to the best of their ability. We clearly understood management's irritation over the wasted time and money and later their disappointment over the study results, but we could not reasonably violate the confidentiality promised.

The research team, composed of well-trained, experienced psychologists, understood and attempted to explain the limits of the study results and their generalizability in operational use. Nevertheless, we had to question whether or not we tried hard enough to convince the management team of the folly involved in implementing a selection procedure with marginal evidence of validity. We also had to ask what we could have done to stop the implementation. We believe we did our best to explain the technical intricacies of a validation study to the management team, but the question always remains, "Could we have done more?"

Work setting

Industrial and organizational psychologists work in many different environments and often go to the client's site to minimize the costs. Although we specify the conditions we need, many prove not feasible to implement, and we must often make compromises just to get the work done. In retrospect, the environment in which we collected these data had a lot to do with the problems that ensued. If we had insisted on testing in smaller groups, would the test administrators have had more control? If we had collected the criterion data from supervisors at some other time and not had them onsite during data collection from the workers, would things have gone better? Worse?

Reflection

Many of the problems we faced on this project stemmed from our ability to manage the relationships with the management team and the labor union more than our ability to make sound research decisions. I toed a narrow line between full disclosure of the chances of insufficient results and talking the management team out of a selection program, and I deferred to the management team with respect to the involvement of the labor union in the project team. The role of an industrial and organizational psychologist usually becomes one of an advisor, and that role limits the extent to which we control the behavior of anyone other than ourselves. Managers and employees often act in ways they perceive to further their own best interest. Our best hope of influencing outcomes often rests on persuasive communication skills few of us learned in graduate school.

Key ethical principles and standards

APA (2002): Standard 1.01 (Misuse of Psychologists' Work), Standard 1.03 (Conflicts Between Ethics and Organizational Demands), Standard 3.04 (Avoiding Harm), Standard 3.06 (Conflict of Interest), Standard 3.11 (Psychological Services Delivered to or Through Organizations), Standard 4.01 (Maintaining Confidentiality).

REFERENCES AND FURTHER READING

American Education Research Association, American Psychological Association, & National Council on Measurement in Education. (1985). *Standards for educational and psychological testing.* Washington, DC: American Psychological Association.
Equal Employment Opportunity Commission, Civil Service Commission, Department of Labor, & Department of Justice. (1978). *Uniform guidelines on employee selection procedures.* Federal Register, 43 (No. 166), 38290–38315.
Society for Industrial and Organizational Psychology. (1999). *Principles for the validation and use of personnel selection procedures* (4th ed.). College Park, Maryland: Author.

PART VI

In Schools and Colleges

27

When in Doubt, Pull Them Out? Ethical Issues Related to Decisions on Child Removal From the Home

Lyvia Chriki

When a disabled child who cannot talk shows up at a day-care center dirty and hungry every morning, despite continual meetings with her parents, do you report the parents to child welfare services, risking the removal of the child from her home, or do you hold back? How do you decide what is in the best interest of the child when the danger to her well-being does not appear imminent, and she cannot express herself? And how much should cultural or socioeconomic factor into this decision?

When I was in the Israeli National Service, I faced this dilemma while caring for a girl in a day-care center for severely disabled children. Nadia was an eight-year-old child born to a Muslim family in Israel. Her family came from a small Arab village known for its community's pro-Israel views. Since most Muslim families in the country did not share their ideology, finding families who would marry into theirs proved difficult. As a result, Nadia's family, consisting of multiple aunts, uncles, first cousins, and cousins once, twice, and three times removed, resorted to marrying within the extended family.

Like many of the children cared for at the center, Nadia came into the world with extreme cognitive and physical developmental difficulties. Most of the children in the center ranged in age between eight and thirteen, although many appeared physically more like four-year-olds, acting and functioning like six-month-olds. These children could not, walk, talk, feed themselves, or go to the bathroom on their own, and mealtime seemed to be the highlight of their day.

It was hard for us, the staff members, to know how these children felt on a daily basis, unless they started crying. As with a newborn baby, even a smile did not necessarily indicate any positive emotions, but sometimes indicated some sort of discomfort or even predicted a seizure. We had no way of knowing how these children experienced their lives, whether they understood anything we said to them, or whether they could read any of our facial expressions or body language.

Nadia seemed fairly happy most of the time—she would laugh a lot in response to tickling or to certain types of food—and she could usually voice when she felt unhappy or distressed by crying. Sometimes, though, it was hard to know what was making her unhappy. All we could do was try various things that might calm her down, such as giving her a bottle, checking her diaper, or making sure she was warm.

In the mornings, we could always tell when Nadia had arrived because we would hear her wailing through the elevator shaft as she came up to our floor. The doors would open, and she would be sitting in her stroller pushed by a staff member, looking very unhappy. She also looked dirty. Her nose ran, her mucus dripping everywhere, and her clothes stunk as though they had not been washed in days. She also seemed especially hungry in the mornings. As a way of trying to help Nadia, Shirah, the other National Service volunteer who worked with Nadia, and I made an effort to bathe Nadia and dress her with a clean outfit every afternoon before she went home, and we let her have an extra serving of food during lunch and snack times. We also made certain the pediatrician checked on her whenever possible. Still, every morning she would show up looking as if we had done nothing the day before.

I would see staff members shake their heads at the sight of Nadia and hear them talk to each other, expressing anger toward Nadia's parents. The other National Service volunteers and I would talk amongst ourselves, wondering if we could do anything to change this situation. We all felt frustrated for Nadia and worried about her, and we felt unsure of what to do. Would reporting the situation to child services as a case of possible child neglect do more harm than good? Perhaps her parents did love her but were too overwhelmed to take proper care of her. Perhaps she liked to go home and calmed down once there, but we did not know this because she could not tell us.

Shirah and I decided that instead of remaining stuck in ambivalence, we would turn to Dina, the social worker at the center. She knew the children, and we thought that perhaps she would be helpful. When we spoke with Dina, she explained that this issue with Nadia had gone on for some time and that it had been brought up before by other staff members. When we protested that more should be done, she explained, "Things are not that simple. If we report this to the authorities, there will be an investigation that could disrupt Nadia's life and make it harder than it is already." She explained that taking a child out of the home did not always turn out better for the child than staying at home, even if the home environment proved far from perfect. She told us we could not possibly know whether Nadia felt truly unhappy at home and whether the care for Nadia at the center could make up for what she lacked at home. "Living with her biological parents may be the best for Nadia, even if she is being somewhat neglected," she said.

Shirah and I did not feel satisfied, and we probably felt a bit horrified at this notion. We wanted to feel that we could do more, and we wanted to feel more certain that deciding not to report the case was the right thing to do. Hearing an experienced social worker tell us there may not be a "right thing to do" did not feel very satisfying. So Dina suggested we invite the parents in for a talk. She told us we could participate at the meeting, and that she would attend, along with one of Nadia's teachers. She would insist that both parents attend, so they would understand this as a serious matter. She explained that sometimes just having the parents come in for a meeting every couple of months acted as a wake-up call for them and reminded them that if they did not care for their child, the consequences could be dire. "Even if in two weeks things go back to the way they were, at least Nadia will be more comfortable for a few weeks," Dina stated.

A few days later, Nadia's parents arrived, and Shirah and I were called into the meeting. Nadia's mother did not speak Hebrew very well, but her father spoke some. Her father talked about having to travel to Egypt for business and to see family quite often, and about having other children to take care of in the house. He said that perhaps this contributed to the difficulty in caring for Nadia and giving her the attention she needed. In the end, the father agreed the family would pay closer attention to Nadia. However, true to Dina's prediction, Nadia showed up better groomed over the next week or two, and then things went back to the way there were before the meeting. Shirah and I decided to take Dina's advice and give her judgment the benefit of the doubt. We worried that risking the removal of Nadia from her home might actually prove more detrimental to her than remaining at home with her parents. We continued to take extra care of Nadia during the hours she spent at the center, and we did not report her parents to social services.

Discussion

Key ethical issues

The primary ethical issue I focused on at the time was doing no harm to Nadia *(nonmaleficence)*. It was unclear to me whether taking Nadia out of her parents' care and letting the welfare system take over was in Nadia's best interests. I felt torn between the drive to act quickly and rid myself of anxiety and the rational understanding that I had no clear answer. I held back from acting rashly because I understood that whatever I decided to do, Nadia would experience the consequences, and therefore I had to deal with the issue thoughtfully. I also felt that since I had no experience dealing with such issues, this decision fell a bit out of my league.

Legally, my obligation, and that of any person of age eighteen and over, focused on Nadia's needs. Israeli law requires that any person who has reason to suspect that harm is being done to a child must report the case to the social services or the police. Because it was not clear to me that Nadia was in danger, and because I did not feel qualified to assess the situation adequately, I felt that the best I could do to fulfill my legal obligation to Nadia as an adult who cared for her involved making my concerns known to her teachers and the social worker. I worried that acting on my own without background knowledge and experience would cause more harm than good, and therefore following the professional's opinion seemed the best that I could do at that point in my life.

Another ethical concern I wrestled with in this case involves the issue of *boundaries of competence*. Nadia's family came from a different culture. The mother in a Muslim household usually holds the responsibility of caring for the children most of the day. Although we all did our best to communicate with Nadia's parents, Nadia's mother did not know enough Hebrew to communicate directly with us. She may not have understood the gravity of the situation, depending on the way her husband portrayed it to her, or she may have felt uncomfortable expressing the struggles that kept her from caring properly for Nadia in front of her husband. Additionally, having a mentally disabled child may have signified something different to this family than it did to us, and perhaps this influenced their attitude toward the problem. Having an Arab translator or social worker in the meeting who came from a similar background as Nadia's parents may have been helpful.

Finally, the ethical principle of *justice* is related to this case on two levels. First, because of the difference in cultures, we needed to remain aware of our own biases as Israeli Jews toward the Muslim and Arab cultures, and we had to make certain that our biases did not interfere with our judgment. Knowing the people I worked with and remembering what went through my mind at the time, I believe we understood the potential prejudices that could have influenced our actions, and I think we did not consciously let them get in the way of our decision-making process. Although the staff felt angry at Nadia's parents because of their concern for her, the social worker and the teachers always told us that we must put ourselves in the parents' shoes and show empathy and compassion toward them, as well as toward Nadia.

Second, when dealing with children and families, defining who the patient is and whose rights must have highest priority can prove difficult. Was Nadia the only patient in this case, or did we owe her parents consideration as our patients too? Balancing Nadia's rights as a child and a human being, and her father and mother's rights as parents, proved a hard task. Overall, since Nadia inherently had essentially no power to advocate for herself, our highest priority involved advocating for her; however, at the same time, the situation also called for us to remain respectful of the parents' judgment and privacy.

Work setting

In Israel, every person is expected to serve his or her country in one way or another after turning eighteen. Men are required to join the army, and women often have the choice of serving in the National Service, which consists of community rather than military service. The expectations of these young people are very high, and the responsibilities put on their shoulders are profound. Soldiers must make life or death decisions on a daily basis, and National Service volunteers often find themselves in settings that require such critical judgment calls as well. Despite the maturity they must show during their service, these young people, still transitioning into adulthood, in many ways still qualify as adolescents.

As in the United States, the welfare system in Israel is inundated with endless cases of individuals, families, and communities who need daily help and interventions, and the system is confronted with a shortage in funds, preventing the system from reaching every person in need. As such, the funds in place for training volunteers and staff members who work in places like Nadia's day-care center are miniscule. The state simply cannot pay to provide adequate training for every volunteer and service provider.

What was expected of me, as a National Service provider, involved helping keep the children I took care of as comfortable as possible, keeping them safe for the eight hours I spent at the center every day, and providing them with some emotional support and nurturing. I had to turn over any problem that required more involvement the social worker or the child's teacher.

Therefore, I had a very limited role. Although the social workers and teachers supervised me, I lacked the training to make well-informed decisions about these issues, and I had to rely mostly on my conscience and sense of what felt right.

Reflection

It is now exactly ten years since I worked with Nadia. I am now twenty-eight years old and a first-year graduate student in clinical psychology in the United States. After earning a BA in psychology, working in the field for a few years, and entering graduate school, I can look back on this case and see its complexities through a different lens. Although I think I would still have been guided by similar instincts and might have still resisted calling child services right away, I might have acted differently.

When I worked at the center ten years ago, I saw the situation as black and white—either we would report the parents to child services, and Nadia would be removed from her home, or we would not report her parents and Nadia would stay at home. I believe that if faced with the same situation today, I might consider a wider range of solutions to this situation.

I would voice the need for a social worker or a psychologist who could speak Arabic and could identify more with Nadia's family's culture and background, so that we could gain more of a genuine understanding of the situation at home and of the family's struggles. Nadia's family experienced different kinds of stressors that we, as Israeli Jews, did not experience on a daily basis. As a Muslim family living estranged from the larger Arab Israeli community on the one hand, and constituting a minority among the Jewish Israeli population on the other, Nadia's parents may have felt vulnerable and afraid that we might judge harshly or report them immediately to social services if they admitted to any family problems or weaknesses. They also most likely lived in poverty with many mouths to feed and children to care for. Although we recognized the differences between the cultures, lifestyles, and stressors, we did not do enough to bridge this gap. Bringing in a translator who spoke fluent Arabic might have proved invaluable in assessing the home environment and in helping the family overcome their own obstacles that stood in their way of providing Nadia's needs.

In helping the family deal with daily stressors and responsibilities, one option might involve asking the family if another relative or a friend in their village could help take care of Nadia. Another possibility would involve asking that the National Service Organization send a volunteer to help the parents with Nadia at home. Finally, counseling aimed at helping the family acquire problem-solving skills, coping skills, and psychoeducation about their daughter's condition may have also alleviated their strain.

Looking back on this case, I am not certain why Nadia's social worker or teacher did not take these additional steps. It seemed clear to me that they cared greatly for Nadia. It may be that they did not see the need for this, or there may have been more to the story than I knew. I remember a brief comment that Nadia had two younger brothers who had been at the center before I came to volunteer there. The social worker might have had more familiarity with the family's situation and with the parents than she let Shirah and I know. I was a volunteer who had only arrived a few of months earlier, and there may have been confidential issues at stake that were not revealed to me.

In addition to having a deeper appreciation for the complexity of the situation, as a graduate student in psychology, I now also have the ability to access and understand the literature that exists on the removal of children from their homes. At the time, I might have felt comforted (or not) to know that in cases where children do not seem in imminent danger, even experts in the field have not reached a consensus on what to do. Studies that have sought to understand social service assessment processes pertinent to child removal from the home show that the patterns in the decision-making processes, and even the decisions themselves, are not consistent among groups of professionals in the field. There do not seem to be specific characteristics that distinguish children who stay in their homes from those who are removed. The factors that influence the decisions often seem related to the parents' or the health professionals' characteristics—not the assessment of the child's development or behaviors. Furthermore, there does not seem to be any standard for "good practice" or any definition of the threshold that constitutes "significant harm," at least enough to remove that child from the family. In my case, the decision became more difficult because of Nadia's inability to express herself, and therefore, we could only rely on our observations and conversations with the parents.

The literature indicates that in cases such as Nadia's, where a "grey area" exists and the harm to the child does not seem imminent, all we can do is our best at assessing whether the child's quality of life will improve or suffer if the child is taken away from the parents. I believe that remaining aware of the complexities involved becomes the most important quality a health professional can have when faced with this kind dilemma and the first step toward an effective decision. As health professionals, we must remain sensitive to different cultures and norms and of the various ways to approach situations—these situations are not black and white. Above all, we must remain aware of our biases, our perceptions, and our reasoning that leads us to such decisions.

As behavioral scientists, we remain far from certain about the "right" answers to these kinds of dilemmas. Only after understanding the motivations within ourselves that move us toward certain judgment calls can we begin to achieve a higher level of clarity and objectivity, allowing us to appreciate the complexities involved and make decisions more likely to serve our patients' best interests.

Key ethical principles and standards

APA (2002): Principle A (Beneficence and Nonmaleficence), Principle D (Justice), Principle E (Respect for People's Rights and Dignity), Standard 1.02 (Conflicts Between Ethics and Law, Regulations, or Other Governing Legal Authority), Standard 2.01 (Boundaries of Competence), Standard 3.04 (Avoiding Harm), and Standard 10.02 (Therapy Involving Couples or Families).

REFERENCES AND FURTHER READING

Ayre, P. (1998). Significant harm: making professionals judgments. *Child Abuse Review, 7*, 330–342.

Davidson-Arad, B., Englechin-Segal, D., & Arieli, R. (2005). Social workers' decisions on removal: predictions from their initial perceptions of the child's features, parents' features, and child's quality of life. *Journal of Social Service Research, 31*, 1–23.

Davidson-Arad, B., & Wozner, Y. (2001). The least detrimental alternative; deciding whether to remove children at risk from their homes. *International Social Work, 44*, 229–239.

Munro, E. R., & Ward, H. (2008). Balancing parents' and very young children's rights in care proceedings: decision-making in the context of the human rights act 1998. *Child and Family Social Work, 13*, 227–234.

Rossi, T. H., Schuerman, J., & Budde, S. (1999). Understanding decisions about child maltreatments. *Evaluation Review, 23*, 579–598.

28

A Near Fall: The Multifaceted Challenges to Work in Sport Psychology and Intercollegiate Athletics

Edward F. Etzel

XU is an inviting NCAA Division II school of 4,500 students, nestled in the rolling hills of western Pennsylvania. Wrestling is big in this hands-on, blue-collar locale. Nearly everyone's dad, uncle, and cousin has wrestled and/or played football at some level in their lives in this neck of the woods—aka "Steeler Country." The gym is full to capacity whenever a match is going on during wrestling season.

Ben was a senior member of the XU wrestling team. He'd grown up in a dying steel mill town, the son of hard-working folks. He was All-Everything going back to elementary school. He had won a state championship and even a high school national championship in his junior year. Although Ben was recruited by the big schools like Iowa, Penn State, and Oklahoma, he decided to "stick around" and attend smaller XU just outside of Pittsburgh.

Over the course of his first four years at XU—he'd red-shirted and did not complete his first season—Ben had done very well in his sport. If not great, Ben was okay in the classroom, achieving Cs and some Bs in school as a physical education major. That was okay with him, his coach, and the compliance office. I'd actually had Ben in my intro to sport and exercise psychology class when he was a second semester freshman. He seemed like a nice kid, rather quiet, sleepy sometimes, but essentially conscientious. I occasionally attend wrestling matches with my wife and 10-year-old son and enjoy the matches.

By the way, I wear more than a one professional hat at XU. I work half-time as a psychologist at the campus counseling center and also teach part-time in the psychology department. For better or worse, I interact with lots of the athletes and coaches on our small campus and in our little town. Like Ben, many athletes take my introduction to sport and exercise psychology class; it appears to have some relevance to their challenging lives. With some frequency, we run into each other in the local Giant Eagle grocery store and other establishments. It is a small world after all!

I occasionally receive a few referrals for personal counseling from the intercollegiate athletics department. Some athletes come in on their own; some are referred by our team physician, one of the athletic trainers, and by a small number of coaches. In general, the rather old-school coaching staff seems unreceptive to psychology and psychologists—except when some sort of crisis or athlete "head-case meltdown" occurs. On occasion, an athlete will visit me to consult on basic sport performance–related concerns such as goal-setting, using imagery, self-talk, etc. Ben had actually popped by my office in the psych building a few times during his sophomore year to chat about these matters, seeking some general information that might somehow help him on the mat. I recall he wanted to talk about mental toughness.

One Thursday afternoon in January, I received a call from the team physician. He was making a confidential referral to me. The call was unfortunately about Ben, my former student and star XU wrestler, now in his senior year and the shining star of the wrestling program. Dr. Andrews, who oversees the drug testing program, indicated that Ben had flunked a random drug screen and tested positive for THC. Under the recently initiated athletic department drug testing policy, the young man was immediately suspended from participation. He was required to do counseling to return to play. The team physician emphasized the "hush-hush" nature of this potentially public case. He indicated that at some time it would likely come to light in the local paper that Ben had "violated team policies" (standard athletic speak) and that his violation would be "dealt with internally." I agreed to see Ben early the next day. Dr. Andrews thought this would help avoid having Ben there when lots of other clients occupy our waiting room. I had a modest amount of training and experience in substance abuse intervention and had worked with several clients from the general student population over the years on these issues.

Ben presented at my office, albeit reluctantly and 20 minutes late, the morning after the call from Dr. Andrews. It was a Friday, a day before a match versus a regional rival college. Ben appeared quite concerned and edgy. In fact, before he had completed the standard set of intake documents used at our service, and before I had actually begun my intake interview, he told me that he'd never gotten into trouble before; he said he drank a little too much in the off-season, but that was about it. Ben insisted that he had gone to an off-campus party and that people in the small apartment were smoking weed. "That's it, Doc!" He told me he was "kinda paranoid" about anyone knowing what happened. I assured him that our work, like that with any client, would remain confidential as spelled out in our informed consent agreement. I spent about an hour and a half with Ben and completed my initial interview with him. He was somewhat anxious, cooperative, and appeared remorseful. We agreed that he would return in a few days to follow up with me. He was to be retested under the supervision of Dr. Andrews in the near future.

I was just about to enter my clinical notes into the computer after finishing my meeting with Ben when the front desk said I had a call on the line from his wrestling coach. Oh boy... Coach Jackowicz wanted to know how it went with Ben. He said he really wanted to do what was best for his star athlete. He said was willing to do anything he could to help me help Ben return to participation "ASAP." Coach J, as he was known, said that he figured Ben would probably not be back for the next evening's match. He thought it best to head off any rumors so he had called Ben's parents earlier and told them what happened and that he'd be seeing me sometime today.

Coach J also said that since people would notice that Ben was not in the lineup on Friday evening, he had revealed in advance to the athletic department's sports information director that Ben was out for "personal reasons" and that he was seeking help at the counseling service from me. I learned subsequently that these athletic department standard practices were apparently part of an annual, preparticipation waiver signed by all athletes so confidential health and educational records could be released to athletic staff who have "need to know." Parental notification of positive screens also came as part of the new drug testing policy.

Needless to say, I felt nearly speechless listening to his revelations. I respectfully indicated to Coach J that while I appreciated any concern he may have for any of his athletes who might seek consultation at our service, I could not confirm or deny any work with Ben, as was the case with any client of the counseling service. As one might expect, he did not seem at all happy, shall I say, with this and hung up the phone abruptly. I took a deep breath or two...

No sooner had he ended our conversation when the receptionist indicated that Ben's father was on the phone to speak with me. A call from a local newspaper reporter was also waiting. I took the call from Ben's father and related the same details of our policy to him. He seemed a bit more understanding, but he still did not quite understand the usefulness of our policy for concerned, "bill-paying" parents. I chose to not respond to the call from the media. I knew I had a challenging day ahead.

Discussion

Key ethical issues

Clearly, every psychologist is faced with ethical challenges—often with great frequency. In this particular situation, many ethical issues appear prominent. These issues are commonly encountered in university and similar sport settings. The reader will undoubtedly identify the avoidance of doing harm to Ben that links to other ethical issues and risks. Ethics codes typically charge us with the considerable responsibility of consistently practicing in ways that allow us to avoid, or at the very least minimize, harm to those we serve.

Another threat to doing good work with Ben involved the potential impact of multiple relationships (i.e., faculty member, consultant, therapist, and possibly being seen as a "fan"). While these overlapping associations do not necessarily or always equate to unethical status, they can sometimes prove tough to avoid and surprising to the psychologist who wears more than one hat in his or her work (i.e., professor and therapist). The variety of calls I received from various people provide ample evidence of the problem.

The reader will also recognize the related ethical risks associated with: 1) maintaining the professional agreements made with Ben through informed consent/informed consent to do therapy; 2) the contract to maintain confidentiality at intake; and 3) well-meaning, but not useful, third party requests for information (e.g., from the coach, parent, and media representative). As discussed below, these are very common practice risks associated with psychological consultation with clients from sport and intercollegiate athletics organizations.

Perhaps not as apparent are important standards that involve potential conflicts with service delivery and differences between one's ethics and organizational demands. I struggled with the delivery of psychological services through an organization—in this instance, to a client associated with a rather small organization (i.e., the department of intercollegiate athletics). Taken together, these issues make a rather standard counseling service referral an ethically uncomfortable one at least.

Work setting

There appears to be a growing number of psychologists and allied mental health professionals (e.g., counselors, psychiatrists, social workers) who have begun to work in sport-related domains. This trend is fueled by the life-skills movement promoted over the past fifteen years by the National Collegiate Athletics Association (NCAA). Today, there are also other, often unlicensed, applied sport psychology consultants and other external consultants (i.e., "mental coaches") who bring to the field a curious mix of credentials and ethics, delivering sport psychology services to athletes, sport teams, and other active people (e.g., exercisers). The wide assortment of professionals involved in sports consultation seems to have created a climate of practice that fosters some ethical confusion and inconsistency of values in this growing field. Many people in sport and athletics (e.g., coaches) do not understand ethical obligations in the way that mental health professionals might.

Professionals working in these settings need to bear in mind that athletes live in a fish bowl. Especially in high profile sports and programs, they are under constant public and department/organizational scrutiny. Incidents in this arena can easily be front page news. Young athletes are often very sensitive to this uncomfortable exposure.

Those professionals who work in the rather unusual world of sport and exercise psychology regularly encounter situations that test their ethical mettle. This necessitates a heightened sensitivity to potential ethical and legal conflicts. The behind-the-scene efforts of sport psychology consultants with clients at professional and Olympic levels of sport and intercollegiate athletics are fraught with unique ethical challenges, given the influence of organizational and departmental practices and pressures, complex NCAA rules, and cultural values bearing on sports, sometimes referred to as "the culture of risk."

In the milieu of sport and intercollegiate athletics, regular contact with athletes, coaches, and other organizational members (i.e., various levels of athletic directors, sports medicine staff) is common. This contact may create the risk of multiple relationships. Although it may be helpful to develop trusting relationships with coaches and administrators, becoming too involved and overidentifying with sports teams (i.e., "bleeding the school colors") can jeopardize one's objectivity and perhaps create unreasonable and unethical practice expectations. In these instances, sport psychologists can be tempted to compromise their professional values to fit better with those of the organization. One can also compromise one's values for some self-serving purpose (e.g., personal gain). This may take the forms of free athletic gear, tickets, travel to playoffs and bowl games, golf outings, etc.—perks that are rather commonplace in business and industry.

Those mental health professionals employed as staff members in intercollegiate athletics and high-level professional sport may have their ethical values challenged by the conservative and controlling values of the culture. For example, confidentiality is often not the coin of the realm when it comes to work with athletes. Many empowered coaches, administrators, sports medicine staff, and managers seem to assume they have a need to know most, if not everything, about "their" athletes or patients. Perhaps to be helpful to their athletes, they may sometimes put pressure on clients or teammates of clients who may confide in them to learn about client issues. Third-party inquiries about athlete clients that compromise privacy and confidentiality are routine. The values of coaches and others in sport organizations may conflict with psychologist's ethics.

Reflection

This case was a novel, personally challenging one to me. I had not faced this type of tricky situation before in my career. Looking back, it seems that I could have been more competent when handling it. I did not have a particularly good grasp of some of the nuances of consultation and referrals from intercollegiate athletics at the time Ben was referred. I did not anticipate how my ethics could be challenged with the inquiries of other unforeseen people directly and indirectly involved with the case.

As a mental health professional who highly values the charge to do no harm to those I serve, the risk to doing harm to Ben came up more than once, rapidly and in unexpected ways. Although I engaged in more or less standard agency efforts to establish trust and protect the confidentiality of my work with Ben at the onset of my contact with him, other people's efforts to be helpful, and in the case of the media representative, simply curious, clashed with my standard practices and expectations. In hindsight, it would have been useful for me to have engaged in some advanced discussions with athletic department staff who might be in a position to refer clients to the counseling center (e.g., sport medicine staff, coaches, administrators). These discussions should focus on how to make referrals, as well as boundary issues such as confidentiality and privacy (e.g., what, if any, information could be shared; how this could happen with the client's consent; and when it might be appropriate). Before accepting this referral, it would also have been useful to have learned more about the drug testing policy of the athletic department, its goals, and the expectations of those who made those referrals before taking on such a referral.

Looking back, it is also clear that it is sometimes difficult to always avoid the ethical challenge of multiple relationships. It is a small world after all! My therapy and teaching roles on a small campus in a small town made that challenge difficult and perhaps unavoidable. While it may have been best to not accept a referral with an ex-student, some degree of trust had been established between me, the athletic department, and Ben. These early efforts may have helped to avoid or at least minimize conflicts with my service provision and differences between my professional ethics and values, expectations, and customary practices of the referring organization—the athletic department. Perhaps some advance communication along these lines with the local sports media would have been useful too.

I have attempted to contribute a case for the reader that reflects an amalgamation of several real, ethically challenging situations I have encountered over several years of work in similar capacities as the consultant discussed above. (I work as a half-time counseling center psychologist paid by intercollegiate athletics and also serve as a half-time faculty member). Work in this setting over the course of time has been rewarding. It is a personal privilege to work with active, high-achieving young college students. Those who seek consultation typically are quite needy; psychological consultation is often the last resort for many new clients, who usually lean on family, peers, and other athletic staff (who may discourage the use of services outside of the athletic "family") before they come to visit. Despite their reluctance to seek help, often inked to their stage of development and the novelty of working with a mental health professional, they seem to appreciate the availability of an objective, caring ear, someone who is out of the athletic and family loop. They also appear to value a helping relationship that fosters trust, respect, and protects the confidentiality of the personal matters that are explored at some risk.

Although gratifying, efforts to practice ethically have also been very challenging and frustrating—from day one. As the reader will likely gather even from this brief case, many of the ethical challenges associated with work in this setting link to the hypercompetitive climate of sport and athletics today. Understanding context becomes critical to skilled, competent practice in such a performance-based culture, characterized by high scrutiny and demanding lifestyles linked to winning, losing, and staying academically eligible. Consultants who venture into this ostensibly attractive milieu need to be sensitive to numerous barriers to efforts to work competently and ethically. They need to know that they will likely be seen as strangers in a strange land. Promoting mental health in an athletic organization does not appear to currently be a high priority endeavor from the perspective of many athletic administrators. Practitioners must remain sensitive to the holistic stress of often year-round training and how this lifestyle takes its toll on athlete's physical and mental health. Resistance to the proactive acquisition of performance-based psychological life-skills that cultivate success on the field, court, pool, and in the classroom will repeatedly fall on deaf ears. Selling psychology in athletics and other sport settings has been described as akin to "selling the plague."

The case of Ben exemplifies many of the numerous ethically challenging factors that can and do impact psychologists' efforts to assist athletes and others in the intercollegiate athletics realm and other sport settings today. Athletics today exists as a complicated, conservative culture with its own customs, values, rules, and idiosyncrasies. It functions as a performance-based business that is rapidly growing within a changing constantly collegiate culture—one likely very different and more complex than the reader experienced. Recent data tells us that more students come to the university with more and more complex psychosocial problems, mental disorders, and growing academic difficulties. Trying to help these young people find their way to adulthood is a significant undertaking for helping professionals. These cultural factors, along with the problems and strengths clients bring to consultation, constantly test professional's competence, energy, and moral character.

Key ethical principles and standards

APA (2002): Principle A (Beneficence and Responsibility), Principle C (Integrity), Principle E (Respect for People's Rights and Dignity), Standard 1.01 (Misuse of Psychologist's Work), Standard 1.03 (Conflicts between Ethics and Organizational Demands), Standard 2.01 (Boundaries of Competence), Standard 3.04 (Avoiding Harm), Standard 3.05 (Multiple Relationships), Standard 3.07 (Third Party Requests for Services), Standard 3.11 (Psychological Services Delivered To or Through Organizations), Standard 4.01 (Maintaining Confidentiality).

REFERENCES AND FURTHER READING

Bennett, B. E., Bricklin, P. M., Harris, E., Knapp, S., VandeCreek, L., & Younggren, J.N. (2006). *Assessing and managing risk in psychological practice: An individualized approach.* Washington, DC: The Trust.

Etzel, E. F., & Watson, J. C. (2007). Ethical challenges for psychological consultations in intercollegiate athletics. *Journal of Clinical Sport Psychology, 1,* 304–317.

Etzel, E. F., & Watson, J. C. (2007). Ethics in sport and exercise psychology. *Ethics & Behavior, 16,* 304–317.

Hays, K. F., & Brown, C. H. (2003). *You're on! Consulting for peak performance.* Washington DC: American Psychological Association.

Koocher, G. P., & Keith-Spiegel, P. (2008). *Ethics in psychology: Professional standards and cases* (3rd ed.). New York: Oxford University Press.

29

Doing Good Versus Avoiding Harm: Resolving Situational Contradictions

Alan G. Green

Malika was a student intern who had taken a group counseling course under my instruction during a previous semester. Malika had become well versed in my professional perspectives regarding empowerment and social justice for students. She knew that I strongly espoused advocacy when working with students, families, and communities marginalized by poverty, racism, and oppression. Malika, a bright and dedicated student, had recently completed her undergraduate degree prior to earning admission to my university's school counseling program. Malika felt justifiably proud of her educational achievement thus far. She was always quick to describe herself as a "product" of the local urban public school system. In fact, Malika took particular pleasure in the fact that she graduated from the notoriously tough inner city middle school where she was currently assigned for her internship placement. For Malika, her background served as evidence to her and others that one could overcome growing up in a tough neighborhood.

My dilemma began one day during the check-in portion of the internship supervision course. Malika began giving the class an update on her work with an eighth grade student named Jasmin. She had previously described Jasmin as a shy but intelligent 14-year-old female referred to the counseling office for excessive absences and low grades. Assigned to work with Jasmin,

Malika had the specific goal of exploring the reasons for her unsatisfactory school attendance. Malika was also asked to work collaboratively with Jasmin's teacher and mother to develop a plan that would keep her on track to graduate and move on to high school on time.

Because Malika was a "product" of this school and continued to maintain ties to the surrounding community, she had very little difficulty building rapport and forming a helping alliance with Jasmin. After getting permission from the student's mother, Malika began to explore the reasons for Jasmin's inability to get to school on a regular basis. During their second session, Jasmin revealed some troubling circumstances that she faced at home, which contributed to her absenteeism and poor academic performance. Malika learned that Jasmin's mother was more than likely engaged in illegal activity involving drugs and prostitution. She also learned of a high volume of traffic at Jasmin's home by her mother's customers, placing her at some risk for harm. The state child welfare service had removed Jasmin from the home on one previous occasion, and she claimed to have experienced a sexual assault while in the resulting foster home.

As Malika shared her update on Jasmin with the class, her verbal and nonverbal responses indicated that she felt troubled by this case. She knew that the student's revelations warranted working with her site-supervising school counselor to report the situation to the local child protective services agency (CPS) within 48 hours. As a school counseling intern, Malika knew about the professional code of ethics as prescribed by the American School Counseling Association (ASCA) and felt committed to the safety of the student. At the same, time she felt troubled because she believed that reporting this case to CPS would result in Jasmin's removal from her home. Based on what Jasmin had told her, Malika feared that Jasmin might run away to avoid CPS, due to her previous experience in foster care. After allowing Malika to share the details of this case, the class offered suggestions on how best to proceed. I noticed that Malika's level of discomfort increased as the conversation progressed. After a while, I decided to end the discussion and offered to talk with her after class.

From the class discussion and my one-on-one conversation with Malika afterward, I learned several salient features of this case that raised my own level of discomfort. First, I learned that Malika felt hesitant about informing her site supervisor, Mr. Wilkes (pseudonym), because she knew he would insist that she file a report with CPS immediately. He was bound by the same ASCA code of ethics. She described him as an older white male who had worked as a counselor at this school well before her time there as middle school student. Although the students liked him well enough, Malika perceived that Mr. Wilkes did not seem willing or able to understand that reporting the case to CPS could possibly create more problems than solutions for Jasmin. Malika felt strongly that Mr. Wilkes did not fully understand or appreciate many of the strengths and challenges faced by the students from this predominantly low-income African American school and surrounding community. To demonstrate her lack of confidence in Mr. Wilkes understanding, Malika related an incident that occurred during her years as a student at the school. Mr. Wilkes had described young Malika and a group of her friends as lazy and not interested in improving their lives, when in fact this was not the case. She noted that Mr. Wilkes seemed to make assumptions about motivation based on perceived behaviors without exploring deeper issues or perspectives.

I also learned that Malika felt very comfortable bringing her concerns to me because she believed that I understood the struggle experienced by students living in an inner city, urban context. She reminded me of how I had lectured and even "preached" about how we in the helping professions must understand the full context of the lives and situations we come across when working with students' families and communities. Malika reminded me of what I taught her about the historical antecedents that led to the current conditions in many urban schools and communities. She recited parts of my lectures about how institutional racism and poverty remain ever-present realities that should stand at the forefront of our efforts to promote sustainable change. Malika also reflected on how liberated she felt when I taught her class that most, if not all, of the public agencies in the inner city lack the capability or interest to break the cycle of poverty, violence, trauma, and overall lack of well-being experienced by its residents. I felt a knot forming in my stomach as Malika pointed out that schools, the police, and CPS all focused on maintaining the status quo rather than offering the kind of liberating and empowering support she felt prepared to offer Jasmin. Malika felt upset that she would possibly have to "snitch" (an unfavorable term used in many urban communities for those who give information to authorities, such as the police or CPS) on her student. She feared that doing so would turn Jasmin into yet another negative statistic coming out of this community.

When asked about her plans to solve this dilemma, Malika told me that she felt prepared to work with Jasmin to stay safe, while empowering her to change her situation. She wanted to help Jasmin develop an awareness of the contextual factors such as poverty and racism that contributed to her problems. Malika wanted to help Jasmin understand that by coming to school and improving her grades in order to move on to high school, she could set the foundation for breaking the cycle of poverty and pain that she currently faced. Malika also wanted to work with Jasmin's mother, whom she had spoken to once over the phone. Malika was well aware that failure to report this case to the proper authorities could lead to a misdemeanor conviction on her record and bar her from earning certification and employment as a school counselor. Nevertheless, she feared that reporting the case would jeopardize her rapport with Jasmin, as well as possibly place Jasmin at risk of further harm in the foster care system.

While brainstorming solutions to this problem that would adhere to the ethical principles in question, Malika informed me that, if CPS became involved, Jasmin had no other blood relatives capable of taking her in. Jasmin never knew her father, and her only blood relative who lived in the area was frequently homeless and challenged with mental illness after returning from service in the Iraq War. She had a godmother, Mrs. Lance, who could possibly provide her a place to stay, but Jasmin knew that foster care would not allow a nonblood relative to have custody of a minor removed from the home.

To complicate matters, Malika seemed to want me to help her "fight the system." She wanted to know how "we" could conceal these revelations from Mr. Wilkes and begin to work with Jasmin and her mother to develop healthier ways of coping. Of course, I knew from my training and practice as a school counselor and a counselor educator what action was required based on the law and our professional code of ethics. However, as I listened to Malika, I felt compelled to follow through on my commitment of not becoming an agent of the "system" and its status quo. I too struggled with how to address this dilemma in a way that spoke to both my ethical responsibilities and my personal commitment to my professional work.

After the meeting with Malika, I consulted with a well-respected colleague about the situation. I told her that, on the one hand, I wanted to do the right thing by demanding that this intern report the situation to Mr. Wilkes. However, I also wanted to live up to my self-imposed image as the great liberator and help Malika "save" Jasmin and possibly her mother from becoming yet another sad story. I shared how I felt that, if given some time, I could help Malika work with Jasmin by inviting her to join a newly forming teen advocacy group. This would offer an opportunity for the young student and her mother to engage in developing a critical consciousness of their life situation and the factors beyond themselves that contributed to it. Malika hoped that such awareness would then lead to their becoming advocates for themselves as they joined with others to pursue accountability from each other and their broader community.

My colleague offered sage, rational, logical advice and integrated sound ethical principles and advocacy for the student. She encouraged me to take a step back from the situation and look at both sides of this dilemma. On the one hand, I wanted to help this student intern do "good," yet our obligation to avoid harm required us to possibly jeopardize the very "good" we intended to do.

The conversation with my colleague allowed me to reflect on the situation from a more objective point of view. I began to realize that avoiding harm and doing good do not have to run contrary to one another. It takes effort and skill, but one can often achieve both. Upon this reflection, a free-flowing brainstorming session followed with Malika that produced several interrelated steps I could take with my intern to address this complex challenge.

In conceptualizing my ethical responsibilities to the intern, Malika; the site supervisor, Mr. Wilkes; the student, Jasmin; her mother; the school and beyond, I realized that each party had the potential for assisting in the balance between doing good versus avoiding harm. My challenge with Malika was to help her understand how to work with Mr. Wilkes to protect Jasmin by reporting the case while simultaneously educating him about the systemic advocacy approach she wanted to take. This discussion led to increasing his awareness and sensitivity to the many stressors existing in Jasmin's world, which further led to his willingness to involve Jasmin in the discussion about why it was important to report the case and how it should be done to protect her. In doing so, Malika, Jasmin, and Mr. Wilkes ultimately reported the case and worked to get the mother more motivated to voluntarily come up with a safer living arrangement for Jasmin. Lastly, we also worked collaboratively to increase the awareness of other school faculty and staff about ways to engage students to identify and address the many life challenges that abound for this population. This included working with a few progressive outside agencies to advocate for more involvement with challenging student issues.

Discussion

Key ethical issues

Avoiding harm or nonmaleficence remains among the core ethical principals relevant in this case. School counselors must inform the proper authorities when they become aware of conditions that present imminent danger to a minor. Under such circumstances, the professional must, when developmentally and contextually appropriate, seek to minimize danger to students by informing them about the need to make a report—in this case to CPS. Allowing for student input on how and by whom the report will be made often proves critically valuable.

Confidentiality stands as an additional core ethical principle intended to protect our client's from harm. We must inform students in developmentally appropriate ways of the procedures, rules, and guiding principles of the counseling process. This includes discussing the way that confidential information will be handled. When discussing limits to confidentiality, counselors must inform students of the obligation to report knowledge of imminent danger or threats to harm oneself or others to proper authorities. Discussing these limits at the outset of the counseling relationship lets the student know what to expect throughout the process. Counselors may find it useful to offer examples of such breaches of confidentiality to illustrate that students' protection and safety creates the priority and rationale for limits to confidentiality.

In addition to avoiding harm, counselors have an ethical obligation to ensure that students benefit from counseling. As such, the school counselor has a responsibility to multiple parties, including the student, her parents, her school, and the larger community where she lives. For students like Jasmin, the professional must treat each as a unique individual seeking to maximize her fullest potential. Responsibility to parents requires that one respects their rights, particularly in spite of cultural and moral differences that may exist, and seek to work with them to overcome challenges on behalf of the student. In the case of Jasmin, this may require examining personal bias toward the actions of her mother. The role of the school counselor in relation to schools and communities requires that collaborative relationships are developed to create appropriate conditions for success within the school setting and beyond, utilizing resources available throughout. For example, Malika and Mr. Wilkes may seek to work with community groups and others to help students like Jasmin successfully face the challenges that exist in their lives.

From an advocacy perspective, each of these responsibilities requires that we broaden the sphere of awareness about the systemic forces that contribute to the threats and opportunities faced by Jasmin and the many students like her. This includes working with the student, her parent, the school, and where possible, the broader community to better understand how the multigenerational patterns of poverty and marginalization have manifested in our everyday lives. These proactive ethical practices, my wise colleague reminded me, complement our responsibility to merely avoid harm by filing mandatory reports with CPS and other agencies.

In addition to ethical standards for school counselors, guidelines for supervising counselors also apply to this case. In protecting the client's welfare and rights, the supervisor roles and program administration roles must remain clearly in focus. School counselors must know the prioritized sequence for resolving ethical dilemmas and must adhere to relevant legal and ethical standards.

Work setting

As a counselor educator and university-based school counseling internship supervisor, I found myself faced with a difficult situation regarding ethical decision-making and advocacy. This dilemma challenged my professional goal of maintaining high ethical standards specifically pertaining to the protection of minors. It also called into question my personal commitment to advocate for the empowerment of marginalized students. School counselor-led advocacy refers to deliberate collaborative efforts to eliminate barriers impeding student development, while working to create learning opportunities and access to quality curriculum in schools. School counselor advocacy expands the traditional role of the school counselor. The advocacy role focuses on empowering students by helping them observe and act upon systemic social injustice as it impacts learning, as well as well-being. This role also represents a shift from the way traditional counseling approaches overfocus on the presenting problem and on the individual student without regard for the broader systemic contributing factors. I felt challenged to uphold these ideals while maintaining my professional obligation and commitment to ethical practice. The entire experience forced me to advance my intellectual acumen and my ability to exercise good judgment.

From a university perspective, supervising a student intern who also reports to a site-based supervisor within a k–12 public school setting presents some unique challenges regarding ethical practice. Given the additional layers of working with minors and parents, these multiple roles and settings require competence, communication, and strategy. Work within the academy becomes characteristically thought-provoking and philosophical in nature. Higher education lends itself to less pragmatism and greater openness to possibility, as compared to the more rigid public school context where the intern has field placements.

Working with a practicing school counselor in a setting bound by the ever-increasing mandates of academic performance and standardized testing, while working alongside multiple professionals trained in different domains (e.g., teachers, administrators, and special educators), proves challenging. Advocating for marginalized groups further complicates this work. These circumstances require that the university supervisor operates with an understanding of the key ethical principles of benevolence, nonmaleficence, and the balance between doing "good" and avoiding harm.

Most school settings place a high priority on compliance with existing mandates, rules, and laws. School counselors operating in these settings over time tend to adopt the administrators' proclivity toward compliance with policies and standards at the expense of taking risks on behalf of the unique needs of individual students. When the high ideals of the academy for doing "good" and promoting change intersect with the rigid practices of the public school, it becomes important that an open, reflective strategy for managing harm and doing good remains in play.

Reflection

I consider myself fortunate when I think of my current professional role as a counselor educator. In many ways, it represents a manifestation of my desire to create the perfect career path based on my likes and dislikes. I enjoy the flexibility of time and reflection my job affords as I teach, supervise, and conduct research and consultation in the higher education setting. No two days are the same. One day I may teach a class of graduate students about how to use group counseling in an urban setting, while the next day I may work with a group of counselors on an applied research project in a school. I truly have one foot planted in each of the distinct worlds of theory and practice. When it comes to ethical practice and the balance between doing good and avoiding harm, I have found that it takes patience, intention, and a willingness to reflect on one's attachment to acting as a "savior."

As I sort through situations similar to the one in the case described above, I must take the time to remain mindful of each of the participants, their contexts, of my somewhat complex mix of roles vis-à-vis each person. In doing so, I find that my personal attachment to changing the conditions of young people living in poverty, if left unchecked, can contribute more to creating harm than it can to doing good. This case affords a prime example of how to seek that balance by slowing down and examining both the details of the dilemma and my own hidden wishes and agendas more closely.

Key ethical principles and standards

The American School Counseling Association (2004): Section A.7. (Danger to Self or Others), Section A.2. (Confidentiality). Ethical Guidelines for Counseling Supervisors from the Association of Counselor Education and Supervision (1993): 1. (Client Welfare and Rights), 2. (Supervision Role), 3. (Program Administration Role).

REFERENCES AND FURTHER READING

Bodenhorn, N. (December 2006). Exploratory study of common and challenging ethical dilemmas experienced by professional school counselors. *Professional School Counseling, 10,* 195–202.

Hipolito-Delgado, C. P., & Lee, C. C. (2007). Empowerment theory for the professional school counselor: A manifesto for what really matters. *Professional School Counseling, 10,* 327–332.

Lee, R., & Cashwell, C. (2001). Ethical issues in counseling supervision: A comparison of university and site supervisors. *Clinical Supervisor, 20,* 91–100.

Murphy, S., & Kaffenberger, C. (2007). ASCA national model[R]: The foundation for supervision of practicum and internship students. *Professional School Counseling, 10,* 289–296.

Stone, C. (2005). *School counseling principles: Ethics and law.* Alexandria, VA: American School Counseling Association.

PART VII

Supervising or Assisting Colleagues

30

The Wink: Ethical Aspects of Encountering Clients in Unexpected Places

Stephen H. Behnke

The following brief vignette[1], presented at a peer consultation group meeting for which I was the discussion leader, provides a deceptively nuanced and rich set of issues to ponder at the convergence of ethics and clinical care. The psychologist presenting the vignette, Dr. V, is a talented, experienced, and clinically savvy psychologist who found herself caught off guard one morning on her way to work. Dr. V's sudden and unanticipated intersection of her private life with that of a client resonated with the psychologists in our consultation group, as it undoubtedly will with many readers. Even a seemingly innocuous encounter outside of a professional context can be fraught with clinical significance and may provoke feelings in the psychologist that are meaningfully explored from both clinical and ethical perspectives. Below, I demonstrate the process I used to think through Dr. V's situation with Dr. V's peer consultation group.

---

[1] Identifying information has been removed from the vignette. Aspects of the situation and the presentation/consultation have been altered and presented as a composite in order to protect confidentiality of both the client and the psychologist.

Dr. V and the wink

Dr. V has a favorite coffee shop in her small town where she stops each morning on her way to work and where she sometimes takes an hour or two to read the Sunday paper on the weekend. She finds the manner in which the baristas top off her latte with cinnamon especially pleasing and the blueberry scones excellent. One weekday morning, Dr. V walked in for her coffee and scone when, standing in line, she noticed her new patient behind the counter. Her patient likewise noticed Dr. V, and with a wink, gave Dr. V the next larger size of latte than Dr. V had ordered and charged Dr. V half price.

Dr. V began her request for consultation with a simple question to the group: "What should I have done?"

I found that my first challenge as the group's discussion leader was to decide where best to begin. Dr. V clearly felt some distress regarding whether she had behaved appropriately—although she had not yet told us what she had done—and her next meeting with the client was to take place the following morning. Rather than focus immediately on Dr. V's behavior, I decided to shift away from asking what Dr. V should have *done* to focus rather on what Dr. V was *feeling* as she stood at the counter. Psychoanalysts might refer to Dr. V's internal experience as her "countertransference." Whatever the terminology, I thought that Dr. V's feelings in that moment would likely provide a window into how she was beginning to frame the issues that emerged with her client in their morning exchange.[2]

I asked other group members to speculate on Dr. V's experience as she interacted with her new client. The group generated multiple possibilities. The primary theme among the likely candidates focused on annoyance; Dr. V simply wanted her morning latte and now found herself "on the clock." Annoyance as an affect in the vignette is interesting because it serves as a cue that Dr. V was experiencing an intrusion into her private life, a crossing of the professional into the personal that she neither anticipated nor desired. The intrusion became highlighted because it potentially extended beyond that one incident; depending on her client's schedule, Dr. V could face the prospect of encountering the client each weekday morning and perhaps even on the following Sunday. Dr. V, with a smile and a sigh, confirmed that annoyance indeed was her initial and primary reaction to the encounter.

---

[2] The longstanding group consisted of a number of colleagues who knew one another very well and so felt comfortable sharing their thoughts and reactions with one another. In a different group, I might have elected to focus less on Dr. V's internal experiences.

At this point in the consultation group meeting, the discussion digressed a bit, away from the facts of the vignette. The group began to explore an issue that underlies our professional identities: Becoming a psychologist involves a commitment. As with any commitment, committing to life in a profession entails making sacrifices. We forgo opportunities, delay gratifications, and sometimes incur significant costs. Along with these sacrifices—in large part *by virtue of* the sacrifices—individuals who make such a commitment encounter enormous professional and personal satisfaction. Yet an issue that remains oddly unexplored in the professional literature involves the nature of the sacrifices individuals make in order to become practicing psychologists: What is it that we ask psychologists to give up in order to enter the profession? This question confronted Dr. V in a mundane yet stark manner as she went for her morning coffee, and the consultation group became curious about their own way of assessing what of their personal lives they routinely gave up in the service of their work.

The group pointed out that it was the unusual psychologist who has not somehow altered or otherwise curtailed behavior in response to the possibility of encountering a client outside of a professional setting. Every psychologist must decide the extent to which he or she is willing to accommodate in this manner, and it can become a fascinating exercise to ask a group of psychologists, as I then did in the consultation group, where they fall on a continuum of "clearly willing to accommodate" to "would not make that sacrifice for my professional life." Although the group had large areas of overlap, distinct individual differences on either end emerged in our discussion. Some psychologists in the group saw sacrificing their morning latte and scone simply as part of the psychologist's role. Others pointed out their agreement with that assessment *if* there were other coffee shops reasonably available. Otherwise they would hesitate to accept such an imposition.

This discussion led into a gentle exploration of how Dr. V managed her annoyance. Managing an affect requires a measure of psychological insight, which is one of the many touchstones where ethics and clinical work meet. Competence is referred to as the cornerstone of ethics because a psychologist can hardly do good or avoid harm—this is Beneficence and Nonmaleficence in Principle A of the *Ethical Principles of Psychologists and Code of Conduct* (American Psychological Association, 2002)—without being competent. A competence essential for clinical work involves the capacity to monitor and regulate one's own internal experiences.

The group reasoned that, although the loss of one's morning latte would not likely trigger terribly intense affects, ethics does not flow solely or even primarily out of high drama. The daily challenges of maintaining a professional stance toward one's work and one's clients forms the "stuff" out of which an ethical psychologist is largely made. How Dr. V managed her reactions in that moment and how she would manage her affects in the subsequent clinical encounters with her client would be well worth her attention, and at this point in the discussion, the group raised the possibility of a continuing case presentation.

Our discussion had explored in detail the relationship between ethics and a psychologist's internal experience in a particular clinical moment. I wanted to get back to the coffee shop. I pointed out that practicing psychologists will almost certainly recognize Dr. V's situation, that of feeling "on the spot" with a client and needing to make a quick decision. All decisions take place in a context, and Dr. V's context involved a bustling coffee shop with people on their way to the office and eager for their morning coffees. As Dr. V considered her options, she must quickly have examined the risks and benefits of various possibilities quickly. Given her experience and clinical talent, I assumed that Dr. V found herself acting out of "instinct," but I pointed out that the word *instinct* masks the many years of training and experience that inform a seasoned psychologist's internal sense of how an encounter will likely unfold and where the dangers and opportunities lie. Dr. V hesitated to respond and said that she would first like to hear from the group what they would have seen as her options as she stood at the counter across from her client.

The group came up with three options they believed best captured the possibilities available to Dr. V. The first involved taking corrective action in the moment by calling the mistake to the client's attention, for example by remarking, "I'm sorry, there may have been a misunderstanding. I asked for a smaller size, thank you." The second response involved accepting the drink and taking corrective action without calling the matter to the client's attention, perhaps by leaving a sum of money on the counter or in the tip jar that would cover the expense of the larger drink. The third and final possibility involved simply accepting the drink and paying the amount requested. The understanding in all three situations was that Dr. V would discuss the incident in the client's next session.

I encouraged the group to discuss the risks and benefits of each of the three possibilities. I asked that they identify and weigh the risks and benefits in order to come up with a *preferred* option, and I asked them to focus on the reasons they would choose one option over the other two. For the purposes of our discussion, I asked the group to imagine themselves standing immediately behind Dr. V in line and so to discuss the options as if in real time, as the action unfolded.

The first option entailed engaging in some form of corrective action at the counter, in the moment. With this option, Dr. V would make clear to her client that she would not accept anything other than the drink for which she paid, in a clinically sensitive manner that did not shame her client. Possibilities included saying, "I'm sorry, there may have been a misunderstanding, I asked for a smaller size, thank you," or "That's a bit larger than I can handle, I'd really prefer something smaller." This option was seen as offering several advantages. First, it makes clear that Dr. V would not become complicit in depriving the coffee shop of its legitimate profits. Second, the option immediately communicates to the client that Dr. V would not collude in an unethical and possibly illegal act. Third, this option interrupts a potential slippery slope involving additional acts of questionable legitimacy. In short, the first option communicates in an immediate and clear manner that Dr. V will not accept what the client offers in that moment.

Along with benefits, the first option entails risks, which I encouraged the group to outline, and to do likewise with the second and third options. According to the vignette, the client is new, which suggests that Dr. V may not have a good sense of how the client will likely experience and react to Dr. V's reaction. The offer of a larger size drink at half price suggests a willingness to cross boundaries, adding to a sense of unpredictability regarding how the client may react if Dr. V refuses the offer. If the client reacts by engaging Dr. V in a verbal exchange, the client's confidentiality is possibly at risk; the stakes grow somewhat higher given that the exchange takes place in the client's place of employment and thus likely in front of coworkers or perhaps even a supervisor. The first option thus risks precipitating an exchange with contours and unpredictable consequences that may have an adverse impact on the client.

The second response entails accepting the larger drink for a reduced price and taking some corrective action without calling the matter to the client's attention in the moment. Possibilities include leaving the correct sum of money on the counter or in the tip jar for the full expense of the larger drink. The advantages of this second option include helping Dr. V not to be complicit in an unethical or possibly illegal act, insofar as she has provided the full price of the drink to the coffee shop. The risk is that the money, although intended to compensate for the drink, may actually end up with the client. Rather than addressing the inappropriate action, Dr. V has now paid the client for having provided her a discounted cup of coffee. Although the second option may address and alleviate Dr. V's own concerns about feeling complicit, this option may do little in the way of communicating her concerns to her client. In short, the second option may prove helpful in Dr. V's managing her *own feelings* about the exchange but may not have the advantages of the first option in terms of an immediate and clear message *to the client* about Dr. V's standards of behavior.

The third and final possibility is for Dr. V simply to accept the drink, pay the amount requested, and move along as she normally would on an average weekday morning. The advantage of the third option is primarily that Dr. V avoids the risks of engaging in an exchange with an unpredictable outcome. These risks are not insignificant insofar as rejecting the coffee, however tactfully done, may have important clinical consequences. In addition, a verbal exchange could result in a disclosure of information, the consequences of which the client would not fully appreciate, even though apparently innocuous at the time. Put succinctly, rejecting the coffee risks precipitating a clinical engagement in a context where Dr. V may not be able to contain the exchange. The third option would avoid this risk.

The group felt reasonably secure that these three scenarios covered the general contours of the options available to Dr. V. Before moving on in our discussion, I asked the group whether they believe Dr. V found herself in an *ethical* or in a *clinical* dilemma at the coffee shop. As the group considered this question, I encouraged them to review the language they had used in setting forth Dr. V's options. The language of the risks and benefits of the three options captured a hybrid quality to Dr. V's situation. From the perspective of ethics, Dr. V did not want to become complicit in an unethical or illegal act at the coffee shop, and she wanted to protect her client's confidentiality. She wanted to avoid the slippery slope that may begin by accepting a small gift. These concerns belong primarily (although not exclusively) to the realm of ethics. From a clinical perspective, Dr. V was mindful that she did not know this new client well and any exchange had unpredictable clinical implications. Dr. V needed to recognize that initiating an exchange, however reasonable and well-intentioned, may have detrimental or complex consequences for the treatment and the professional relationship. These latter concerns seemed to the group more clinical in nature. The group concluded that both clinical and ethical considerations were central to Dr. V's situation.

At this point, over half the group's meeting time had passed, and I wanted to accomplish two additional tasks. First, I wanted the group to examine the significance of the client's wink. Finally, I wanted Dr. V to tell us what she had done in the coffee shop, what she expects might happen in the next session, and whether she planned to visit the coffee shop again that week. I invited the group to begin by discussing "the wink," a behavior fraught with meaning under virtually any circumstances.

The wink

In a very short discussion time, the group offered six possible meanings for the wink:

1. The wink had an erotic tinge and signaled an attempt to flirt with Dr. V.
2. The wink invited Dr. V to engage in an illicit, "forbidden" act.

3. The wink acknowledged a secret relationship that they shared and that no one else in their immediate surrounds shared or was even aware of.
4. The wink recognized that the client and Dr. V shared a bond, perhaps that they were both hard at work early in the morning.
5. The wink offered a note of acknowledgement and gratitude that Dr. V understood and supported the client in a unique way.
6. The wink signaled that the client recognized Dr. V so that Dr. V did not need to do anything further to acknowledge the client's presence or role in preparing Dr. V's coffee.

The group noted that none of these meanings are mutually exclusive and this list of six was by no means exhaustive. Some of these meanings strongly suggest a measure of Axis II (American Psychiatric Association, 2000) involvement, others much less so. I suggested that an interesting exercise in ethics workshops would be to vary client characteristics—gender, age, sexual orientation, life circumstances—and see which of the above meanings of the wink seem more plausible to participants. At this point, with the group's time drawing to a close, I asked Dr. V to tell us what happened in the coffee shop and to speculate about the next session or two with the client. Members of the group also asked when, or if, she planned to return to the coffee shop for her daily latte and scone.

Dr. V directly linked the wink and her response. She thought that the group had provided very plausible meanings for the wink and explained that she did not know her client well enough to know which of the possibilities was more likely, although she felt reasonably certain that Axis II factors played some role. Because of her uncertainty regarding the meaning of the wink and her general sense of not yet knowing the client, Dr. V had decided that the third option identified by the group was best, and that was indeed the option she had chosen the previous day in the coffee shop. I asked Dr. V to say in detail what she had done, and she explained that she had nodded her head and said "Thank you" to her client, accepted her change, took her latte, and left the coffee shop as she normally would.

I asked Dr. V if she could tell us how she imagined beginning next session with the client and if she would share her thoughts on returning to the coffee shop in the immediate future. Dr. V said that she intended to begin the next session by directly inquiring about the exchange, and she had in mind an opening such as, "Let's talk about what happened at the coffee shop the other morning," or "Help me understand what was going on there." Other psychologists in the group suggested they might hesitate at the outset of the session in order to see whether the client would initiate a discussion of the exchange. The group felt clear that regardless of which option was chosen, discussing what occurred at the coffee shop would be an important part of their next meeting.

Finally, Dr. V said that she intended to forego visiting the coffee shop until she felt that she better understood the exchange. When I pressed her on how long she felt working through the exchange might take, Dr. V smiled and replied that it depended on how deeply the exchange "spoke" to the client's conflicts; it could take weeks or longer. In returning to the group's initial discussion, I asked Dr. V if she would share a final thought on how it would feel for her to miss her morning lattes and scones. Dr. V smiled and replied that a coffee and a scone seemed a very reasonable price to practice her profession up to her standards.

As the group ended, Dr. V asked me to comment on whether her behavior was satisfactory from the perspective of ethics. Psychologists often press for the "right" answer to an ethical dilemma. In many, if not most, instances, however, there simply is no single, demonstrably correct course of action. What becomes important is the psychologist's willingness to engage in a thoughtful process of reflecting on the various possible courses of action and on the risks and benefits inherent in each. From that perspective, I felt Dr. V's performance had been outstanding. And I told her so.

Key ethical principles and standards

APA (2002): Principle A (Beneficence and Nonmaleficence), Principle C (Integrity), Principle E (Respect for People's Rights and Dignity), Standard 3.04 (Avoiding Harm), Standard 2.01 (Boundaries of Competence), Standard 2.06 (Personal Problems and Conflicts), Standard 3.05 (Multiple Relationships), Standard 3.06 (Conflict of Interest).

REFERENCES AND FURTHER READING

American Psychiatric Association. (2000). *Diagnostic and Statistical Manual of Mental Disorders* (4th ed., text rev.). Washington, DC: Author.
American Psychological Association. (2002). Ethical principles of psychologists and code of conduct. *American Psychologist, 57,* 1060–1073.

31

Can You Help Us? Supervising Graduate Students in a Crisis Situation

Clark D. Campbell

It all began with the best intentions. I was teaching doctoral students in a professional psychology program, and part of my faculty duties involved supervising students' research and dissertation projects. I had a group of about eight graduate students on my research team at various levels of training, but mostly third- and fourth-year students who had already earned an MA in clinical psychology. My team had become cohesive, and the students seemed genuinely interested in helping each other succeed in their research and clinical skill development. I tried to perpetuate this cooperative team environment because it created a positive outlook toward research and resulted in productive outcomes.

One fall, a student suggested to me, and then to the research team, that we consider providing some psychoeducation in a rural part of northern California. She told us that her father served as the pastor of a large church in a small rural community, and that the church provided an annual health fair for community residents. She further described the community as isolated, but in need of health and mental health services. The community had faced hard economic times, significant poverty, and unemployment. Two areas of research on our team included social responsibility and rural psychology. This seemed like an ideal opportunity to put our values and research interests into practical action.

The students became very interested in this opportunity and described this as a team "road trip," somewhat reminiscent for all of us of grade school field trips. Only one of the students on the team couldn't go on the trip because of prior scheduling commitments, but the other seven agreed at once. I contacted my student's father to gain more information about the educational services that we could supply. He said the health fair took place in the church parking lot on a Saturday, and it had become a big hit in the community. In fact, the city council had endorsed it as a positive event for the town and commended the fair in the local newspaper. In previous years, professionals volunteered free medical, dental, hearing, and vision screenings. Organizers also provided free haircuts, food, and household goods to these needy families. Children, single parents, and elderly residents were among the several hundred attendees of these annual health fairs. However, even though the pastor knew that many people in the community had unmet psychological needs, no one had offered psychological services at the health fair. I made it clear that we could not provide therapeutic services, but that we could provide basic psychological information to those who desired it. He thought it sounded like a great idea and welcomed us to the community event.

Our research team grew more excited about this prospect as we discussed the ways in which we could offer practical services. Students researched the kinds of psychological problems likely to exist in a rural community where many residents lived in lower socioeconomic conditions and had little access to health and mental health services. Further consultation with the pastor revealed that depression, substance abuse, and domestic violence were significant problems in the community. My students researched these areas and looked for existing psychoeducational materials on these topics. They prepared materials and made copies of information sheets they could hand out to those seeking such assistance.

We received permission to use a university van for our field trip, and the church agreed to help pay for our lodging at a local motel. With excitement and a bit of regressive giddiness, we embarked on our 300-mile journey to the rural location. When we arrived, it became clear that the health fair organizers at the church were delighted to see us. They prepared a generous meal for us and were glad to see "the outsiders" who cared enough to assist with their outreach into the community. They described their plan for the health fair and showed us all of the groceries, clothing, and other materials they had organized to facilitate easy pick-up by local residents.

The following morning, we arrived at the church parking lot a couple hours early so we could help with the final set-up. The parking lot was large and effectively organized so people could walk to various stations to receive care, consultation, or goods. My students set up our table and laid out various packets of information for people to pick up. Local residents gathered by a fence at the edge of the parking lot and waited for the gates to open at 9:00 AM. The crowd grew, and there were a couple hundred people waiting to enter the parking lot when the gates opened.

About 15 minutes after the gates opened, and as many people worked their way through the parking lot, we heard a loud noise and mass confusion erupted in the parking lot. I stood about 20 feet away from my students and our table when a car came careening through the parking lot at a high rate of speed and crashed into the side of the church. Tables were strewn about, people were lying on the ground, and panic developed in the crowd. It took all of us several minutes to comprehend what had happened—an elderly woman driving to the health fair had lost control of her car and stepped on the gas rather than the brake. As a result, she drove haphazardly through the parking lot, hitting several attendees before crashing into the church building. She felt shaken, but only had minor injuries.

My first response was to gather all of my students to check on their safety. I felt a great deal of panic, wondering if any of the students had been injured or perhaps killed. I quickly contacted each of them and saw that none of them was hurt, although they felt seriously shaken by the event. We quickly began assessing the injured and doing what we could to assist with basic first aid. Although two ambulances and a fire truck arrived from the volunteer fire department, it became apparent that the community emergency resources had become overwhelmed, and they could only treat the most seriously injured. In the final assessment, about twenty-five people suffered significant injuries and were taken to the local hospital, and one woman died as a result of the accident.

About an hour after the accident, the pastor of the church found me and asked if the graduate students and I could provide some psychological help to those who had just survived the tragedy. He indicated that the police and fire departments did not have the resources and that the local hospital had already become overwhelmed with the injured residents. Furthermore, the fire department contacted a Red Cross representative and learned it would take several days before they could dispatch a team to the rural area. The pastor made a desperate plea for some help for his church and community members.

This situation created quite a dilemma for me. What had started out as a way to help students learn about providing useful information to a rural community had turned into a request for psychological services. I was the only licensed psychologist present, and I was not licensed in California. The graduate students had all completed foundational courses in assessment and counseling interventions, as well as some practicum experiences, but none had the clinical competence to practice independently in such a situation. To complicate matters more, we also qualified as victims of the tragedy. As witnesses to the accident, we had all been affected by the accident and were processing it in our own ways. Some were obviously emotionally numb and seemed distant, while others seemed to compartmentalize the event and appeared to be functioning well. Overall, we were all affected by the event to some extent and were not in an optimal emotional state to provide help to others. At the same time, there was a huge need, and there were no community psychological resources. Because we had more training than anyone else around, it seemed appropriate for us to try and help in some way.

I gathered the students together and briefly talked about their experience of the accident. None of them had incurred physical injury, but all had witnessed the disaster. I asked each one to simply describe what they had experienced and try to put their observations and feelings into words. This appeared to be very helpful to them, and they all expressed fear, anger, frustration, and sadness for the injuries and loss of life, as well as for the sudden change in plans. I told them about the request of the pastor and asked if any of them had any experience in crisis intervention. Interestingly, one of the students had completed a continuing education course on this topic a few months earlier. I had received training from the Red Cross and from other continuing education sources as well, and I had worked with a number of patients who had experienced trauma. All of the students expressed a desire to help in any way possible. However, I was concerned about their competence to practice without direct supervision, my competence and ability to supervise these students in this situation, the perception of the recipients of their care regarding the students' competence, and the degree to which our own mental health had been compromised by this event. Despite these concerns, I decided that it was most important for us to try to help in ways that we could.

I described an intervention format that was supportive, but not intrusive or forceful in the sense of imposing ourselves on others. We wanted to be sensitive to the fact that many people had not come to the health fair to process traumatic feelings but rather to receive economic and physical assistance, and therefore it was important to me that we were sensitive to that fact. I thought that it would be most helpful to simply be available to listen to those who wanted to talk and to not push anyone to say anything unless they expressed an interest in doing so. I stated there was evidence that a supportive environment was important and that victims could simply be asked if they would like to describe their experience. I cautioned against efforts to draw out deeper feelings and instead encouraged students to merely normalize the experiences others shared. I asked students to divide into groups of two or three and to make themselves available to those who continued to meander about in the parking lot and inside the church.

The students responded well to this approach and began talking with some of the victims. Many of them formed small groups with some of the chairs that were in the parking lot. Others met with some of the church members who were there to help with the health fair. I slowly moved through the groups and listened and offered support to the students if they needed it. I was amazed by the students' clinical skills and professionalism in this situation. They seemed to garner immediate respect from the victims and were gently supporting these victims in normalizing their thoughts and feelings.

That evening, we gathered for dinner and discussed the unexpected events of the day. Although it was emotionally draining, the students described an energized feeling of having helped others in ways they had not anticipated. They felt gratified by the many kind words from the people with whom they spoke. Many of them expressed some surprise at their own—heretofore unknown—clinical skills, and the students felt they had made a difference in many people's lives. Additionally, they described how challenging it was to compartmentalize their own pain and empathize with those around them.

The next day was Sunday, and our group was asked to stay for the church service and be available to anyone who requested help. There were a few hundred people in attendance, and the pastor asked me to make some remarks to the congregation, which I did. The students and I decided the night before that we would try to offer some small debriefing groups on Sunday for various age groups: children (with parents), adolescents, and adults. Again, we broke into small groups and provided a voluntary context for people to express their thoughts and feelings. Interestingly, many parishioners posed rather difficult theological questions such as, "How could God let this happen?" and "Why did this have to happen in our community?" and "How will people trust us to provide for this community in the future?"

George Fox University is a Quaker institution, and the Doctor of Psychology (PsyD) program was developed upon this historic and theological foundation. As such, these theological questions were ones that our students were prepared to respond to from an academic perspective, but they had not had to deal directly with these questions in practice. Additionally, they were in a doctoral psychology program and not a pastoral program, so their competence to respond to these theological questions was enhanced by their training, but they were still psychology graduate students under supervision and not prepared to respond independently. Of course, the question for me was how the "clients" (in this case the people who showed up for the health fair) perceived the students. Did they see them as pastoral counselors or graduate psychology students, and how would this blurring of professional boundaries be a potential ethical conflict for the students and clients? The students also observed how trauma was processed by different people and in different ways. Some of the people who attended these groups had clear underlying psychological disorders that were exacerbated by the trauma. In those situations, we tried to make referrals back to the community mental health center for the following week.

The students and I continued processing our own responses in the van on the trip home, and the following week I arranged for all of us to express ourselves with a trauma specialist at our community hospital. This one group session seemed to be helpful to all of us in bringing some closure to our experience of the traumatic event. The students continued to express surprise at their ability to apply their clinical skills in a crisis situation.

Discussion

Key ethical issues

There are several ethical issues present in this case including: boundaries of competence; informed consent; supervision; practicing without a license (legal and ethical implications); beneficence; providing services in emergencies; delegation of work to others; personal problems and conflicts; avoiding harm; and documentation of scientific and professional work. Psychologists have an obligation to not harm others in the provision of psychological services. The onus is on the psychologist to be aware of his or her competence and not act outside that area of competence. Furthermore, we inform clients about our services and the potential risks involved with the services. However, such standardized informed consent was not possible in this emergency situation, and the requirements of the emergency pushed the boundaries of our professional competence. But with a desire to help and not harm others, professionals have to make calculated decisions in these situations regarding the cost/benefit of psychological services in an emergency.

This situation had the added complexity of supervision of students. It was not just me trying to deal ethically with a crisis, but it was the necessity of supervising students simultaneously that created increased concern. I did not have the luxury of time to determine their specific competence to provide such services. Furthermore, I was not able to provide ongoing supervision for each of them as they interacted with the "clients." Additionally, we were not completely sure if our "clients" were in an emotional state to provide reasonable consent to such emergency psychological services.

Work setting

Faculty members are often called upon to provide clinical supervision for graduate students. However, supervision typically occurs in a controlled setting, such as an office, where the faculty member can focus on the clinical material and the student's responses. In this situation, the students and the supervisor were witnesses of the same traumatic event, and the supervision took place in a field setting where the supervisor had little control. When supervisors and students work in highly controlled situations, there is often time to reflect upon the possible crisis or emergency situations that could arise. For example, providing psychological services in a correctional facility, some military and hospital triage units, or crisis centers are work settings in which psychologists can anticipate emergencies and prepare for them. Psychologists have an obligation to prevent harm to students and clients, and they need to have protocols in place to anticipate responding ethically when harm may occur. However, we were completely caught off guard in this situation. I had not anticipated an emergency situation and therefore had not prepared myself or the students for this possibility.

Reflection

Although this "road trip" proved to be a very difficult and sad situation, it did exemplify the nature of isolated, rural communities. When tragedies happen in an urban setting, we typically see news coverage and have some psychological resources available to deal with the tragedy. However, in rural settings this may not be the case. Interestingly, a catch-22 (Heller, 1961) or no-win situation exists in rural communities. When a crisis exists, few resources exist in place, so outside help is needed. However, many rural residents feel very suspicious of outside help and would prefer aid from those in their own community (Bock & Campbell, 2005). As a result, many rural community crisis situations may go unattended by the professional community. How can we prepare graduate students for rural practice without placing them in rural training sites where there are typically few supervisors or broader psychological resources? Perhaps telehealth supervision can prove helpful for training students in rural areas.

Going through this situation with my students reminded me of the basic toolkit that most psychologists should have. We never know when we may be called upon to assist in a crisis situation. We are trained in general and specific treatment modalities, and it may prove useful to consider the basic ways in which we could be of service to others when called upon for such duty.

Basic training for crisis response could be beneficial for all mental health professionals to facilitate this readiness to serve.

Finally, knowing our competence and the limits of our competence is important for all mental health professionals. There are certainly situations in which we should say no to requests for help out of the concern that we may do more harm than good. Many of us are aware of the limitations of our competence when sitting in our offices, but when called upon to respond in a crisis situation we may not be so reflective. The situation described here is a reminder that we may have the intention to do good, but we run the risk of harming others if our skills do not match our intentions.

Key ethical principles and standards

(APA, 2002): Principle A (Beneficence and Nonmaleficence), Standard 2.01 (Boundaries of Competence), Standard 2.02 (Providing Services in Emergencies), Standard 2.05 (Delegation of Work to Others), Standard 2.06 (Personal Problems and Conflicts), Standard 3.04 (Avoiding Harm), Standard 7.06 (Assessing Student and Supervisee Performance), Standard 10.01 (Informed Consent to Therapy), Standard 10.03 (Group Therapy).

REFERENCES AND FURTHER READING

Bock, S., & Campbell, C. D. (2005). Crisis intervention in rural communities: A cultural catch-22. *Journal of Rural Community Psychology, E8*. Retrieved from http://www.marshall.edu/jrcp/8_1_Bock_Campbell.htm.

Heller, J. (1961). *Catch-22*. New York: Simon & Schuster.

32

Doing It by the Book: Ethical Issues in Teaching a Group Didactically and Experientially

Gerald Corey

Ron, a new assistant professor in a counseling psychology master's program, contacted me for consultation at the conclusion of his first semester of teaching. Ron felt dispirited, confused, and was contemplating resignation from his job. When I inquired as to the source of Ron's dejection, he relayed that the department chair had assigned him a group counseling class with a required experiential lab component. Although initially excited about the course, things had gone badly—so badly that several students had complained vigorously to the dean that the course and the professor were unfair. I agreed to consult with Ron and try to help him better understand what might have gone wrong. In the details that follow, I provide a summary of the group's evolution from Ron's perspective.

Ron met with his group counseling class of 12 students during the first day of the semester and spent most of the time going over the syllabus and the requirements for the class. He had hoped to create a climate that would be conducive for students to learn basic concepts of group work from an academic perspective and also provide a safe place for students to learn experientially about group process. Ron explained that the first half of each class meeting would focus on didactic content based on his lectures about various aspects of group process, discussion of the assigned reading, viewing of videos of a group in action, and some interactive group exercises. The second half of the class, designed as experiential in nature, would involve the students as group members. Ron explained that he would facilitate this group for the first four weeks of the semester, and then from the fifth group meeting to the end of the semester, the students would have an opportunity to function as coleaders of the group, under his supervision. Everyone in the class would have a chance to colead their group at least one time, and the rest of the time he expected students to function as members in the group. He explained that he expected students to identify personal issues and concerns they would willingly explore in this group and stressed his belief that they would best learn about how groups function by experiencing the process of a small group. When I asked Ron how he had prepared the students for the group by offering a rationale for experiential work and explaining the potential risks and benefits of the experience, he appeared perplexed and said, "I didn't want to influence the process with too much direction; my group professor taught us that some ambiguity is good for eliciting members' issues."

Ron began the first group by sharing something about himself, including the fact that this was his first time teaching group counseling. He added that in his own doctoral studies he had only one group course that consisted almost exclusively of lectures and discussions. He stated that he felt some misgivings about his ability to orchestrate an experiential group, yet he felt ready to take the risks involved in learning something new. He looked forward to learning along with his students. When Ron asked students to introduce themselves and say something about how they could become personally involved in this experience, he encountered considerable hesitation and caution on their part. They made only general comments about themselves, showing some reluctance to participate in a personal way from the initial class session. Ron attempted to counter this reluctance by emphasizing that one cannot learn group counseling simply by reading a book or by listening to lectures. At the next class, Ron made it clear that he expected the students to become actively engaged in the significant and meaningful self-disclosure necessary for a group to function well. Furthermore, he reminded them that part of the grade for this course would depend on their participation in the group. When I queried, Ron acknowledged that he did not review basic ground rules such as confidentiality, appropriate boundaries, the multiple roles he would occupy in this group, and guidelines for participation in the group as a member and as a cofacilitator. He admitted he was concerned that "too much information" would make members wary about participation.

When Ron asked his students for their questions and reactions, the students raised some concerns and expressed surprise that he expected them to disclose personal matters in an academic class. Some did not like the idea of revealing their personal problems or concerns in a group with their peers and with an instructor. Some stated they had enrolled in the class to learn about conducting a group, not to do their personal work. Others believed they might face judgmental criticism if they openly shared their personal lives and wondered if what they said (or did not say) would have a negative impact on successful navigation through the master's program. Others expressed concerns about the influence their level of participation might have on their grade in the course. Students raised anxieties about expectations of cofacilitating a group composed of their peers, especially since they had no experience.

When I asked Ron how he responded to these concerns, he said that he did not think it appropriate to directly address negative reactions but rather reiterated that students would learn a great deal from struggling. He reminded students that in their work settings they might find themselves leading groups comprised of members who did not sign up voluntarily. Thus, it would be good for them to experience how they themselves deal with challenges posed by participating in a required group.

During the next four weeks, students listened and took notes as Ron lectured about group process concepts. When he tried to get a discussion going based on the readings, the students tended to remain quiet and had little to say. During the second half of the class session, when he facilitated their small group, the level of disclosure tended toward superficial content. People did not seem willing to talk about what it felt like for them to participate in this group or what they wanted from this group experience. Ron felt dissatisfied with their level of involvement, so he tried to increase involvement by calling on people individually, which produced only strained responses. He introduced structured exercises to promote interaction and personal sharing, but the energy in the room typically was low. Ron did not deal with the lack of energy that became obvious within the group.

At the seventh meeting of the class, a number of critical incidences surfaced during the small group session cofacilitated by students. Nell expressed her resentment about the expectation that she must share her personal life in this kind of group. She said, "I am a private person, and I want to choose the time and place where I will get personal with people." Another member, Ruth, exclaimed, "I am with Nell, because I feel I am being forced to dig up and reveal secrets. I don't see the point in airing our dirty linen in a classroom setting." Allen joined in with Nell and Ruth and added, "I know I am holding back any criticism of the instructor/supervisor of this group because I am afraid that my grade will be jeopardized if I say what I think." Matthew chimed in with, "If I could drop out of this group, I surely would. I am here putting in my time because this is a required course, but I am not getting anything from the group.

I'm hearing nothing but psychobabble and complaining, and I don't see the point of listening to petty problems." Susan, who had spoken up before Matthew, interjected with, "I feel attacked by Matthew, and the instructor is not protecting us." Susan began to cry and left the room. After several minutes, Susan returned to the group, still crying. When Ron asked her to talk about what was going on with her, she refused and said she wanted to be left alone. Matthew sat with his arms crossed and said, "I'm not saying anything because when I do I get put down for being honest about the way I see things in here." Darcey, who rarely participated verbally, sat quietly during this conflict, looking puzzled. When called upon by Ron, she said she saw no point to all this conflict. Twyla tried to express what she regarded as her overarching concern. She reacted negatively to the entire structure of this course: "I feel pressure to talk about my private life in this group. This goes against everything I have been taught in our law and ethics course, where we have been repeatedly cautioned about keeping personal and professional boundaries separate. I feel a bind in this training experience because I think my boundaries are being violated."

As I began to help Ron engage in a postmortem exploration of the group, it became apparent that he had not explored the reactions by his students, preferring instead to "let the process unfold without interference." Ron never invited students to focus on what they wanted from their group experience and never directly addressed their worries and questions about boundaries, expectations, confidentiality, and the contours between the group experience and the larger course. Instead, Ron interpreted his students' behavior as resistance and cautioned that without more active personal engagement, they would be unprepared to function as group leaders themselves.

Discussion

Key ethical issues

The main accreditation body in counselor education, the Council for Accreditation of Counseling and Related Educational Programs (CACREP), addresses training in group work and requires programs to provide an experiential component to assist students in acquiring the skills necessary to function as effective group leaders. The CACREP accreditation standards specify that students should participate in a small group activity for a minimum of 10 clock hours over the course of one academic term. Instructors handle this small group component in many different ways, and therein lay some potential ethical issues.

The case of Ron's group class illustrated several of these ethical issues: providing informed consent to students during the orientation process prior to admission to a program; providing informed consent and preparing students for the experiential aspects of the course at the first meeting (or earlier) of a group counseling course; discussing matters of rights and responsibilities of students; exploring confidentiality concerns; clarifying how grading and evaluation will be handled; establishing appropriate boundaries and clear expectations from the beginning; establishing group norms and ground rules necessary for the effective functioning of this group course; addressing matters such as dual and multiple relationships as they apply to this course; addressing the multiple roles of the instructor; explaining ways of sharing power in a group course; and considering the competence of the instructor in teaching group courses.

Work setting

Students graduating from a counseling program will likely find themselves expected to design and facilitate groups in various work settings. Those who work in schools may find themselves asked to organize a structured group around a particular theme for children or adolescents. Those working in agency settings may find themselves expected to design a psychoeducational group, a group for adults struggling with a particular life issue, or a therapy group for people who have experienced trauma. In order to competently lead any therapy group or psychoeducational group, practitioners must have basic knowledge of group process and specific skills that are basic to competent group facilitation. They need to have had supervision as they facilitate a group, and it is crucial that they do not exceed the boundaries of their competence.

For all these reasons, it becomes important that, during graduate work, students have opportunities to learn about group dynamics from both the vantage point of membership and leadership. I strongly endorse participation in a group as part of a leader's training. Learning from books and lectures has an important role, but it has limitations as well; we learn certain skills best through experimentation and actual supervised practice. Struggling with trusting a group of peers, risking vulnerability, receiving genuine support from others, feeling a sense of cohesiveness, and experiencing confrontation all comprise vital learning experiences for future group leaders. If for no reason other than providing an understanding of what clients face in groups, I think a group experience for trainees who will lead groups is indispensable.

As a group psychotherapy instructor and leader for the past 36 years, I know that it can prove challenging to combine both didactic and experiential components in a single group course, yet I find it possible to create a climate wherein students can learn a great deal about group process and simultaneously achieve greater understanding of how they function interpersonally. But combining the didactic and experiential aspects of learning requires that faculty members address a number of ethical considerations. Professionals who lead didactic/experiential courses must manage multiple roles while fulfilling numerous responsibilities to trainees.

Reflection

I find it essential that instructors remain aware of the potential dangers inherent in multiple relationships when teaching group courses, and they must have the competence necessary to balance didactic and experiential educational components. I have ethical concerns about a faculty member such as Ron who begins teaching a group course, but who has not experienced participating as a member of a group himself and lacks adequate preparation for the task. I think that the department chair was remiss in asking him to take on the course when he did not have the education and training required to meet the task in a competent way. At the same time, Ron had an obligation to recognize the limitations of his training and decline the assignment. He might have asked for another course that he was qualified to teach.

Faculty who teach group courses often function in multiple roles: facilitator of a group, teacher, evaluator, and supervisor. At various times, instructors may teach group process concepts, lead a demonstration group in class, set up an exercise to illustrate an intervention in a group situation, and evaluate students' work. Faculty members who teach group classes often assume a supervisory role, observing trainees as they facilitate a group and giving them feedback. Ron would have done well to identify for the class the multiple roles he would strive to balance in this course. It would have proved useful for Ron to talk with his students about the rationale for his performing multiple roles in this course and address any of their concerns about his many roles. Ron also might have opened a discussion about the multiple relationships involved with participating as a member in a group with fellow students. At times, students worry about what others will think of them and how their peers may react if they make themselves known. However, as students come to know one another in a personal way, they can often identify with each other's struggle, which facilitates building a cohesive group. They develop solid relationships to use for mutual support throughout the program.

If training programs expect students to disclose personal information as a requirement, then the program or training faculty must clearly identify this requirement in its admissions and program materials. The program must make explicitly clear from the outset any expectations that students will share personal information in their courses. Students have a right to know the rationale for any kind of required personal work, and they need to be adequately prepared to involve themselves in a meaningful way in experiential learning. The code of ethics of the ACA and the APA insist that students have a right to know the specific nature of course and program requirements *before* they enter a program. [See ACA, 2005, F. 7.a., F. 7. b; See APA, 2002, 7.02, 7.04, 7.05.] Ron's program was remiss in not providing complete and accurate information regarding expectations of students by way of self-reflection and participation in experiential and personal learning.

In addition to informed consent at the time students matriculate in a program, instructors in the various courses need to inform students about matters such as the benefits and risks involved in experiential aspects of their courses. Faculty members need to clarify how students will be evaluated in the course. Ron made a crucial error in not addressing informed consent as it pertained to his group class. He made only a general comment that he expected students "to become actively engaged in significant and meaningful self-disclosure, necessary for a group to function well." He could have explained what he meant by this and talked more about how students might make decisions about ways they could involve themselves personally. Students can share some personal content in a group and at the same time retain their privacy and maintain appropriate boundaries. Ron could have stressed their right to decide what they would disclose or not disclose. He needed to inform his students that some personal topics could be more appropriately dealt with in their own individual or group therapy apart from this class group. It would have been useful for Ron to provide more information and examples of what constitutes appropriate personal participation. The classroom group is not a place to work extensively on personal problems; rather this group can help members identify areas of their lives they need to further explore in their personal therapy.

Another ethical concern relates to Ron's use of the experiential group as a part of his students' grade. There is consensus in the field of group work training that students not be graded on their functioning in an experiential group. Thus, apart from requiring that his students attend the group sessions, Ron should have separated their participation in these groups from their grade in the course. He could have based their grade solely on factors such as papers and tests. He might have used a combination of essay questions and objective tests as a basis for grading. When using subjectively graded questions (e.g., essays or term papers) he could have students identify the paper with an identification number, so he would not know the identity of the student as he read each paper. This would prevent any subtle bias from behavior in the group from creeping into the grading process.

Finally, Ron should have addressed the conflict that surfaced during the seventh session openly as it occurred. Ron had the responsibility to actively intervene to encourage members to talk more about themselves, rather than putting the focus on others. Ron's lack of training to serve as an instructor in a group course most clearly showed up with his inability to effectively address the conflict that surfaced and the negative reactions expressed by many students in the group. From my perspective, all of the comments made during the seventh session were highly relevant topics for exploration, since they all pertained to happenings within the here-and-now context of the group. Even if students were not talking about their personal concerns outside of the group, they could have greatly benefited by focusing on their personal reactions to the here-and-now themes emerging within the group. Groups become energized when the members willingly express what they are thinking and feeling as it pertains to participating in a group.

My colleagues and I have found that most serious students who are sincerely interested in qualifying professionally as group practitioners will invest themselves by participating in such groups. Our challenge as educators is to provide the best training available, keeping in mind safeguards that will prevent students from harm. If a therapeutic group is offered as a resource for the personal development of counselors, and if students are given the freedom to determine their goals and the structure of the experience, most students will be eager for and will appreciate such a resource.

Key ethical principles and standards

APA (2002): Standard 3.04 (Avoiding Harm), Standard 3.05 (Multiple Relationships), Standard 7 (Education and Training), and Standard 3.10 (Informed Consent). ACA (2005): Standard F.7 (Student Welfare: Orientation and Self-Growth Experiences).

REFERENCES AND FURTHER READING

American Counseling Association (2005). *Code of ethics.* Alexandria, VA: Author.
American Psychological Association (2002). Ethical principles of psychologists and code of conduct. *American Psychologist, 57,* 1060–1073.
Association for Specialists in Group Work. (March, 2004). Special issue on teaching group work. *The Journal of Specialists in Group Work, 29,* 1–154.
Corey, M., Corey, G., & Corey, C. (2010). *Groups: Process and practice* (8th ed.). Belmont, CA: Brooks/Cole, Cengage Learning.

Council for Accreditation of Counseling and Related Educational Programs (2009). *CACREP: The 2009 standards.* Alexandria, VA: Author.

DeLucia-Waack, J. L., Gerrity, D. A., Kalodner, C. R., & Riva, M. T. (Eds.). (2004). *Handbook of group counseling and psychotherapy.* Thousand Oaks, CA: Sage Publications.

33

So, How *Exactly* Did You Get Interested in Eating Disorders? Confronting a Colleague's Unhealthy Behaviors

Jennifer L. Derenne[1]

Morgan caught my eye as the ritual began. Half a turkey sandwich, no cheese or condiments. A Ziploc bag of carefully portioned unsalted pretzels. A can of V8 juice. A Diet Coke. A month after beginning work on the unit, I could recite the contents of Lauren's lunch from memory. Because we held team rounds over the noon hour, I had a pretty good sense of the types of foods my colleagues favored. Jim ate whatever was on special that day in the cafeteria, Morgan usually brought specialty vegan meals from Whole Foods, and as much as I tried to pack a lunch each morning, I often ended up spending outrageous amounts of money on foods that I could have easily brought from home.

When you work with eating disorders, food is the center of everything. Our break room was often filled with specialty chocolates and other treats. Talking incessantly about self-deprivation can bring out the hedonist in just about anyone. So it wasn't

---

[1] The author would like to acknowledge the tremendously helpful editorial assistance of Dr. Laura Roberts in the preparation of this manuscript.

terribly surprising to me that we all eagerly attacked our lunches each day as we prepared to discuss the progress of our patients.

However, Lauren was a bit different. A registered dietitian, she was responsible for determining the caloric needs and meal plans for each of the young women under our care. Young and attractive, she was also quite thin and appeared to be losing weight. Each day, she waited until fifteen minutes had passed before opening her lunch bag. She carefully removed each item and set it on the table. Five minutes later, she slowly began to nibble at her sandwich. Lauren made sure to finish one item before starting the next. Sandwich, then pretzels, then juice. She finished her meal precisely 45 minutes after the first bite, seemingly hours after the rest of us were done eating. Before and after work, she headed to the gym for hour-long running sessions.

Eating disorders are fairly common, and the field does sometimes draw individuals who have struggled with anorexia or bulimia themselves at some point. Some may still have low-level disordered eating behaviors. Of course, this occurs commonly in many other areas of medicine; many health care professionals have also had personal battles with depression, anxiety, cancer, or other disorders. All of us have experienced adversity and hardship at some point in our lives. However, therapists generally agree that we should not assume that a patient/client's experience in a given situation will mirror our own. The pros and cons of disclosing one's personal eating disorder history are hotly debated at academic meetings and through listserv entries. Some therapists believe that personal disclosure of one's struggle with an eating disorder can prove very powerful and beneficial in therapy.

As a young, female therapist who works predominantly with children and adolescents, I am asked personal questions quite frequently. Parents often want to know how long I've been in practice, where I was educated, and whether I am married or have children of my own. One look at the diplomas on my office wall (or a quick trip to www.google.com) tells them the location and dates of my medical school and residency training. I do believe that patients should feel confident that their clinician has the appropriate credentials to provide the care they need. But my age, marital, and reproductive status really have little to do with my ability to treat children. Often, when people ask if I have children of my own, I find that people are really asking me whether I will be able to understand them and their experience.

So it should come as no surprise to learn that I am quite frequently asked whether I have struggled with an eating disorder. Years of training in psychodynamic psychotherapy have taught me that it is generally best to explore the meaning of the question (i.e., "What do you imagine my experience has been? What would it be like for you if I had struggled with an eating disorder?").

I'll admit that I haven't always felt thrilled with their responses, such as the time a new patient's mother looked me up and down before replying, "Well, you clearly don't have one *now*. . ." But even after we've discussed the transference issues, some patients still want to *know*. So I tell them, quite honestly, that while I have never experienced an eating disorder, I *have* had the experience of feeling unhappy with myself at times. The reality is that every individual's struggle is different, and having experienced an eating disorder myself would not necessarily help me understand their situation any better. While I may not have shared their exact experience, I tell them I will do my best to understand the issues that led to their symptoms. To be truthful, if I had struggled with an eating disorder, I'm not sure I would disclose it to my patients, as I do believe it is a boundary crossing that introduces some risks in the therapy.

They say that "When you're a hammer, everything looks like a nail." When you are surrounded by patients struggling with eating disorders, it can be tempting to attribute every self-deprecating comment or concern about the caloric content of a piece of pie to a budding eating disorder. Unfortunately, it has become culturally normal to worry about body shape and weight. All in all, most people who obsess about their weight do not have a diagnosable eating disorder. Not all people who work in the eating disorders field have eating disorders. However, sometimes there *are* nails lying around.

Lauren had become quite the topic of conversation around the unit, and although I was new to the team, I knew that the concerns would need addressing sooner rather than later. In this case, we were not debating the ethics of personal disclosure in eating disorders treatment. We felt concerned about a colleague with an active eating disorder that potentially had implications for the care of all of our patients. Team members worried about her. Patients commented on her noticeably gaunt figure, and families began to wonder aloud how we could trust an anorexic dietitian to determine their daughter's meal plan. We all joked that we couldn't win when it came to our own weight. Our patients were acutely aware of any fluctuations. Jim, a very attractive and fit man in his early forties, once admitted that he went home and ran seven miles after Molly told him he had a "beer belly" during group. Patients didn't want to work with anyone who could be considered overweight because they feared that following that person's recommendations would make them fat. Those who were deemed too thin were accused of having an eating disorder. We became used to discussing their concerns and spoke at length about the importance of trusting the treatment team's recommendations. But when patients on the unit commented on Lauren's weight and shape, we could easily see why.

One afternoon, Dana, a quiet 16-year-old with severe anorexia, burst into tears when Lauren increased her meal plan due to inadequate weight gain.

"This isn't fair! I know you don't eat that much! Why are you allowed to be so skinny? You just want to make us all fat!" The rest of the young women, who usually averted their eyes at any sign of conflict, nodded knowingly as Dana stomped off toward her room. Later that day, they circulated a petition requesting that Lauren be admitted to the unit as a patient herself.

I found myself questioning whether I should approach Lauren. I felt worried, and I cared about her health, but was it really my place to inquire about a medical condition? I was new to the team, and a confrontation could prove awkward, even if done gently and in a supportive manner. I wanted to consult with my colleagues, but worried that I could be viewed as gossiping. What if I were wrong? So one day following the after-lunch process group, I summoned all of my courage, followed her into her office, and shut the door. "I'm worried about you," I began. For a second, Lauren looked as though she might cry, but then she clenched her jaw and glared at me. "What for?" she asked. Lauren went on to explain that she had been ill with the flu and had been having some stomach issues, but that she felt fine. She was tired of everyone making a big deal out of her weight. "We tell our patients that every body is different, and that they shouldn't fixate so much on weight. Why is everyone so concerned about me? I've always been thin. I don't have an eating disorder!"

I wasn't sure what to say. In a purely therapeutic relationship, I wouldn't have gotten rattled so easily. In fact, Lauren's response did not seem much different from that of many of my own patients. But things definitely do become more complicated when you are talking to a colleague. While I did encourage her to have a medical check-up, I found myself backing down very quickly. Wanting to believe her, I felt pulled to explain away all of the red flags that I knew pointed toward a diagnosis of anorexia nervosa.

Despite wanting to believe there was nothing wrong, I started looking at the nutrition notes on our mutual patients to make sure Lauren had calculated their caloric needs correctly. I listened even more attentively during rounds to make sure that patient care was not being compromised. I worried that malnutrition might impair her ability to make medical decisions, and I wondered if I might need to report her as an impaired clinician. Item 17 of the code of ethics of the American Dietetic Association states, "The dietetics practitioner withdraws from professional practice under the following circumstances: a. The dietetics practitioner has engaged in any substance abuse that could affect his/her practice; b. The dietetics practitioner has been adjudged by a court to be mentally incompetent; c. *The dietetics practitioner has an emotional or mental disability that affects his/her practice in a manner that could harm the client or others.*"

Fortunately, her patient care and documentation seemed in impeccable order. It was interesting that she could make good decisions regarding meal planning for others, but seemed to have difficulty believing that the principles of nutrition also applied to her. I became a bit concerned when Lauren argued during rounds that we should consider lowering Dana's goal weight range, but she let the issue drop almost immediately when other team members questioned her rationale. Being careful to protect Lauren's identity, I talked with my own supervisor about my concerns. We agreed that because the weight loss could potentially affect patient care, the concerns warranted formal assessment and documentation. When I spoke with our medical director, I felt relieved to know that others had expressed concern as well, he had made contact with the dietetics licensing board, and that a plan was being put into place.

After a couple of days, the entire team met to discuss how best to proceed given our concerns. The team was somewhat divided on what to do. There were those who felt that Lauren, as an adult capable of making her own decisions, should have her autonomy respected. Others believed she should not be allowed to work on an eating disorder unit at all. Despite the fact that we all wanted to support Lauren emotionally, the fact remained that her weight loss and inability to stabilize her weight had a negative impact on the unit's therapeutic milieu. The drama surrounding Lauren's health distracted our patients and the staff from focusing on the recovery process. The medical director met with Lauren and insisted that she take some time off to address her medical concerns. In a very supportive manner, he empathized with her concern over all of the speculation about her health status. Importantly, he did not engage with her in a debate about whether or not she indeed had an eating disorder. He made it clear that Lauren could return to work once she had sought medical care and was more stable.

Unfortunately, Lauren chose to resign her position and did not return calls or email from those of us who tried to check in with her to see how she was doing. One of the other team members heard that she later took a job with an obesity clinic, but it was unclear whether she had sought her own treatment.

Discussion

Key ethical issues

This case illustrates a number of ethical issues: beneficence and nonmaleficence, autonomy and privacy, professional boundaries, and the problem of overlapping roles. The problem of the potentially impaired (or "at risk") clinician incorporates a number of these ethical tensions. The definition of impairment is the inability to provide clinical care with reasonable skill and safety due to physical or mental illness or substance abuse.

Clinicians have a responsibility to "do good" or "to do no harm" when caring for patients. Lauren's case was not clear-cut; those of us in the eating disorder field felt fairly confident that she had anorexia nervosa, but it was possible that her symptoms had an alternate explanation. Despite the disruption on the unit, her work seemed clinically appropriate. However, most would agree that an addiction specialist who actively abused substances should not be allowed to practice (even if he or she were treating patients appropriately), due to concerns about patient safety. While Lauren's clinical judgment appeared sound, the concern remained that malnutrition might adversely affect cognition, which could impair judgment. Further, distorted body image and excessive comparing of weight and shape could potentially lead Lauren to make inappropriate decisions regarding the care of her patients. In addition, widespread concern about her weight loss on the part of patients and fellow staff members (whether or not it was related to an eating disorder) proved distracting from the active treatment process and therefore had a significant adverse affect on patient care.

Another important theme in this case relates to the issues of privacy (the right to not have others intrude on one's body or mind) and autonomy (self-determination). One might argue that, as a legally competent adult, Lauren has the right to make medical decisions for herself that others might not find appropriate. However, in this work setting, disordered eating has numerous potential negative effects for patient care, and the issue requires addressing. Privacy is a right, while confidentiality is a privilege. When a concern about potential clinician impairment arises, the need for safety outweighs the privilege of confidentiality.

The ethical issue of professional boundaries in clinical work also emerges in this case. Boundaries are important in that they allow the therapeutic relationship to feel safe and predictable. Self-disclosure does impact on transferential issues in psychotherapy, no matter what modality is being used. Therefore, the therapist needs to remain very thoughtful about the potential therapeutic effects, both positive and negative, of disclosing personal information, and he or she should examine whether the disclosure is truly therapeutic or whether it gratifies the therapist's own interests. At the extreme, inability to maintain boundaries may suggest evidence of clinician impairment. While many health care providers have the choice of whether or not to self-disclose, Lauren was forced to publicly entertain the question of whether or not she currently suffered from an eating disorder. Behaviors can be kept private, but dramatic weight loss to the point of emaciation is difficult to hide. Public knowledge of her own current eating disorder would most certainly impact her work with patients and her professional relationships with colleagues, who might change their referral patterns based on knowledge of her illness. The problem of overlapping roles arose in relation to the fact that Lauren was practicing on a unit with other eating disorder professionals who also stood in the position of trying to determine whether she met criteria for an eating disorder.

Work setting

This case raises the importance of managing group dynamics and the potential conflict of overlapping roles in the work setting . The multidisciplinary team members on the eating disorder unit provide care in a highly acute setting, which can bring out intense group dynamics. In spite of the focus on working together as a team, there *are* power differentials between professionals. Reality dictates that the MDs on the unit carry more responsibility than do the dietitians. Members of the team may have blind spots in their approach to patient care based on both professional training and personal experiences. For example, primary care physicians may tend to think about eating disorders in a way that differs from the dietitians or mental health professionals. No matter what the discipline, every professional has personality traits that affect his or her ability to interact with both colleagues and patients in the work setting. Finally, personal experiences or interactions with friends and family members affected by the illness may also shape one's approach to patients. Team decision-making can become clouded by any of these variables. For this reason, an ethically robust approach to care would involve transparency around the ways in which decisions are made, with regard to both patient care and the handling of a situation in which a health care professional seems "at risk."

The problem of overlapping roles also becomes evident in the discussion of the work setting. Health care professionals are not immune to illness. However, being ill does not necessarily mean that one has become impaired. Clinicians have a responsibility to limit their practice when a medical condition negatively affects their ability to provide safe care, and colleagues who become aware of impaired practicing clinicians have an obligation to report such individuals to the appropriate licensing board. Lauren was in a unique position—she was losing weight and appeared to exhibit the cardinal symptoms of an eating disorder while working on an eating disorder unit and caring for individuals struggling with severe eating disorders. While she showed occasional glimpses of concerning behaviors, her ability to provide care was not clearly impaired. Nonetheless, her colleagues found ourselves in the difficult position of needing to confront a coworker about the very behaviors that we treated in patients on a daily basis.

Mental health professionals deal with difficult patient interactions on a daily basis, and therapists receive special training in dealing with transference and countertransference issues. Talking with a colleague about clinical concerns can become more difficult for a number of reasons. Even when they fall ill, our colleagues are *not* our patients; they are our coworkers, and often, our friends. Knowing someone in a nonclinical capacity makes it nearly impossible to remain objective about concerning behavior. We may feel pulled to make excuses or explain away issues we would otherwise address. As such, it generally proves best to respect the boundaries of the work relationship and rely on independent clinicians to make clinical decisions.

Reflection

The skills of the ethical clinician have been described by Roberts as: the ability to identify the ethical features of a patient's care; see how one's own experiences, attitudes, and knowledge shape the care of the patient; identify and work within one's scope of clinical competence; anticipate ethically risky situations; gather additional information and seek consultation to clarify and resolve the conflict; and enact a plan for conflict resolution while building ethical safeguards into the patient care situation.

In order to think through the ethical dilemmas in this situation, it was important for me to be able to bring my concerns to an off-site supervisor. This also enabled me to reflect on the ways in which my own experiences shaped my reactions to Lauren and the situation overall. Since I felt concerned about the potential for an adverse patient care outcome, I made it a point to closely observe Lauren's work and review her documentation, and I did some research into the code of ethics for registered dietitians. Because my supervisor did not know Lauren and was not familiar with her work or reputation, we were able to explore my reactions to her in a more objective way. While my colleagues on the unit had a lot of experience and provided very helpful consultation for my work with eating disorder patients, it did not feel appropriate to discuss Lauren with them. However, once I felt confident that the issues warranted more formal attention, I didn't hesitate to talk with Lauren's supervisor, who was also the medical director of the unit.

Despite the fact that events did not go as well as I would have hoped, I felt glad that I chose to talk with Lauren directly about my concerns. It did not seem fair to discuss the situation behind her back without letting her know I had become concerned. I worried that she would feel angry with me, and she did at the time. Over the long term, though, I hoped that she would appreciate that I cared enough to risk her anger.

In retrospect, it would probably have been helpful to have been more thoughtful about how to broach my concerns with Lauren. Had I been more prepared, I may have more ably articulated my concerns, which might have persuaded Lauren to seek treatment faster. Because I felt concerned about the potential for impaired clinical decision-making, I probably should have involved unit leaders immediately, rather than attempting to talk to Lauren on my own. As with most ethically complex situations, there was not one "right" way to manage this situation. Fortunately, the appropriate people were alerted relatively quickly, and the situation was handled as empathically and discretely as possible.

Key ethical principles and standards

American Psychiatric Association (2008): The Principles of Medical Ethics With Annotations Especially Applicable to Psychiatry. *Section 2:* A physician shall uphold the standards of professionalism, be honest in all professional interactions, and strive to report physicians deficient in character or competence, or engaging in fraud or deception, to appropriate entities. *Section 4:* A physician shall respect the rights of patients, colleagues, and other health professionals, and shall safeguard patient confidences and privacy within the constraints of the law. *Section 8:* A physician shall, while caring for a patient, regard responsibility to the patient as paramount.

REFERENCES AND FURTHER READING

Giordano, S. (2007). *Understanding eating disorders: Conceptual and ethical issues in the treatment of anorexia and bulimia nervosa.* New York: Oxford.

Petrucelli, J. (2007). When a body meets a body: The impact of the therapist's body on eating-disordered patients. In Anderson F. S. (Ed.), *Bodies in treatment: The unspoken dimension* (pp. 237–253). New York: The Analytic Press/Taylor & Francis.

Lowell, M. A., & Meader, L. L. (2005). My body, your body: Speaking the unspoken between the thin therapist and the eating-disordered patient. *Clinical Social Work Journal, 33,* 241–257.

Roberts, L. W., & Dyer, A. R. (2004). Concise guide to ethics in mental health care. Washington DC: American Psychiatric Association.

34

Knocked Off Kilter: Supervising in the Wake of Sexual Boundary Violations

Janet T. Thomas

As I opened the door into the waiting room, my new supervisee leaped from his chair smiling and bounded into my office before I finished introducing myself. I reached out to greet him and was surprised when he lifted my hand as if to kiss it, then bowed and said, "It is an honor to meet you." Startled, I withdrew my hand and invited him to sit on the couch. He walked to my desk and began to slide the chair across the room, stating, "This one looks like more fun." I directed him to return the desk chair and choose the couch or another available chair. With a deep sigh and a wounded look, he shoved the chair in the direction of desk, dropped onto the couch, and apologized effusively. His tone vacillated between irritation and deference. He then explained how *he* allowed his clients to choose where to sit, noting that perhaps I was unaware of research supporting the efficacy of "client choice." He promised to fax me a related article. This eventful 60 seconds marked the beginning of my 18-month supervision of Dr. More.

Dr. More, a Caucasian man who appeared to be in his 60s, had recently left his job as an academic advisor in a small, rural community college. Following two complaints from student-advisees, his licensing board required him to undergo a mental health assessment. This evaluation resulted in several recommendations, including a period of supervision—Dr. More then contacted me. The licensing board concluded that Dr. More had violated the sexual boundaries of both complainants. One woman alleged "inappropriate touch." She reported, for example, that on two occasions, he had embraced her tightly as she got up to leave his office. Another time, she said he had lifted her necklace to admire it and, in the process, touched her breast. And, despite her squirming and moving away to convey her discomfort, she said Dr. More often massaged her neck as they sat looking at his computer screen during advising sessions.

A second complainant, a freshman, reported that she met with Dr. More to discuss her concern that she might have a learning disability. Before he could help her, Dr. More allegedly asked her to complete an "intake questionnaire," which included questions not only about her academic background but also about her personal life, including her sexual habits and history. When she questioned him about whether she really needed to respond to those items, Dr. More told her he practiced "holistic psychology" and could be most helpful if he had "the big picture."

These behaviors clearly represented departures from practice standards, and I wondered just how a psychologist could have come to believe them legitimate. Dr. More's personal and professional history, I would learn, had set him squarely on a trajectory for the boundary difficulties that developed.

Our initial meeting began with informed consent. I highlighted points from the materials I had sent him, emphasizing confidentiality and its limitations. I explained the fees and cancellation policy, accessibility between appointments, and my expectations of him. I asked that he agree, as a condition of supervision, keep me apprised about his clinical work and tell me immediately should any of the following occur:

- impasse or conflict with a client
- allegations of unethical behavior
- suicidal thoughts, gestures, or attempts by clients
- threats of violence or violent behavior
- possible mandated reporting triggers (e.g., suspicion of abuse of a child or vulnerable adult)
- departures or contemplated departures from standard practice
- boundary challenges by clients (gifts, requests for disclosure, or favors)
- personal problems that might compromise professional objectivity.

Finally, I reviewed other possible risks and benefits associated with supervision. Dr. More signed a release authorizing my communication with the licensing board, a fee agreement, and an agreement to participate in supervision in light of these policies.

At several points in the process, Dr. More interrupted and suggested we forgo the discussion because, as a professional, he already knew the rules. Further, he was paying for the time and felt he should have input into how it was spent. I explained that the informed consent process was an ethically required part of any new professional relationship and that I wanted to ensure his understanding of all the parameters before we began. He squinted, folded his arms across his chest, sat back on the couch, and said, "Fine." I continued.

I asked Dr. More to summarize his career as a way to begin the process of identifying factors that contributed to his violations. He completed his doctorate in the late 1960s and subsequently enrolled in a training program focused on innovative forms of psychotherapy. After a few sessions of psychotherapy with the program's director, he realized he had grown up in a "sexually repressive" family. The director encouraged him to attend the weekend sexuality seminar that he facilitated with his wife, a former student in the program. Dr. More described the seminar as "life changing," adding that it led to the discovery of his desire to specialize in helping others find joy in fully embracing their sexuality. As part of his training, he facilitated psychoeducational sexuality groups for undergraduate students, one of whom he began dating and eventually married.

Dr. More later moved to the Midwest, where he searched unsuccessfully for full-time work as a psychotherapist; he ultimately settled for a teaching position. Hoping to return someday to clinical work, he became one of the first in his state to get a license as a psychologist in the mid-1970s. Although not psychotherapy, he said that teaching gave him opportunities to "informally" counsel students when they seemed distressed. He also enjoyed reading the journal entries and sexual histories he assigned. Dr. More reported that students in his history of psychology course especially appreciated his slide show of himself in earlier years, accompanied by his favorite music and poetry from the 1960s.

Unfortunately, he found his department chair was "rigid and controlling." Dr. More claimed that his chair repeatedly tried to interfere with his academic freedom by dictating how he could teach. After years of episodic conflicts, she confronted him with "a few bad course evals from some uptight students" who didn't appreciate the unique opportunities he offered. She subsequently assigned him to work in the academic advising center.

Although initially angry, Dr. More considered that this new assignment might give him some longed-for autonomy and a chance to use his clinical skills. All went well for more than a year, he said, until the "overly controlling" father of one of his advisees complained to the college that Dr. More was "coming on" to his daughter. The next day, he found himself summoned to a meeting with the department chair, the dean, and the director of human resources. Following an "unpleasant discussion" with them, he decided that perhaps the time had come to retire from the college. Shortly thereafter, a colleague asked Dr. More to join the staff of a local private clinic. Although a bit apprehensive given that he had not actually done any "formal" counseling in 30 years, he was eager to give it a try. He practiced there about three months when he was notified about the board complaint.

At the conclusion of our first meeting, I asked Dr. More about his retrospective insights. He said he knew he had "made mistakes" and that he had done wrong, but he could not elaborate beyond saying he felt sorry that he had "apparently offended somebody." He just wanted to do whatever I needed him to do to keep his license.

Throughout the months that followed, we passed many milestones—both in Dr. More's clinical work and in the supervision. Finding myself challenged in unprecedented ways by his behavior and revelations, I agonized over the often-conflicting ethical responsibilities I carried as I attempted to balance the best interests of Dr. More, his clients, the profession, and the board. My legal liability for his actions weighed heavily. For his part, Dr. More had moments of anger, indignation, remorse, and shame. In the end, he reached a difficult, but I believe sound, decision—one that I came to admire.

Course of supervision

The primary goal of the supervision focused on helping Dr. More modify his practice to reflect ethical and practice standards, particularly with respect to boundaries. It soon became clear, however, that he also lacked current understanding of standards for record keeping, informed consent, and client privacy. At one point, he off-handedly remarked about how much things had changed since he last read a journal—in graduate school. In the wake of that revelation, I became further alarmed to learn that he belonged to no professional associations and had not seen a professional newsletter in years.

I assigned him to revise his practice forms, read related publications, and present electronic recordings of psychotherapy sessions. I reviewed all of his records, and together we watched and discussed video vignettes on professional boundaries. To address competency deficits, I recommended he attend various clinical skill-building workshops. I highlighted parallels between current clinical challenges and problems that led to the complaints, and ultimately, Dr. More began to note these connections as well.

Recognizing the need for further reconnaissance, I arranged to visit Dr. More's work site. I asked to see the waiting area, his office, where he kept records, and so forth. The first thing I noticed upon entering the office was what appeared to be a water bowl on the floor. Dr. More indicated that he usually had his dog with him, adding that all of his clients loved her. I noticed a couple of files on the desk, the names visible from the door. He had a large family photo displayed next to his diploma, political buttons adorning the bulletin board, and a wall calendar featuring picturesque beaches and women in swimwear hanging over his desk. With the door closed, I could clearly hear the waiting room radio, evidencing inadequate soundproofing. I did not know where to begin.

Not surprisingly, the boundary confusion evident in his teaching and advising reverberated in his clinical work. My persistent inquires about any hint of nonstandard practice uncovered numerous unconventional practices, such as his plans to send his family's holiday card to clients, provide marital counseling to his cousin, and shop at his client's garage sale. Similar challenges emerged in the supervision. At times, Dr. More seemed intent on supervising me, suggesting modifications to my policies and practices. At other times, his behavior became more characteristic of a client: He would abruptly shift to expressing strong emotions, blurting out highly personal information. It also was not uncommon for Dr. More to behave like a psychotherapist, making personal inquiries and presumptive comments about my well-being.

In short, I found myself frequently invited to replicate the dynamics so familiar to him by diverging from my role as supervisor and becoming his supervisee, psychotherapist, client, colleague, or friend. These challenges required constant vigilance to ensure that I gave consistent messages about the nature of our relationship, my expectations of him, and about what he could expect of me. More than once, I unconsciously stepped into one of these other roles and had to work hard to regain my balance.

I often wondered whether supervision would prove sufficient to remedy the wide range of competence deficits so evident in Dr. More's work. With frequent assistance from my peer consultation group, I pondered whether Dr. More was qualified to practice, whether the supervision could adequately address his ever-emerging problems, and whether I felt willing to continue supervising him.

Despite a slow start and many setbacks, Dr. More's perspective on the complaint cases did evolve. Initially, he had tried to convince me that his unique approach to students was beneficial. He felt confident they appreciated his physical affection and willingness to listen to their problems. Together, we reexamined these assumptions using the strategies described above. Dr. More gradually began to entertain the possibility that he may have misread social cues, made some irrelevant and offensive inquiries, invaded students' privacy, and diverged from his assigned role. We considered his role models. His mentor had married one of his students and engaged in multiple roles with Dr. More, functioning simultaneously as his psychotherapist, employer, supervisor, and friend. Although this behavior was probably not inconsistent with the zeitgeist of the late 1960s, Dr. More's lack of subsequent clinical experience and related continuing education, along with years of professional isolation, had left that model intact and unchallenged.

One theme resonating throughout the supervision involved Dr. More's difficulty in distinguishing his own needs from those of his students and clients, and his difficulty determining which of those needs would be appropriately addressed in the context of a professional relationship. Because he enjoyed reminiscing about his history, exploring his sexuality, expressing physical affection, and working in the company of his dog, he assumed his students and clients shared these desires and that he should gratify them. Examining the elements of his job description and, more generally, his role as a psychologist, represented a new concept to him. Over time, he considered these issues, identified common themes in his struggles, and made significant modifications in his problematic practices. Dr. More's ability to generalize his learning to novel situations, though variable, steadily improved.

In light of the myriad challenges facing Dr. More, I often wondered whether he had considered relinquishing his license and commencing with his retirement. Near the end of the supervision, I decided to raise that issue. I commented on his tenacity in the face of so many obstacles. He became tearful as he told me, "Being a psychologist is who I am. My wife and kids are proud of me. When I die, I want to know that I ended my career as a member in good standing of my profession."

Dr. More completed the supervision, and five months later, when his license was due to expire, he notified the board that he did not intend to renew it. Shortly thereafter, I received a note from Dr. More. He said he had reached the conclusion that the profession had evolved so much that he did not want to continue to do all of what it would take to stay current with the changes. Yet he felt good about having completed the supervision and other requirements and was proud to be fully licensed once again. Enclosed with this note he included a copy of a letter to colleagues announcing his retirement.

Discussion

Key ethical issues

Providing board-ordered supervision requires careful attention to ethical issues on several levels: the supervisee's past ethical violations, the ethical issues arising in his or her concurrent practice, and those ethical challenges facing the supervisor. The most salient issues in this case—evident in all three levels—pertained to boundaries, informed consent, confidentiality, and competence.

Dr. More's concept of boundaries in professional relationships grew from his education, training, and supervision acquired some three decades earlier when practice standards differed markedly. As described, he had related difficulties in his past and concurrent work, as well as in the supervisory relationship.

Informed consent and confidentiality have special application to any board-ordered supervision. Supervisors must inform supervisees about risks and benefits, including the limits on their privacy. For example, supervisors typically have the responsibility of preparing periodic evaluative reports for the licensing board and for notifying the board of imminent concerns about the welfare of the supervisee's clients. If the supervisee shares something personal, the supervisor may or may not disclose that information in a report, depending on its perceived relevance. Any information provided to the board by the supervisor may ultimately affect the supervisee's licensure status in ways that may or may not prove favorable. Filing a criminal complaint or civil suit may result in discovery of supervision reports that may be ordered into evidence and used to the supervisee's advantage or detriment. Clearly, in addition to the limitations to privacy, supervisees must have full information about any aspects of the supervision that might reasonably be expected to influence their decisions about whether and how to participate.

Competency also has multiple levels of relevance. First, I needed to continually assess whether my supervisee had adequate skills to provide the services and treat the types of clients he accepted. Second, I, as the supervisor, had to ensure that I maintained competence in these areas of practice. Finally, I needed to have adequate education, training, and experience in general supervision, as well as specialized knowledge of the unique challenges of board-ordered supervision.

Although every area of psychological practice requires minimum skills, competency is a goal requiring sustained effort. This quest for competence represents a dynamic ideal to which we aspire and continually strive.

This supervisee had not kept current with professional literature or obtained relevant training. For me, the complexity, degree of responsibility, and legal liability required that I regularly review relevant literature, reflect on and critically evaluate my work, and obtain consultation from competent colleagues willing to challenge my perspectives and decisions.

Work setting

I supervised Dr. More in an off-site independent practice. Therefore, he either had to conceal the identities of his clients or seek client authorization to disclose identifying information. The recording of sessions also required specific client authorization. Further, supervising from an off-site location requires creative strategies to ensure adequate oversight. Thorough review of practice forms, treatment and administrative records (redacted if necessary), and electronic recordings often becomes necessary for monitoring an individual's practice. Site visits can also provide important information that one would not otherwise have available. When the work site has an administrative supervisor, authorizations allowing communication between supervisors becomes necessary to coordinate supervision.

Another way in which supervision in a private, independent setting differs from typical supervision flows from the fact that the supervisee generally selects (with board approval), hires, and pays the supervisor. Conversely, when supervision occurs as part of an internship, practicum, or employment arrangement, the supervisor is assigned by the organization, and no fee comes from the supervisee. Independent supervisors must remain aware of the potential influence of hiring by supervisees and ensure that their business interests do not corrupt their objectivity in making supervisory decisions.

Reflection

Supervising colleagues whose behavior has harmed clients and compromised the public trust in our profession has significant potential for countertransference. My experience with Dr. More was no exception. I found the work challenging, educational, and humbling. There were many moments in which I contemplated terminating the supervision, and I consulted with trusted colleagues about whether and how to do this. When I realized how far out of line he had stepped, I had to ask myself whether my work would prove adequate and whether the overarching goal of the supervision, helping him meet current practice standards, was realistic. I lacked the authority to require other remedial strategies (e.g., graduate course work) but could only inform the board of my concerns.

Throughout the supervision, I experienced a range of feelings and reactions that I needed to contain and examine with an eye to distilling what might inform rather than contaminate the work. I had moments of frustration when the supervision seemed futile. At times, I felt angry at or embarrassed by his behavior. Other times I felt sympathetic, protective, or even worried about him. Occasionally, I remembered one of my own clients who had left angry or dissatisfied. I thought of mistakes I had made over the years and of cases that, with hindsight, I would have handled differently.

It was important for me to acknowledge these responses, to process them in my own consultation when necessary, and to ensure that I did not allow them to compromise my objectivity and effectiveness or distract me from my primary responsibilities: to guard the welfare of my supervisee's clients, assist in his rehabilitation, provide a service for the licensing board, and serve as a gatekeeper for the profession of psychology.

Key ethical principles and standards

APA (2002): Principle A (Beneficence and Nonmalfiecence), Principle B (Fidelity and Responsibility), Standard 2.01 (Boundaries of Competence), Standard 3.05 (Multiple Relationships), Standard 3.10 (Informed Consent), 4.02 (Discussing the Limits of Confidentiality), Standard 4.10 (Maintaining Confidentiality).

REFERENCES AND FURTHER READING

Celenza, A. (2007). *Sexual boundary violations: Therapeutic, supervisory, and academic contexts*. Lanham, MD: Jason Aronson.

Falvey, J. E. (2002). *Managing clinical supervision: Ethical practice and legal risk management*. Pacific Grove, CA: Brooks/Cole-Thomson Learning.

Thomas, J. T. (2005). Licensing board complaints: Minimizing the impact on the psychologist's defense and clinical practice. *Professional Psychology: Research and Practice, 36*, 426–433.

Thomas, J. T. (2007). Informed consent through contracting for supervision: Minimizing risks, enhancing benefits. *Professional Psychology: Research and Practice, 38*, 221–231.

Thomas, J. T. (in press). The ethics of supervision and consultation: Practical guidance for mental health professionals. Washington, DC: American Psychological Association.

PART VIII

Religious Concerns and Settings

35

Of Course It's Confidential—Only the Community Knows: Mental Health Services With the Old Order Amish

James A. Cates[1]

The hiss of white gas lanterns served as a backdrop to the steady murmur of conversation in the crowded basement. Seated on benches normally used in the Sunday morning service, 46 members of my client's Old Order Amish church waited expectantly, women to my left, men to my right. The bishop gave a nod, and with heart pounding, I said, "Good evening. My name is Jim, and I'm a counselor working with John and Anna."

My work with the Old Order Amish had not prepared me for the ethical dilemmas posed by this outwardly quiet couple. Together thirteen years, John began married life with a solid future as a carpenter in a small shop, crafting cabinets for the tourist trade. Prepping his buggy for the ride home one evening after work, an unfortunate blow from a horse's hoof caught him in the right forehead. Unconscious for several days, he emerged with amnesia for the event, impaired fine motor skills, and an impulsivity and ease to anger that had not existed before the accident.

---

[1] The author would like to acknowledge Chris Weber, LMHC, clinical director of the Amish Youth Vision Project, Inc., an advocate and keen ethicist for the Amish in his care.

Still, it was not the injury per se that led me to counsel John and Anna. The community adjusted to his disability as best it could, providing financial and emotional support to the family. And yet a darker side to John's personality change had begun to emerge.

Beginning several months after his return from the hospital, John began sexually molesting his two young daughters. The abuse continued for some time before discovery; one child, attending public school, told a teacher, and Child Protective Services intervened. The standard service protocol for an adult male sex offender came into play.

Unfortunately, the protocol did not consider John's Amish background. A primary focus was intensive group treatment; in the group available, John was the only Amish client. The presence of those denying their offense and requiring confrontation, the use of obscene, profane, and sacrilegious language, and the multiplicity of spiritual beliefs represented were discomfiting at best and counterproductive at worst in the effort to provide effective intervention. The program also isolated John from his community. Providers cast a suspicious eye on the request that his bishop be apprised of his progress and that his ministers attend a treatment team meeting. Rapidly, it became clear that he would not benefit from this typical approach.

As a psychologist familiar with both the Amish and sex offender treatment, I was asked to assume John's counseling. Some immediate dilemmas required addressing: his relative lack of supervision in the community and my responsibility for his care; the efficacy of sex offender treatment with a man who could quite conceivably—given the theological views of some Amish—parse partial blame to his older daughter in particular and receive community support in so doing; the sequelae of a closed head injury, with unknown permanent impairments in judgment; and the prejudice against counselors that exists as a frequent undercurrent in the Amish community.

Nevertheless, based on the options available, my intervention with John seemed the closest to an ethically appropriate response. Due to the expense of transportation to my office, I agreed to meet with him in the home; his wife Anna normally participated in these sessions as well.

To my relief, I found John willing to accept full responsibility for his actions. He did not seek to deflect responsibility to the victim, as sometimes occurs, and no apparent support for any such deflection surfaced from the community: one cultural hurdle crossed! He also appeared less impulsive and more emotionally stable than I had been led to believe, although traces of the injury at times became discernable in his rash statements or actions and irritable outbursts.

As we met week after week around their kitchen table, sessions continued to go well. I felt comfortable in my niche, although one nagging doubt pushed at the back of my mind. It would be important at some point to visit with John's bishop, the ultimate temporal authority in his church and his life. Before I could raise this possibility, however, Anna prodded me into action.

"The bishop doesn't understand," she said. "And the ministers don't either. They keep coming here and trying to help, but all they do is make us feel as if we're outcasts. Would you talk to them?" With further conversation, I learned that the sense of ostracism had actually begun with John's head injury and worsened considerably following the revelation of his sexual offending and its report to the authorities. Church leaders appeared unsure how to respond to this problem.

Several weeks and multiple voice mails later, the meeting was arranged. I found myself sitting in still another Amish kitchen flanked by the clergy responsible for John, Anna, and their family. Clients and counselor had made a prior agreement on what could I could share (everything), and the meeting went well. The clergy asked no "pointed" questions about dynamics, marital stresses, or other ticklish issues; they merely wanted to understand the effects of a closed head injury, the type of supervision that might best assist John, and ways they could effectively respond to the family's needs. We left with a common respect for a new "team" approach to John and Anna that would include infrequent meetings to stay updated. A breach in confidentiality had certainly occurred, but the information shared had minimal significance. When I next met with John and Anna however, they had another surprise request.

"Things are going so well with the bishop and ministers," John said, "we want you to meet with the whole church."

"And just how many people is that?" I asked.

"Oh, about fifty adults" came the reply.

At this point, we began processing. Or perhaps more accurately, *I* began processing, and John and Anna began patiently playing along. They had absolutely no concerns about sharing—with the entire church—anything and everything that had happened and that we had discussed, planned, or would be planned in terms of treatment. They felt that their fellow members were isolating them, and such distance had become an intensely painful and bitter experience. After the meeting with the clergy, they saw me as the person who could change that. My issues with client confidentiality, including the confidentiality of their children, seemed simply irrelevant from the perspective of their cultural background.

I, on the other hand, experienced significant reservations. I felt I could handle one bishop and three ministers as a "committee," but 50 church members became an unwieldy number to allow free rein into the psyches of my clients. With that many participants, the group would probably include some who had experienced sexual abuse as children, or who had close friends and relatives who had experienced sexual abuse; I could not predict the extent to which they had effectively resolved their issues. Likewise, both John and Anna had grown up in this community, although not in this church; there were potential long histories with individuals who would be present that had nothing to do with the current situation. In addition, no semblance of confidentiality could exist when dialoguing with this many individuals.

With the exception of suicidal clients, I do not believe I have ever so earnestly advised a client in my professional career, all to no avail. John and Anna remained determined. They wanted their church to know—*to understand*—their situation. They believed it would provide healing. And did I understand the Amish "community psyche" well enough to tell them flatly it would not?

Within this cultural context, the request to speak to the full church became justifiable, if outside my comfort zone as a therapist. John and Anna already hid very little; every neighbor who passed their home when my car was in their drive knew "the counselor" was there; and John had made a full confession of his sins in church, so all members became aware of what had occurred. I was the one who struggled with confidentiality; not the client. Thus my meeting in that bishop's basement with a full complement of church members on a starlit fall evening, to discuss the most intimate aspects of a client's treatment, seemed a natural outgrowth of their culture, even if it violated my sacred expectation of ethics.

At this point, it would be wonderful to write an elegant paragraph that describes the power and beauty with which I handled that evening. Honestly, I felt so terrified that my memory remains a blur of passive or potentially hostile faces. I felt keenly aware that I was sharing the case history of two individuals (and indirectly their family) in an open forum, laying bare for any interested party the emotional experiences that had driven these clients to ask for this meeting, and the psychological and emotional impact of treatment. This decision would have consequences no one could fully foresee; I stood quite literally as a guest in another culture, laying aside an approach to ethics that had served me in situation after situation and believing in that moment in the wisdom of my client. The questions tended to the generic once again, focusing on closed head injuries and the experience of sexual abuse. I do know that John and Anna reported an increased sense of inclusion in their church following the meeting, but whether that stemmed from their perception that "something" had been done, or a true change of attitude among their fellow church members, I live too far outside the Amish world to know.

Discussion

Key ethical issues

Federal and state statutes across all mental health professions mandate confidentiality. Both statutes and ethics recognize that the client holds the right to breach confidentiality at will; however, both originate with the individualistic, privacy-oriented mindset of the 21st century American. They do not align with the community-oriented mindset of the Old Order Amish (or most Plain People communities, for that matter).

To understand this viewpoint requires an understanding of the Old Order Amish. Most casual observers may recognize their plain dress, their use of horse and buggy for transportation within their settlements, and their refusal to use external sources of power in the home. Still, these are mere symbols of the underlying spirituality that defines them as a Christian sect. They remain separate from the world and take pride in a perception as a "peculiar people" (1st Peter 2:9). As such, their primary allegiance focuses on God, followed by community. They maintain cohesion by the leadership of the clergy; and with this understanding, "privacy" seems minimal in comparison with their non-Amish American and European counterparts. Confession of sin occurs as a public ritual, and the anticipation exists that all will share emotional distress in order to obtain the prayers and support of the larger community.

The authority of the bishop in the Amish church also involves an experience that is alien to the large majority of mental health providers (I have used the alternative term "counselor" to describe providers throughout this case study because it is the term most commonly used by the Amish themselves). Although far from omnipotent, his word carries tremendous weight, and the church members take his role as overseer, appointed by God, quite seriously. As such, his decisions are often considered much more influential than the decisions of the state. Legal and ethical mandates regarding confidentiality, then, are of far less importance than these expectations. Effective treatment with Amish clients may require at least tacit approval of the clergy, and such approval may require their awareness of the broad parameters of a treatment plan. Again, this cultural expectation violates the normal boundaries of confidentiality from the perspective of mainstream American society.

Thus, mental health professionals intervening in these communities may find themselves working in a confidentiality funnel. At one end, facing "the world," is a tightly controlled channel of information about the client, consistent with familiar expectations. At the other end, the funnel widens and empties into the client's community, sharing information with what may appear (despite the client's implicit consent) alarming abandon.

This attitude of openness also comes with a caveat. Situations do arise with Amish clients, as with any others, in which they prefer that information *not* be shared with the clergy or the community. At these times, the normal strictures of confidentiality remain in force. These situations often involve behaviors or emotional experiences that extend beyond the pale of acceptable behavior within the community and feel deeply shaming.

Work setting

In my years of counseling the Amish, I have found benefits in working at their homes whenever possible, rather than asking them to meet at an office. One practical reality involves the cost of transportation; another involves the potential curiosity they inevitably garner in a public setting. Any mental health professional who sees clients outside the office recognizes that the power differential changes. The client remains in her or his home, or a neutral location. In the case of the Amish, "the world" has come to them, and a level of comfort results. Such comfort evaporates when they must enter an environment that they learn from birth is at best dangerous and at worst evil. An unabashed balancing of ethical demands occurs here: Amish families average six children, so "confidentiality" always becomes somewhat compromised as I meet in kitchens, basements, bedrooms, on back porches, sitting in the car, and on occasion even in the barn. Nevertheless, the client feels comfortable, regardless of the anxiety for confidentiality that pervades the observer-therapist in my mind who accompanies me to every session.

Perhaps the greatest challenge in the work setting involves the effort to balance cultural respect with advocacy for basic human rights as the majority of mental health providers perceive them—an issue referenced but not specifically addressed in this article. Among the Amish, the most glaring issue that counselors may confront is the subjugation of women. Their role is perceived as subservient to men. This case study alludes to at least one difficulty that role creates: projecting blame onto the victim. I have no easy resolution to this dilemma, for to insist that the victim is indeed fully a victim, and may not bear any responsibility for her role in a sexual encounter (at least in some settlements and/or churches), may doom her to the very type of distance and lack of support that John and Anna experienced.

Reflection

Involvement in another culture—any culture—expands one's self-awareness. For me, mental health intervention with the Old Order Amish has been one of the greatest challenges and greatest rewards of my professional career.

I have focused on the ethical issue of confidentiality in this chapter, but many other ethical issues demand consideration in work with this population: multiple relationships, competence to practice, and appropriate assessment and therapy. The ethical demands increase because of the basic premise of the Amish in regard to treatment. A common statement counselors will hear from Amish clients is, "We don't care how much you know until we know how much you care." At one level, it becomes a profound and moving testament to the need for empathy and compassion in the therapeutic process; at another level, it testifies to the disregard for critical thinking that characterizes much of Amish life: most leave school after the eighth grade, believing further formal education unnecessary for the plain life they pursue. Because these clients will provide minimal critical assessment of the treatment they receive, it places an often overwhelming burden on the therapist to remain aware of, and advocate for, their ethical interests.

Although not specifically discussed in any ethical standards, I also find the struggle to balance respect for the beliefs of the sect/culture against a desire to become parental in my interactions. The question of sharing with John and Anna's church consumed many a sleepless night, not only with the issue of advocating for their best interests, but painful introspection into my own motives: Did I trust them to make appropriate decisions? Or did I wish to assume the mantle of the "wise therapist" and divest them of the respect they deserved as clients because of their educational and life experience "limitations"? I felt cold comfort in tossing this issue back and forth with other professionals working with the Amish, only to find ourselves agreeing: we have no rational answer to that question. The only rationality we can find is that working with the Amish, particularly in their own communities, engenders many unique situations, and as they arise, we are forced once again to confront the ethical demands they place upon us with an understanding that the designers of ethical principles and ethical codes of our respective professions never had this cultural impasse in mind.

That said, the apparent naiveté of the Amish in regard to ethical expectations does not mean they are uniformly naïve. They are insightful clients, highly sensitive at an interpersonal level, and skilled at interpreting subtle nuances of behavior. Unfortunately for the therapist, they are also skilled at distancing themselves from the world; only with time and trust will they share their observations.

Key ethical principles and standards

APA (2002): Standard 3.10 (Informed Consent), Standard 4.02 (Discussing the Limits of Confidentiality), Standard 4.05 (Disclosures), Standard 10.02 Therapy Involving Couples or Families).

REFERENCES AND FURTHER READING

APA Council of Representatives (2002): Guidelines on Multicultural Education, Training, Research, Practice, and Organizational Change for Psychologists.

Kitayama, S., & Cohen, D. (2007). *Handbook of Cultural Psychology*. New York: Guilford Press.

Kraybill, D. (2001). *The Riddle of Amish Culture* (Revised). Baltimore: Johns Hopkins University Press.

Nolt, S. (2003). *A History of the Amish* (Revised and Updated). Intercourse, PA: Good Books.

Zur, O. (2007). *Boundaries in Psychotherapy: Ethical and Clinical Explorations*. Washington, DC: APA Books.

36

Working Out One's Salvation in Fear and Trembling: Ethical and Spiritual Dilemmas Around Therapeutic Boundaries

Andrew Michel

I first met Sandy when she found herself in the midst of a life crisis and presented for an urgent care evaluation. She had many storms in her life, including difficulty with subordinates and a supervisor at her publishing firm. She had recently lost her temper and yelled at coworkers in an angry outburst that had put her job at risk. The frustrations surrounding this pattern in her work life led her to seek help. However, she also felt frustrated in relationship to her husband, who she accused of being passive and disengaged. Perhaps related to this disconnect with her husband, Sandy had on occasion connected emotionally with other men in her work environment, leading to a different level of interpersonal complication.

Sandy was engaging and often funny, though her biting sarcasm could sometimes leave me (and others) feeling off kilter, uncomfortable, and on edge. She was smart, ambitious, and involved in numerous projects, including book writing and research. However, she frequently had severe internal storms, including moments of intense despair when she would cut or burn herself. She felt chronically depressed and occasionally suicidal.

Diagnostically, Sandy presented as a person with a borderline personality organization based on her impulsivity, disruption in self- and other-perception, self-harming, feelings of worthlessness, numbness, dysphoria, and occasions of intense rage. She showed some signs of a cyclic mood disorder in addition to the borderline character traits, intermixed with occasions of binge drinking.

Our early work focused on crisis management, safety, decreasing self-harming behavior, and building at least some tenuous alliance. I encouraged her toward a referral for dialectical behavior therapy, but she consistently refused to pursue this, saying I was the only one she could trust. At her initial intake, on social history screening, she said she had grown up Catholic but felt "antireligious," implying that overtly religious or spiritual concerns did not constitute a focus of attention.

About three months into the work, she become very interested in my personal life, a common response of patients, and she had actually uncovered my association with a nonprofit agency with religious values. She said that a colleague of mine had revealed this to her (though I actually did not know the person she named). Later she said she had discovered it by Googling me on the Internet (a search that I could not replicate at the time). In any case, she brought in the text from a website connected to the nonprofit and read excerpts from it aloud, including a statement of orthodox Christian beliefs. She then accused me rather angrily of "deceiving" her and "withholding" from her.

She queried, "How can you be a Christian and a psychiatrist? That doesn't make any sense!"

Admittedly, Sandy hit a nerve in me with this question. Indeed, it is one I have asked myself repeatedly, and my fumbling response to her was a likely giveaway. As is well known, those with a borderline personality organization can be very interpersonally perceptive and have a remarkable capacity to hone in on elements of conflict. She next asked me, "Does this mean you can't see me anymore?" I asked her if she felt uncomfortable being seen by me given her discoveries, but she said she wanted to continue in therapy with me. I simply explained that I did not see a reason to discontinue therapy together, though we would need to attend to these developments in our ongoing work. Overall, I wanted to display my willingness to remain available to her and not overreact by rejecting her and missing out on the underlying dynamic at work in the moment between us. I was mindful of an admonition from one supervisor who would say, "Don't do anything; just sit there." I sought supervision with two colleagues who both encouraged me to continue working with her in therapy and also provided ongoing assistance along the way.

Sandy and I clearly entered together into somewhat uncharted territory. My willingness to walk into this with her rather than rejecting her allowed

Sandy to develop some trust in my capacity to sit with the overwhelming turmoil she struggled with. Perhaps this even helped bring some calm to her storms. Her understanding of me and my religious beliefs had a decided impact on the course of her therapy and the kinds of questions she began to pursue in our shared work together.

Sandy began attending church, reading Christian books, and discussing her religious experience in therapy. Her doing these things certainly related to her identification with me, but also related to other simultaneous movement in her life. She found renewed relationship with a brother who had maintained a religious life, dialoging with him about this development in her life, and established a relationship with the pastor of a local church. She also found opportunity in session to process some of her early life experiences, largely negative, with religious representatives and institutions, especially focusing on the way her primary family had embodied these beliefs and practices.

She asked profound existential questions about life that seemed to transcend her psychological difficulties. I focused on my role as her psychotherapist while not tampering unduly with the normal questions all of us as humans ask and seek answers to. There remains a lot of mystery in how to do this well. It feels a lot more like improvised jazz music than rote classical and doesn't fit neatly under solely rule-based ethical systems.

After several more months, Sandy reported that she had become a Christian and invited me to her baptism, saying that I had served as an important part of this movement in her life and that she wanted me present.

I again felt on the spot. I sought the council of colleagues in a supervision group. My colleagues expressed a palpable antagonism even to the idea that I might consider going to the baptism. I felt acutely sensitive to concerns about boundaries in this case, especially given the nature of borderline character pathology, and I could understand the admonition to keep roles tight and boundaries crystal clear.

I then sought the counsel of several pastors in my religious community. "Of course you should go. What's the problem?" replied one. The pastors could not understand how I could turn down this invitation. The more nuanced of them sympathized with my internal turmoil but admittedly couldn't fully appreciate the uniqueness of a therapeutic relationship nor the clinical perils typically encountered when caring for those suffering with borderline character structure, both of which made me hesitant to attend.

Beyond these concerns, Sandy had improved clinically in relation to her spiritual transformation. She had ceased cutting or burning herself, no longer felt suicidal, her depression improved, and her relationship with her husband and family had stabilized. She, self-admittedly, still had some rough edges and difficult traits, but she had also experienced a substantial change in her behavior and disposition toward the world and others. From a pragmatic perspective, even a health perspective, why not encourage this transformation?

As a person of religious belief, I felt the acute conflict of sorting out how best to care for her in my role as her psychotherapist at a secular academic institution, while at the same time having integrity to my own deeply held sacred beliefs and values. Sandy had clearly invited me into her storm, and I found my ship tossed and turned. I felt accountable to secular colleagues within the tradition of psychiatry but also to my faith tradition. My attention remained focused on *her* care. As a clinician, I wanted what was best for her psychologically, yet as a person of deep religious conviction, I also wanted what was best for her spiritually.

I ultimately decided not to attend.

Discussion

Key ethical issues

Key ethical questions raised by this case include when to cross boundaries and allow for extra-therapy contact with a patient, how to respect and support a patient's personal system of values while not unduly influencing the patient, and how much flexibility there is in the role of a therapist to attend to spiritual or religious matters.

Regarding extra-therapy contact, I would argue there are appropriate instances to cross a boundary and make extratherapy contacts. As Gutthiel and Gabbard (1998) have articulated regarding boundary crossings, the context is very important. In general, the length of treatment, particular kind of psychological pathology, focus of the work, and role of the clinician (whether social worker, CBT therapist, or psychodynamic therapist) all matter in deciding. I could imagine situations in which attending an important event in the life of a patient, such as a baptism, right of passage, or performance, could further the work of therapy, especially if the therapy had persisted over a relatively long period of time, in a person without personality pathology, and where the focus of the work had been largely supportive.

One particular question each clinician should ask herself around these decisions is "What is best for the patient?" The needs of the therapist should not be the primary reason for extra-therapy contact. (In Sandy's case, two potential sources of clinician need are the need to avoid guilt for not meeting the asssumed expectations of one's religious identity and the allure of receiving praise for religious accomplishment, such as conversion to the faith.) In this particular case, the patient's personality organization, as well as the focus of the work, which was around modeling and discovering personal boundaries, made attendance at a baptism complicated and may have distracted from the overall good of the patient, psychologically and spiritually.

The American Psychiatric Association's Religious/Spiritual Commitments and Psychiatric Practice resource document (2006) says, "Psychiatrists should foster recovery by making treatment decisions with patients in ways that respect and take into meaningful consideration their cultural, religious/spiritual, and personal ideals." It is increasingly acknowledged that spirituality and religion are often an important source of hope, meaning, identity, morality, inspiration, and practical support for those suffering with mental illness. Psychiatrists are now generally encouraged to investigate a patient's spiritual and religious history and to take into account how these elements may be involved in a patient's current presentation and overall mental health.

What makes this case unique is the way in which the patient adopted a new spiritual direction partially as a result of information obtained about the treating clinician in the midst of treatment. While I did take time to examine the psychological import of her having sought personal information about me, it would have been overly rigid and perhaps impossible to avoid the religious and spiritual questions that she subsequently raised in our sessions. Given Sandy's personality constellation, I tended toward a more structured, matter-of-fact style, erring on the cognitive side, while remaining present and available within limits. There was room within this style for allowing the patient to bring up theological topics, scriptural insights, and pastoral guidance she had begun to recieve. I am sure my acceptance of her spiritual wonderings and my comfort with these topics was obvious to her given my naturalness in response to her. I did not see it as my main task to stop this movement in her life or correct doctrine, though her understanding of her beliefs may have been clarified, perhaps deepened, by questions asked. I routinely encouraged her to seek guidance and teaching from her pastor and religious community.

I did ask questions about the elements of her religious movement that were an identification and perhaps idealization of me. One of my other main roles was to help her navigate a new relationship with a pastor and church community, as well as adjust to other transformations in the way she viewed her life. We routinely processed her relationship with her pastor, especially her feelings toward him and amount of time spent with him, and how this related to prior relationships that had started ideally and intensely and then been devalued and discarded. We wondered together about what had made it difficult to sustain relationships with others in the past and how this may impact on the present. I also addressed at points our therapeutic relationship and this pattern of idealization and occasional frustration and dissapointment that led to attempts to disrupt our work together.

Work setting

This case also invites a fresh look at the dynamics involved in addressing spiritual and religious concerns for both patients and clinicians in contemporary work environments. This therapy proceeded in a large academic medical center with historic religious foundations but no overt religious practice in the daily culture or work of the place. It would be accurate to say that its ethos was largely secular. While there has been an obvious shift over the last generation to include as relevant spiritual and religious concerns for mental health, it remains somewhat unclear how these concerns are to be integrated into care. There are now whole texts devoted to spiritually oriented psychotherapy. The range of stances proceeds across generic understandings of spirituality to particular faith-informed traditions. One guideline from the American Psychiatric Association's Religious/Spiritual Commitments and Psychiatric Practice resource document (2006) says, "Psychiatrists should not impose their own religious/spiritual, antireligious/spiritual, or other values, beliefs and world views on their patients." This statement rightly aims to protect from coersion patients who may be in vulnerable states and prevent an abuse of power. However, it also assumes practitioners *can* somehow stand outside of a value-laden point of reference, imposing no influence.

Don Browning, in his oft-cited *Religious Thought and the Modern Psychologies* (1988), argues cogently that schools of psychotherapy are "practical moral philosophies" with histories that form cultures with religious and ethical dimensions. Do not institutions and traditions of practice, even secular ones, start and end with certain assumptions about how the world works and how people can get along well in it?

In recent decades, a confluence of factors, including scientific evidence suggesting that religious life is important for physical and mental health, as well as an increasing awareness that even the secular has its underlying biases, sometimes intensely held, has opened the door to further exploration of these concerns.

Cases like Sandy's do seem to call on all of us to acknowledge as best we can our underlying assumptions and potential biases. They raise questions for those with sacred leanings about how to be responsible, especially underneath secular authority and in working with those who are in vulnerable states, so as to avoid an abuse of power.

How can a clinician pursue right relationship with those he cares for, with himself, with the institutions he is accountable to (including both those of medicine and religion), and with the divine? Can secular academic settings tolerate the conflicts that may arise for individual practitioners who find themselves deeply committed to particular religious beliefs, especially those of an orthodox sort?

It is increasingly acknowledged that spiritual concerns are relevant to all areas of health care and that the physical, psychological, and spiritual realms are not easily quarantined from one another such that they can be conveniently attended to by specialized practitioners in each distinct area. Just as primary care physicians sometimes are the only source of care for mental illness and the psychiatrist can never neglect to rule out organic etiology for symptoms of emotional distress, there is a need for a somewhat expanded and flexible role for mental healthcare professionals to attend to the spiritual life of people without forgetting one's primary role as psychiatrist or psychotherapist. Just how to work within this expanded model is an open question and likely requires delicate balance. Though working within such a model at this point in history admittedly feels tenuous and uneasy, avoiding spiritual exploration altogether misses out on critical elements influencing what it means to be human and on the unique ways in which we suffer and pursue healing.

Reflection

This case continues to challenge me. While Sandy found help and healing and marked transformation, I continue to find my role and responsibility deepened and clarified by the challenges she presented.

Psychological, spiritual, logistical, and intuitive factors all influenced my ulitmate decision to not attend the baptism. I considered the potential confusion Sandy might experience regarding how much I influenced her religious decisions. Perhaps she had some need to become like me (as she understood me), to please me, or to have my approval. It seemed important for Sandy to realize that she had initiated and carried out her own religious movement rather than her feeling connected to a real or imagined identification with me.

Logistical circumstances also played a role in my discernment. I had engaged in no other extra-therapy contacts, and the treatment relationship qualified as still relatively young at roughly six months. Furthermore, Sandy knew that I would relocate from the area in three more months, and our therapy relationship would terminate. One colleague reminded me of how difficult it can be for patients to transition to new therapists, especially when they recall "special treatment" by the prior clinician. I was aware that Sandy would need to continue the concrete work of therapy after my departure and was already preparing alongside her for what I knew would be a difficult transition. Finally, my experience with Sandy told me that while sides of her wanted me present at her baptism, my actual in-the-moment presence may have been somehow awkward for her, perhaps even distracting from the primary significance of her baptism.

After sitting with my initial leanings to not attend, I began to sense that not going might actually allow for psychological and spiritual growth for Sandy. It would model clear boundaries and give space to her personal agency while highlighting her responsibility for her spiritual decisions. The downside of this decision was Sandy's potential perception that she was unsupported in this significant life event. But as best I could discern, I ultimately felt that not attending was paradoxically the best way to support her ongoing psychological and spiritual growth.

At Sandy's visit following her baptism, she reported that her pastor had expressed feeling "very disappointed and couldn't understand" why I had not attended. The displacement to her pastor of her own frustrations allowed an entrance for us to process her disappointment with me and the significance of her baptism.

REFERENCES AND FURTHER READING

Browning, D. S. (1988). *Religious Thought and the Modern Psychologies: A Critical Conversation in the Theology of Culture*. Minneapolis: Augsburg Fortress Publishers.

Guidelines on religious/spiritual commitments and psychiatric practice. (2006). Arlington, VA: American Psychiatric Association.

Gutheil, T. G., & Gabbard, G. O. (1998). Misuses and misunderstandings of boundary theory in clinical and regulatory settings. *American Journal of Psychiatry*, 155, 409–414.

Sperry, L., & Shafranske, E. P. (Eds.). (2005). *Spiritually Oriented Psychotherapy*. Washington, DC: American Psychological Association.

PART IX

In the Public Arena

37

A Psychologist in Congress: Ethics, the Constitution, Politics, Clinical Judgment, and the Case of Terri Schiavo

Brian Baird

What is the right thing to do when you are faced with a decision having life and death consequences, have limited information to guide the decision, do not really believe the decision should be yours to begin with, are confronted with conflicting demands, and know you will be judged publically for whatever choice you make with no ability to fully explain your choice to anyone's satisfaction?

Terri Schiavo

Terri Schiavo was a young woman who had survived in persistent vegetative state for fifteen years after a cardiac arrest and subsequent anoxia. Following a protracted series of events, well detailed on Wikipedia, Ms. Schiavo's husband Michael succeeded in legal efforts to have her feeding tube removed as he said she would have wished. Ms. Shaivo, however, left no signed living will to confirm this wish, and her parents, Robert and Mary Schindler, vehemently opposed Mr. Schiavo's efforts. The Schindlers argued that their daughter would not have wanted to die in that manner and in their judgment she had a real chance of recovery, if she received alternative treatment.

Through a variety of legal challenges, eventual intervention by the Florida State Legislature and then-Governor Jeb Bush, and a public campaign that made the case a national cause for the self proclaimed "pro-life" political movement, Ms. Schiavo's parents sought to challenge Schiavo husband's guardianship and insisted on keeping their daughter alive.

As a psychologist who has spent years working with severely brain injured patients, I found the case interesting from a clinical perspective and followed it from afar as it worked its way through both the court of law and the court of public opinion. This role of interested observer suddenly changed when President Bush and conservative Congressional leaders took up the cause and sought to transfer jurisdiction from state courts, which had ruled the feeding tube could be removed, to federal courts for further review.

The United States Senate, then controlled by a Republican majority, convened on an exceptionally rare Palm Sunday session and passed by "unanimous consent" a voice vote allowing the transfer of jurisdiction to federal courts. Among those voting with the unanimous Senate was then Senator Barak Obama, who later expressed regret over that vote. Following the Senate action, the House then took up the bill and passed it at 12:41 a.m. the next day. The final tally for that recorded vote was 203–58 with 174 members not voting. That is where my involvement occurred. In addition to being a clinical psychologist, I also served as a member of the House of Representatives and cast one of those votes.

When the measure passed and President Bush signed it into law, the case entered the federal court system. The federal judge acted quickly, sustained the state court's earlier decisions to deny appeals of the parents, and the Supreme Court refused to take the case. Following some last-minute maneuvering within the state of Florida, the decision of the state courts was carried out, the feeding tube eventually removed, and Ms. Schiavo died on March 31, 2005.

Discussion

Key ethical issues

The case raised many ethical issues, and they become particularly interesting when considered along with constitutional matters, legal precedents, political considerations, and personal values. All of those questions and more weighed heavily as I pondered the case throughout the day and participated in the debate and voting late into the evening.

To begin with, the case raised a host of thorny constitutional questions concerning separation of powers, intrusion by the legislative branch into the functions of judiciary, etc. The very fact that I choose to begin this discussion of ethical concerns with constitutional issues itself highlights the potential conflicts one faces when serving in an official capacity for which responsibilities and judgments may conflict with professional ethics and clinical judgment. Yet as a member of Congress sworn to uphold the Constitution, that is where I must begin.

In that capacity, my belief going into the debate was, and still remains, that Congress crossed boundaries between branches of government by inserting itself and directing the case to federal court. I felt particularly concerned in this case because information became public indicating that, for at least some of the public and elected officials involved, political concerns and opportunism seemed a primary driving factor in bringing the case to the Florida legislature and then on to Congress.

Those motivations notwithstanding, I acknowledge that cogent arguments came forth during the debate citing precedents and constitutional language that permitted Congressional involvement in judicial affairs under certain circumstances.

One of the most compelling of these arguments asked rhetorically if members of Congress on the liberal side would willingly intervene if there were reason to believe that racially biased state courts had sentenced a black person to death under questionable circumstances and had denied any appeals. If a human life is at stake, and a miscarriage of justice may have occurred, which is more important—preserving strict separation of powers or being as certain as one can be that due process was fully followed and the case fairly heard before allowing someone to die?

Shifting now to ethical standards and clinical issues in psychology, the case also proved challenging. Among the ethical issues I faced were questions about who is the client—or better said, who are the clients and what obligations did I owe to each? What principles from what professional roles should guide decisions? How do clinical judgments interact with other obligations, and what constraints exist on clinical judgments formed in the absence of direct contact with a patient? Finally, how do personal values and personal issues interplay with clinical and other judgments?

With regard to clinical considerations, based on my professional training, clinical experience, knowledge of the literature, and reading of the information presented in legal proceedings on this particular case, I believed it highly unlikely that someone in Ms. Schiavo's circumstances would ever likely regain any significant return of higher-level cortical function. At the same time, however, because I had not had an opportunity to visit with or assess Ms. Schiavo personally, I felt ethically compelled to refrain from offering any public clinical opinions about her specific individual situation or prognosis.

That same compunction apparently did not constrain some of my Congressional colleagues, including certain prominent members who offered well-publicized professional medical opinions on Ms. Schiavo's status and promising potential for full recovery. A similar lack of restraint was also evidenced by nonmedical members of Congress, several of whom cited apocryphal tales describing putative cases in which people had supposedly survived in persistent vegetative states for many years, then suddenly awoke and returned again to a normal life. Based on such "evidence," these members argued in favor or referring the case to federal courts in an effort to maintain use of the feeding tube in the hope of a similarly miraculous recovery for Ms. Schiavo.

This created a rather odd situation. With twenty some years of prior clinical experience and specialization in work with brain injured patients, I purposefully refrained from commenting about this case in particular, yet people who had no professional background or knowledge whatsoever readily opined about clinical matters completely beyond their ken or, in the case of those with actual medical backgrounds, beyond what I believed ethical practice should allow.

There is yet another side to this story of clinical judgment, experience, and ethical silence. Having worked in the field of brain injury as long as I have, there have also been opportunities to observe cases in which certain family members of severely injured patients have seemed more motivated by desires for financial compensation from legal settlements than by genuine concern for a patient's well-being. In the case of Ms. Schiavo, there was a large malpractice settlement, and many of those opposed to Mr. Schiavo's decision to remove the feeding tube regarded his motive as pecuniary, not genuine concern for his wife.

Once again, I had not had an opportunity to meet with Mr. Schiavo directly, but I did read extensively about the case and did have a chance to observe him during numerous interviews on television. As with any judgments I might have had about his wife's prognosis, I felt it most prudent and responsible to keep any thoughts about his motives or other matters to myself as well. Those issues did, however, factor into my final vote.

Yet another factor, this one personal, must have also influenced me at the time of the debate and vote. Several years before this case came to Congress, I had been present as my own father died of idiopathic pulmonary fibrosis. My father believed strongly in death with dignity, as do I. As he neared the end of his life from this dreadful disease, my father had insisted to his family that heroic measures not be employed to keep him alive. As such, in the end I held him in my arms as he died. It was the most difficult, painful experience of my entire life and in many ways still haunts me to this day.

That personal experience with the death of a loved was compounded by my wife having given birth to premature twins just a few weeks prior to the vote on the Schiavo case. Indeed, part of the reason I was in DC at the time of the vote, rather than back in my district as were many other members of Congress, was to help care for my wife and our sons, who were at the time still in need of constant heart and respiration monitoring. Thus, not only had I dealt with the death of a loved one under difficult end-of-life circumstances, I also had become a new parent of two boys who faced some real challenges to their survival in the first few days and weeks after their birth. Hence, I knew something deeply personal about the feelings that surround these sorts of cases.

Finally, I must also mention that any controversial vote in Congress carries with it political ramifications. I long ago decided that as a member of Congress my first and only priority in critical instances would be to focus on doing what I think is right and not worrying about the political fallout from friend or foe. I held to that perspective in this instance as well, but even though I may vote based on such principle, it does not escape me that votes will have political consequences. One side or another may form impressions about what a vote means; there tends to be a default assumption that every action an elected representative makes is solely politically motivated. Whatever we do of course will impact how constituents decide to cast their own votes in upcoming elections.

In this instance, what felt particularly difficult was knowing that for professional ethical reasons, I might not be able to fully explain all the considerations that went into my vote and, even if I could have done so, those reasons might not have seemed either persuasive or even accepted as truth by those who would disagree with my vote.

Reflection

With these factors in mind, as I sat in the House of Representatives and listened to the debate late into the evening, I felt an obligation to speak on the issue. As I mentioned, I would have preferred that the issue be left to the courts and not have been brought to the legislative branch to decide. I strongly disagreed with the political agendas of those who brought the measure to the Congress to begin with, I am a proponent of death with dignity, and I had grave reservations about Congress taking up a measure such as this and directly intruding into what had begun as, and I believed rightfully should remain, a judiciary matter.

Those positions notwithstanding, once the matter did come before us, I could not escape taking a position and recognized that the choice we would make that evening would likely determine whether or not a young woman would die. More accurately, our decision would likely determine whether or not a woman would die with or without having her case reviewed one more time to determine if all factual and procedural stones had been turned and fairly, thoroughly reviewed.

Relative to many colleagues, I do not speak on the floor of the House very often, but in this instance I determined that I should do so. My intent in speaking did not seek to sway votes one way or another or to explain or defend how I intended to vote myself. Rather, I hoped to in some way that evening to deepen the debate, take it out, for a moment, of the political boxing match it had become and offer some general clinical facts in contrast to some of the fanciful and misleading statements that some of my colleagues had made. Most importantly of all, I wanted to try in some way to acknowledge the profound existential difficulty that such circumstances and choices present to each and every one of us as human beings.

With that goal in mind, I prepared no written remarks but spoke from the heart in the moment. This is what I said in the brief time members had to speak individually during the debate.

This following text comes from the Congressional Record, "For the Relief of the Parents of Theresa Marie Schiavo" (3/20/2005, page 1,715–1,716):

> Mr. BAIRD. Mr. Speaker, I thank the gentleman for yielding me time. I do not know what to do tonight. I honestly do not. If Terri Schiavo were here, she could tell us what she would like her fate to be under this circumstance. Those who say that we are condemning her to death by starvation, that may be so if action is not taken tonight. But it may also be so that you may be condemning her to a life that she might not choose were she here to choose that.
>
> Some of us have spoken on both sides of the aisle of holding our loved one in our hands as they died, having made the decision not to have heroic measures. For 23 years before working in this body, I served as a clinical neuropsychologist. I have been with many patients in persistent vegetative state. I wish life were different. I really wish it were. I will tell Members that the stories like the gentleman from Arizona (Mr. Franks) and others about sudden recoveries, where people almost miraculously or magically are better and return to their former state, are apocryphal for the most part. After years of coma, people do not return to who they

were before. What happens is we have a brain stem that is miraculously robust at protecting breathing and heart rate, but it is our cortex that makes us who we are, and that cortex dies when it is deprived of oxygen and we effectively die with it. And I am sorry about that. It is so tragic. I honestly do not know what to do. But for anybody to try to imply that people on one side or the other do not care about this woman is not right or fair, on either side. This is an American tragedy, but more importantly, it is a personal tragedy. And people on both sides are pro life in the richness and complexity and difficulty of it. Some are trying to do their best to honor what they believe are this woman's wishes to not live condemned to a bed where she cannot speak or enjoy the higher virtues of life she might choose. And if she did indeed say "I would not choose the fate of being condemned to this bed," then we are denying her that right to make the choice. That is the challenge here tonight, my friends. But let no one who leaves this body somehow imply that whichever the vote is taken, one side or the other does not respect life in its richness. We are all pro life. We all feel for this family. And also let no one believe that we are somehow saving this woman from a horrific fate whichever route we choose.

Key ethical principles and standards

Principle A: Beneficence and Nonmaleficence, Principle B: Fidelity and Responsibility, Principle D: Justice, Principle E: Respect for People's Rights and Dignity, 1.02, Conflicts Between Ethics and Law, Regulations, or Other Governing Legal Authority, 1.03, Conflicts Between Ethics and Organizational Demands, 2.04, Bases for Scientific and Professional Judgments, 3.04 Avoiding Harm.

REFERENCES AND FURTHER READING

Abeles, N., & Barlev, A. (1999). End-of-life decisions and assisted suicide. *Professional Psychology: Research and Practice, 30,* 229–234.

Haley, W., Larson, D., Kasl-Godley, J., Neimeyer, R., & Kwilosz, D. (2003). Roles for Psychologists in End-of-Life Care: Emerging Models of Practice. *Professional Psychology: Research and Practice,* Vol. *34,* No. 6, pp. 626–633.

Kleespies, P. (2004). *Life and Death Decisions: Psychological and Ethical Considerations in End-of-Life Care.* Washington, DC: American Psychological Association.

Werth, J. L., Welfel, E. R., & Benjamin, G. A. H. (2008). The duty to protect: Ethical, legal, and professional considerations for mental health professionals. Washington, DC: American Psychological Association.

38

Isn't This Against the Law? Boundary Problems in Police Psychology

Gerald Sweet

I began the trip into my career as a psychologist from traditional and somewhat conservative origins. The path included a university-based, APA-approved doctoral training program in clinical psychology, followed by internship and postdoctoral fellowship programs with similar pedigrees. My first job took me to a medical school–affiliated teaching hospital in suburban Boston. When the need for new challenges became irresistible, I completed a postdoctoral fellowship in forensic psychology and then engaged in a combination of clinical and forensic practice. All through these years, I took a reasonably conservative and cautious approach to my clinical and consultative work. My profession's code of ethics and several senior clinicians in the Boston mental health community provided mentoring, professional guidance, and direction.

About a dozen years ago, I made another midcourse correction and took a full-time position as a psychologist in a major city police department. The idea of practicing police psychology seemed an appealing blend of the clinical and consultative skills I had practiced up to that time, but doing so in a new work environment. I joined a group of police psychologists who serve as civilian members of the department whose job involves providing a variety of clinical services to the officers and civilian employees of the department. In addition, the members of the psychological staff are actively involved in the training of police officers, organizational and management consultation, critical incident response, collaboration with sworn SWAT negotiators in hostage/barricade situations, and on-call emergency mental health coverage for the entire department. The diversity of the job responsibilities and the "action" associated with them seemed like the kind of change I wanted at that point in my career. Working with police officers, for me a new and largely unknown patient population, and doing so in a large dynamic organization in a new city, seemed an attractive professional challenge. The possibility that I would be walking into a job situation with difficult ethical dilemmas had not occurred to me. However, I assured myself that my experience as a psychologist who had worked in a variety of diverse clinical and forensic settings, and had dealt with or heard about many ethical challenges, would serve me well.

As time passed in my work as a police psychologist, I realized that the demands of the job put me in situations that raised frequent questions about dual relationships, boundary crossings, and boundary violations. On a relatively frequent basis, I would have contact with an individual officer in more than one professional role. For example, I could potentially see an officer clinically for evaluation or psychotherapy, have him/her in a class where I served as an instructor, and encounter him/her in a geographic area where they are assigned and I work as the division psychologist. All of these circumstances could also apply to the civilian employees who work for the department.

Many possible combinations of contact between a police psychologist and his or her patient(s) come up as a normal occurrence. When I first confronted one of these uncomfortable situations of blurred boundaries, the answer I got from my more experienced police psychologist colleagues did not seem helpful. Their most frequent response to me typically included, "That's what it means to practice police psychology in a department like this." For a psychologist with my background, who believed it essential to adhere to traditional ethical guidelines, this did not offer much help or reassurance. Yet the nature of the job responsibilities and the organization repeatedly put me in such uncomfortable positions.

Adding to the complexity of this situation is the bifurcated nature of the clinical role in which police psychologists may find themselves. Most of the referrals to police psychologists in the department are initiated by the officer. These referrals qualify as voluntary, and the patient enjoys the same assurance of confidentiality he or she would have in the office of a licensed practitioner anywhere in this state. In addition, the practice guidelines for me and my coworkers align fully with the Health Insurance Portability and Accountability Act (HIPAA) privacy rules. Our group has modified its clinical, consent, and record-keeping procedures so we are now fully HIPAA compliant. The psychological staff members routinely review these issues with patients during their first clinical interview, and the patients sign a detailed document regarding informed consent. Police psychologists adhere to the same statutory mandatory reporting guidelines regarding dangerousness to self and others, child abuse, and elder abuse as do other mental health practitioners.

The other category of referral to police psychologists occurs as a result of a directed or management referral. In such situations, a commanding officer orders one of his or her officers to consult a police psychologist. A variety of reasons may trigger such referrals: an officer-involved shooting, a serious use of force by an officer, involvement in a critical incident, below-average job performance possibly related to mental health issues, substance abuse, a commanding officer's concern about a subordinate's well-being (stress, anxiety, depression, illness), and/or exposure to a blood-borne pathogen. In directed referrals, which may involve one interview or more often a series of sessions, the psychologist must provide limited verbal feedback to the commanding officer. These guidelines are also based on statute, and the feedback is limited to work-related issues. Specifically, we advise the commanding officer about issues regarding general well-being and officer safety, return to current work assignment, and recommendations for follow-up interviews with a psychologist.

In this organizational context, I encountered one of the most complex ethical challenges of my career. An officer I will call Bill for purposes of this chapter came to me as the result of a referral by a mutual acquaintance from outside of the department in which Bill and I worked. Bill's psychological concerns included multiple professional and personal issues. The seriousness of Bill's problems led the person making the referral to tell Bill that he would call me on his behalf and would notify Bill's commanding officer if he (Bill) did not set up an appointment to see me. When I received the call from the mutual acquaintance, I agreed to see Bill promptly and said I would call him if Bill did not reach me within a few days. While Bill initiated the contact voluntarily, he did so in this somewhat coercive context.

Bill called the next day, and I saw him for an initial interview two days later. He presented as a tall, healthy-looking man in his early fifties. He spoke in an articulate, but somewhat hesitant, manner about a series of professional and personal issues. These included disruptive conflicts with his immediate supervisor, marital and family conflicts, financial problems, and on off-duty business that was failing. He informed me that he had served as a police officer for over fifteen years and for the last several years had worked in an administrative assignment. One of Bill's issues included an off-duty situation that, as a police officer, he should have reported to the department. He had not done so and that fact, as well as the incident itself, could result in an investigation by Internal Affairs. He also told me about a significant health issue that would require him to undergo extended evaluation and treatment. He seemed understandably emotional and overwhelmed by all of these life circumstances. As the interview progressed, Bill came across as tired and stretched almost to the limit. He worried about losing his job and his marriage. He expressed strong interest in involving himself in psychological treatment. We agreed to begin a treatment relationship and started meeting on a weekly basis. I reviewed with him, as I do with all new patients, the limits of confidentiality. Since he initiated the relationship, standard patient/psychotherapist confidentiality would apply, although we acknowledged that our mutual acquaintance had played an important role in facilitating the referral.

Several weeks later, I received a call from the captain of a division within the department where I served as the psychologist consultant. He talked with me about a directed referral. The officer in question was Bill. In fact, a personnel complaint had been initiated, and the captain wanted a psychological opinion about Bill's mental well-being and other related issues. He asked if I could see Bill, as Bill had informed his captain that he had been seeing me on a confidential basis. Bill had also told the captain about the general nature of the psychological issues for which he had sought treatment. Although it is not unusual for a psychologist in our department to undertake what is usually a time-limited directed referral with an officer who is also a patient in confidential individual psychotherapy with the same psychologist, this role shift required some careful discussion with the patient. Bill had requested that I be assigned to handle the directed referral and acknowledged his understanding that this would require limited communication between me and his captain. A treatment situation that had begun with a somewhat unusual referral had now taken on an additional dimension of complexity. I completed the directed referral in the usual manner and without any complications. I gave the captain the verbal feedback that is allowed in such management referrals, and my sessions with Bill reverted back to confidential treatment. The Internal Affairs investigation led to a disciplinary suspension of moderate length. Bill remained in the same work assignment and was counseled by his captain about the relevant work-performance issues. The interruption of the directed referral appeared to have no detrimental effect on my therapeutic alliance with Bill or the treatment itself.

The same captain called me three months later to ask that I make a presentation at a divisional training day. When I agreed to the request, I knew that my patient, Bill, would most likely be in the audience. The subject that I was asked to present related to one of the issues that had brought Bill into treatment. I discussed the request with Bill during his next therapy session. He assured me that he felt fine with my making this presentation, and he would, in fact, be in the audience. On the day of the presentation, I arrived early to set up my laptop and other equipment. When I asked the captain who might assist me with this, he said, "Bill is our high-tech guy. He'll help you." I had the impression the captain gave no thought to my previous and ongoing therapeutic relationship with his high-tech expert. Bill assisted me, and I made my presentation. The next time we met, I asked Bill about our interactions at the divisional training day. He answered unhesitatingly that he felt fine about them and had no problem with what had occurred. I saw no effect, positive or negative, in subsequent sessions.

Several months later, the same captain called and told me about a major change in the working conditions of one of the units within the division. He thought that a psychological debriefing would prove helpful and asked if I could meet with the involved officers. I knew that Bill was a member of this unit and initially hesitated when talking to the captain. I discussed the request with Bill later that day. He was not aware of the captain's call to me, but he indicated that he had no problem with my responding to the request. He indicated that he intended to be present for the debriefing. The debriefing occurred a few days later and was completed without difficulty. The next time Bill and I met, we reviewed the boundary issue that had arisen. He again confirmed that he had no discomfort with seeing me in a setting outside the psychotherapy office. Once again, I saw no negative effects in subsequent sessions.

Discussion

Key ethical issues

Role shifts and blurred boundaries do not always equal an ethical violation or compromise the care of the patient. At times, the blurring that occurs when the therapist and the patient work within the same subculture can foster the development of therapeutic alliances. The sequence of events reported here illustrates the "small world" phenomenon that can occur when a psychologist has several roles within a particular work environment. Because I served as a consultant in Bill's assigned division, our relationship began with a degree of familiarity and mutual understanding. At the same time, I had to make a series of decisions that departed from the usual adherence to and respect for boundaries in the psychotherapeutic relationship. Traditional boundaries became temporarily blurred when our customary confidential relationship intersected with a management (directed) referral in which prescribed limits of confidentiality applied. Certain professional contacts occurred between me and the patient in the workplace, yet outside the therapy office, with advanced discussion and consent. In this case, the professional and clinical worlds of the therapist and the patient overlapped in a number of different ways.

When considering any decision about the practice of psychotherapy, the ethical therapist is taught to ask, among other things, "Whose needs are paramount in making this decision? How will doing (or not doing) this help or harm the patient?" Additionally, what impact will a decision to depart from standard practice have on the therapist/patient relationship? Does any therapeutic benefit seem likely from a boundary crossing?

In this case, as in many others, I had multiple roles with some members of the department. In addition to my direct clinical role with Bill, my consultative relationship with the captain of the division where Bill worked became an issue. When I debriefed Bill's unit, I had a professional role with some of the other officers in Bill's division. While these relationships received serious consideration, my psychotherapeutic relationship with Bill held the primary and enduring importance in the development of consultation and treatment strategy and decision-making.

Throughout the course of Bill's treatment, which continues as I write this case, I made decisions about boundary issues based on furtherance of the goals that brought him into treatment. I did this by considering his complex psychological and family history, preservation of the therapeutic alliance, and my best judgment about the impact my decisions would have on his progress. I could not, however, make these decisions exclusively on the basis of our psychotherapy relationship and the relevant ethical principles. I also had to take into account the realities of the police organization.

Work setting

Police departments with thousands of sworn and civilian employees have unique organizational characteristics that psychologists rarely confront outside the five branches of the military. Working as a police psychologist in a large law enforcement agency compelled me to deal with these organizational qualities. These include the paramilitary nature of police departments, the existence of a prominent chain of command, the ever-present concern about issues related to officer safety and fitness for duty, the cultural uneasiness of having psychologists as part of the organization, and the issue of stigma faced by officers who utilize mental health services.

Police psychologists work to become integrated into the fabric of the law enforcement organization. We want to earn acceptance as members of the team and recognition for the contributions we can make to the organization and to individual officers. One part of our job involves promoting the health and well-being of the officers, the civilian employees, and the organization itself. We feel pressured to fit into the law enforcement culture while we strive to maintain our ethics, standards, and professional identities.

The realities of the law enforcement organization require flexibility to adapt to a culture and a set of "rules" quite different from traditional clinical settings. Where else would therapists accept as standard practice that most of their patients come to psychotherapy appointments with a loaded handgun on their belts? In what clinical or work environment would a therapist expect to see his/her patient in the office on Monday, in a classroom on Tuesday, at a crime scene on Wednesday, and at a SWAT callout on Saturday night?

Most police psychologists begin their careers in clinical psychology training programs. For me, that was followed by training and work in hospitals and emergency rooms, clinics, forensic settings, the courts, and a private practice office. None of those work environments prepared me for the demands of working in a big city police department. I have experienced a gradual but relentless process of adjustment to law enforcement culture, the paramilitary environment, and the unpredictability of not knowing what will happen next and what I may find myself expected to do.

Reflection

As I consider the work I have done with Bill, I think about the serious professional, personal, and medical issues he brought to the psychotherapy process. In any traditional clinical setting, this combination would have proved to be a challenging endeavor. In the larger law enforcement context, it became more so and, at times, felt like the experience of swimming in deep and occasionally turbulent waters.

Bill had been dealing with a set of circumstances that threatened his career, his family, and his health. He had serious expectations of me and the psychotherapy process: symptomatic relief, emotional support, psychological growth, career survival, increased professional effectiveness, and improved physical health. All of this occurred in an organizational environment that has its own expectations of me and my psychologist coworkers. Police psychologists are expected to find a way to balance the needs of the officers who are patients, the needs of the organization, and the welfare of the community. These organizational needs include promoting the health and well-being of the individual officers and the operational effectiveness of the department as a whole. Operational effectiveness involves individual officer safety, collaborative workplace relationships, respect for the chain of command, and fitness for duty.

The decisions that I made during the course of Bill's treatment consistently held his best interests as the paramount consideration. I always viewed this as a non-negotiable ethical obligation that overrode any organizational expectations of me as a psychotherapist operating in an internal mental health unit within a police department. As my time as a police psychologist has passed, I understand that the needs of the two are more compatible than I had previously realized. The goal in law enforcement focuses on maintaining public safety and sending every officer home safely at their end-of-watch. To do so requires that the police psychologist strive to meet the individual and organizational needs discussed earlier.

The boundary crossings that I agreed to during the course of Bill's treatment represented responses to my assessment of his needs and to the expectations of the organization in which we both worked. As a clinician trained in the psychodynamic tradition who has functioned comfortably in that theoretical orientation throughout my career, this has proved to be a challenge.

At times, I wondered if the culture of the police department would permit the psychological wellness and healing that police psychologists were hired to promote. Bill has made good progress during the time I worked with him, as had many other officers treated by me and by the other police psychologists I have worked with over the years. I have learned that intelligent, caring, ethical decision-making is rooted in a firm commitment to doing what is best for the patient, not blind adherence to a code of ethics.

I am reminded of something a clinical supervisor taught me earlier in my career. The state I worked in after completing my first postdoctoral fellowship required regular supervision prior to obtaining a license to practice as a psychologist. During one meeting, we talked about a difficult patient who was not doing well and whose psychotherapeutic needs I was struggling to identify and meet. We discussed various possibilities for how to move the therapy forward. As we concluded our conversation, my supervisor said, "The longer you are in this profession, the more you will understand when to follow the rules and when, for the benefit of your patient, to make an exception." Her words have been more and more helpful to me as I have worked in this profession and as a police psychologist.

Key ethical principles and standards

APA (2002): Principle A (Beneficence and nonmaleficence; Principle E (Respect for people's rights and dignity; Standard 1.03 (Conflicts between ethics and organizational demands); Standard 3.04 (Avoiding harm); Standard 3.05 (Multiple relationships); Standard 4.04 (Minimizing intrusions on privacy).

REFERENCES AND FURTHER READING

Barnett, J. E., Lazarus, A. A., Vasquez, M. J. T., Moorehead-Slaughter, O. & Johnson, W. B. (2007). Boundary issues and multiple relationships: Fantasy and reality. *Professional Psychology: Research and Practice, 38,* 401–410.

Blau, T. H. (1994). *Psychological Services for Law Enforcement.* New York: John Wiley.

Gutheil, T. G., & Gabbard, G. O. (1993). The concept of boundaries in clinical practice: Theoretical and risk management dimensions. *American Journal of Psychiatry, 150,* 188–196.

Smith, D., & Fitzpatrick, M. (1995). Patient-therapist boundary issues: An integrative review of theory and research. *Professional Psychology: Research and Practice, 26,* 499–506.

Index

Abandonment
    anti-Semitism issues and, 25–31
    ethical issues related to prospect of, 37
    fears of, 9–10
Abuse. *See also* Child abuse; Sexual abuse
    anger and, 50
    of elders, 337
    statistics, 135
    women and, 127–36
Abusers, 135
Acute care setting, 170–72
Acute situational distress, 180
Adaptive functioning, deficits in, 86
ADD. *See* Attention-deficit disorder
Addiction specialist, 292
Adolescents, socializing strategies of, 154
Afghanistan, 194
    military, 202
Alienation, 131, 135, 136
Allegations, 135
Alliance, 58, 60, 162
    development, 339
    forging, 168
    preservation of, 340
    therapeutic, 58, 60, 162
Ambiguity, 278
American Dietetic Association, 290
American Psychiatric Association, 295
    Religious/Spiritual Commitments and Psychiatric Practice (2006), 321, 322
American Psychological Association (APA), 55, 99, 219

American School Counseling Association (ASCA), 250
Amish. *See also* Old Order Amish
    church, 313
    theology, 310
    women, 314
Amnesia, 309
Anger
    abuse and, 50
    illness and, 65
    loss of control, 27–30, 56–59
    resentment, 10
    toward client, 19
Annoyance, 262
    managing, 263
Anorexia nervosa, 288. *See also* Eating disorders
    diagnosis of, 290
Anti-Semitism
    abandonment issues and, 25–31
    case study in, 25–29
    ethical issues in dealing with, 28–29
    ethical principles and standards, 31
    work setting and, 29
Antisocial behaviors, 208
Anxiety, 49
    among MHPs, 2
    suicidal patients and, 37
APA. *See* American Psychological Association
Appearance, 123
Appelbaum, P. S., 142–43

Arab-Israeli Six-Day War, 26
ASCA. *See* American School Counseling Association
Assessment, competent, 37
At-home nursing, 159
Atkins v. Virginia, 86
Attention-deficit disorder (ADD), 41
Attorney
 dilemma created by, 109
 domestic violence and, 114
 forensics expertise of, 108
 for health care decision making, 145
Autonomy, 79, 291, 292
Axis II factors, 267

Baptism, 319, 323, 324
Behavior
 antisocial, 208
 assumptions about determinants of, 125–26
 changes for clinicians to ensure well-being, 107
 of colleagues, unhealthy, 287–95
 ethically questionable, 220–21
 guidelines when dealing with another professional, 218
 in institutional settings, 221–22
 low-level disordered eating, 288
 morality/immorality of, client, 125
 obsessive-compulsive, 73, 74
 responsibility for others', 215
 sexualized, troubled, 111
 suicide, 33, 37
Behavioral functioning, 36
Behavioral Health Services, 184, 186
Behavioral science
 ethical principles and standards in, 202
 in national security settings, 197–203
Behavioral scientists, 200
 role of, 199
Behavior therapy
 cognitive, 168
 dialectical, 318
Beneficence, 79, 96, 263, 274, 291
 principle of, 160
Best interest, 45
 legal counsel and, 109
Betrayal, 36
Binge drinking, 318
Blackmail, suicidal, 33–40

Blood-borne pathogen, 337
Board ordered supervision, 303
Body image, distorted, 292
Borderline character traits, 318, 319
Borderline personality organization, 318
Boston Center for Refugee Health and Human Rights, 26
Boston University, 25
Boundaries, 12, 21, 303. *See also* Overlap, client/boundary
 with abused women, 127–36
 blurring of professional, 273–74
 of competence, 236, 274
 confidentiality and, 21
 in emotionally intense contexts, 167–72
 with former client, managing, 119–26
 group, 278
 issues, 122, 124
 military psychologists and, 179–80
 norms surrounding, 122
 in police psychology, 335–43
 professional, 291–92
 role shifts and blurring, 339–40
 sexual, violations, 297–305
 spiritual/ethical dilemmas around, 317–24
 violation of, 13, 101–2
 work setting, challenges and, 122–23
Boundary crossing, 13
 agreement, 342
 context, 320
 military psychologists and, 179–80
 therapeutic benefits from, 340
Brain injury, financial compensation, 330
Browning, Don, 322
Bulimia, 288
Burnout, job-related, 145
Bush, Jeb, 328

CACREP. *See* Council for Accreditation of Counseling and Related Educational Programs
Cancer
 pancreatic, 63–64
 psychology of, 67–68
Capital punishment. *See also* Death penalty litigation
 forensic psychology and, 85
 values and, 84–85
Catastrophic thinking, 177
Caution in group therapy, 278

Certificates, in office, 29–30
CF. See Cystic fibrosis
Chain of command, 340
Cheating spouses
  case study, 41–44
  ethical issues in dealing with, 44–47
  ethical principles and standards when working with, 48
  work setting and, 47–48
Child abuse
  police psychology and, 337
  sexual, 111–13, 127–35
  statistics, 135
Child protective services (CPS), 133, 250
  school counseling and, 249–56
Child removal from home, 233–40
  alternatives to, 238
  ethical issues concerning, 233–40
  ethical principles and standards, 240
Children. See also Custody; Pediatrics
  in custody litigation, 96–97
  disabled, 233–40
  divorce and separation issues related to, 41–48
  divorce during treatment of, 93–100
  environment and, 97–98
  Ethical Principles of Psychologists and Code of Conduct and, 99
  parental conflict impact on, 116
  separation anxiety during divorce, 111–12
  transplant evaluation for, 157–64
  work setting and, 97–98
Child welfare services, 233
Chronically ill. See Terminally (or chronically) ill
Client(s). See also Human immunodeficiency virus (HIV) clients; Overlap, client/boundary
  anger toward, 19
  athletic, 245–46
  authorization, 304
  best interest, 109
  boundaries with former, 119–26
  choice, 297
  clarifying primary, 45
  confidentiality with suicide, 75–76
  dependence on clinician, 13, 50, 52
  dislike/disgust for, 18
  encountering, in unexpected places, 261–68
  gratifying desires, 302
  identifying, 97
  initial decline of, 29
  military as, 186
  morality/immorality of behavior, 125
  obligation to, 3, 52
  in prison, 123
  privacy, 300
  record, 180
  sexual relationship with, 120
  violent, 189–93
Clinical skill-building workshops, 300–301
Clinician
  behavioral changes for, to ensure well-being, 107
  challenge practice of, 146
  child custody evaluation role, 136
  dependence on, 13, 50, 52
  on Facebook, 149–50
  hospitalizations and, desire for riddance, 37
  impaired, 290–93, 295
  medical condition of, 293
  self-disclosure, 29–30
  skills of ethical, 294
Coaches, 245–46
Cognition
  enhancing, 197
  malnutrition and, 292
Cognitive-behavioral therapy, 168
Cognitive functioning, 142
Colleagues
  in-house, 106
  as patient, 294
  supervising/assisting, 261–305
  unhealthy behaviors of, 287–95
Collegiate culture, 248
Combat environment, 189–96
Commitment, 263
Common knowledge, skills, abilities and other characteristics (KSAOs), 224
Communication, with former client, 121–26
Community
  mental health care, 75

Community (Cont'd)
  psyche, 312
  rural, 275
  small, 21–22
  transplant, 161
Competency, 294, 303
  assessment, 37
  to be executed, 86
  boundaries, 236, 274
  cultural, 184–87, 315
  deficits, 300–301
  ethics and, 263
  judging, of prior MHP, 133
  practitioner, 169–70
  professional, 37
  of supervision, 303
Complaint, filing, 134
Concrete goals, 36
Confidentiality, 20–22, 96–97, 131–32, 300
  board ordered supervision and, 303
  boundaries and, 21
  breaching, 310, 313
  breaking, 79
  after death, 63–69
  forensic evaluation and, 104
  in group, 278
  at GTMO, 186–87
  imminent danger/threat and, issues, 55–59
  of inmate clients, 123
  job analysis and, 226, 228
  laws, 55
  limits of, 56, 59–60
  Old Order Amish and, 309–16
  on police force, 338
  privacy *vs.*, 292
  protection and, 52
  social networking and, 152
  of students, 253
  with suicide clients, 75–76
  when spouses cheat, 41–48
Confirmatory bias, 87
Conflict resolution, 294
"Conflicts Between Ethics and Organizational Demands," 221
Congress, psychologist in, 327–33
Congressional Record, 332–33
Contracts
  "no harm," 37
  "no suicide," 37
  research, 201
Co-parenting, 171
Corrective action, 264
Cortex, 333
Council for Accreditation of Counseling and Related Educational Programs (CACREP), 280–81
Counseling course, 249–56
Counselor educator, 252, 280–81. *See also* Group counseling class
  role of, 256
Counter-transference, 294
  anti-Semitism and, 25–31
  "mother bear" stance, 19
  supervision and, 304
Co-worker, problematic, 215–18
CPS. *See* Child protective services
Crisis management, 318
Crisis situation
  MHP response, 276
  providing services in, 274
  in rural communities, 275
  supervision in, 269–76
Criterion oriented validation, 225
Critical incident, involvement in, 337
Critical thinking, 315
Cultural competency, 184–87, 315
"Culture of risk," 245
Custody, 46, 114–15
  dispute, 111, 171
  forensic standard of, 136
  sexual abuse and, 132–35
  sole *vs.* joint, 115
Custody litigation, 94–95
  ethical issues in, 96–97
Cyclic mood disorder, 318
Cystic fibrosis (CF), 157–64, 167

Danger to self/others, 60–61
  confidentiality issues and, 55–59
  ethical issues, 59–60
  ethical principles and standards, 61
  suicide and, 72
  work settings with patients who impose, 60
Data privacy laws, 109
Death. *See also* Deceased patient, disclosure of information about
  confidentiality after, 63–69
  with dignity, 330–31

Death penalty litigation
　confirmatory bias and, 87
　ethical issues in, 84–88
　ethical principles and standards in, 90
　forensic psychology and, work setting for, 88–90
　forensic psychology in, 83–92
　mental retardation/illness and, legal contours related to, 86–87
　testifying in, 88
Deceased patient, disclosure of information about
　confidentiality and, 63–69
　ethical issues, 66–67
　ethical principles and standards, 69
　work setting and, 67–68
Deception, detecting, 197
Decisional capacity, 142
　assessment, 143–44
Decision making, 4
　attorney for health care, 145
　ethical, 2
　ethical model, 78
　high-stakes, 2
　impaired clinical, 295
　military policy, 181
　structured model of, 14
　team, 293
Decorations, in office, 29–30
Department of Defense (DoD)
　behavioral research programs, 197–203
　policy, 198
Dependence, 124
　on clinician, 13, 50, 52
Depersonalization, 56
Depression, 73, 269
Dialectical behavior therapy, 318
Dialysis refusal, 141–44
　ethical issues, 144–45
Didactic education, 277–85
Dietetics licensing board, 291
Dietitian, registered, 288, 293
　anorexic, 289
　code of ethics for, 294
Diplomas, in office, 29–30
Direct management referral, 337, 338, 340
Dislike/disgust for clients, 18

Disruption in self- and other-perception, 318
Dissociative-like experiences, 56
Divorce
　children and, 41–48
　ethical issues in high-stake, 113–14
　high-conflict, 111
　post, co-parenting, 171
　separation anxiety of children during, 111–12
　during treatment period, 93–100
Doctor of Psychology (PsyD) program, 273
DoD. *See* Department of Defense
Doll play, 112
Domestic violence, 269
　attorney, 114
　ethical principles and standards in, 117
　investigation of allegations of, 111–17
　work setting and, 114–15
Do no harm principle, 193
"Door-in-the-face," 200
Drawing, 112
Drug testing, 242
　ethical issues concerning, 244
Dual relationships, 67, 126
Dysphoria, 318

Eating disorders, 287–95
　diagnosable, 289
　low-level behaviors, 288
　personal history disclosure, 288
　unit work setting, 293–94
Electronic recording, 300
Elie Wiesel Center for Judaic Studies at Boston University, 25
E-mail, 151
EMDR. *See* Eye movement desensitization and reprocessing
Emergency psychological services, 269–76
Emotionally intense contexts
　boundaries in, 167–72
　ethical issues in, 169–70
End-stage renal disease (ESRD), 141
Environment
　children and, 97–98
　combat, 189–96
ESRD. *See* End-stage renal disease

Ethics
  committee, 134
  competence and, 263
  decision making and, 2
  decision-making model, 78
  duty, of legal counsel, 109
  internal experiences and, 264
  obligation vs. organizational
    policy, 207–13
  responsibilities, conflicting, 300
  safeguards, 294
Ethical dilemmas, 317–24
Ethical impropriety, 123
Ethical issues
  abandonment, related to prospect
    of, 37
  anti-Semitism, in dealing
    with, 28–29
  cheating spouses, in dealing
    with, 44–47
  of child removal from home, 233–40
  in communication with former
    client, 121–22
  in Constitution, 327–33
  cultural competency and, 185–86
  in custody litigation, 96–97
  danger to self/others, regarding
    imminent, 59–60
  in death penalty litigation, 84–88
  dialysis refusal, 144–45
  of disclosure of information about
    deceased patient, 66–67
  in emotionally intense
    contexts, 169–70
  in forensic psychology, 105–6, 108
  gifts, in responding to offers of, 12–14
  group counseling, in required, 280–81
  in high-stake divorce, 113–14
  impaired clinicians, 291–92
  in informal treatment of
    friends, 178–79
  law and, conflict between, 59
  Old Order Amish and, 315
  in organizational standards, 211
  organizations and, 218–19
  patient care and, 294
  with patient who fails in self
    protection, 50–53
  in pediatric transplantation, 160–63
  in police psychology, 339–40
  of practicing graduate students in
    crisis situation, 274
  in prisons, 123
  of professional boundaries, 292
  school counseling and CPS
    reports, 253–54
  in sexual abuse of children and custody
    litigations, 132–35
  of social networking, 152
  in sport psychology, 244
  in suicide issues, 36–37
  with terminally ill suicide clients,
    75–76
  in test validation, 223–29
  themes in, 3
  work setting, context and, 126
Ethical principles and standards
  in acute care settings, 172
  adhering exclusively to, 3–4
  in anti-Semitism issue, 31
  in behavioral science, 202
  cheating spouses, when working
    with, 48
  in client overlap issues, 23
  communications with former client
    and, 126
  confidentiality after death, 69
  in custody case with abuse, 136
  danger to self/others and,
    imminent, 61
  in death penalty litigation, 90
  deceased patient and, 69
  domestic violence allegations
    and, 117
  when encountering clients
    unexpectedly, 268
  in experiential group course, 284
  gift offer responses, 15
  GTMO treatments and, 187
  impaired clinician and, 295
  managerial/leadership positions,
    221–22
  modification of practice for, 300
  Old Order Amish and, 316
  overlap, in client/boundary, 23
  with patients who fail in self
    protection, 54
  patients who impose danger to self/
    others and, 61
  for pediatric transplantation, 164

in police psychology, 343
in politics, 333
psychological testing for organizations, 213
refusal of treatment and, 146
removal of child from home, 240
in school counseling, 256
in sport psychology, 248
in suicide issues, 40
supervision, 305
terminally ill suicide clients, 78–79
test validation and, 229
of treatment within friendship, 181
violent patient, when dealing with, 196
Ethical Principles of Psychologists and Code of Conduct (APA), 55, 99, 219
Ethical silence, 330
Ethics in Psychology and the Mental Health Professions (Koocher & Keith-Spiegel), 2
Evaluations
  court ordered, 104
  custody, 136
  for Federal Bureau of Prisons, 85
  structures, 108
  transplant, 157–64
Evidence-based methods, 200
Execution, legal qualification for, 86
Executive officer (XO), 192
Experiential group course, 277–85
  benefits and risks involved in, 283
  ethical principles and standards in, 284
  grading, 283
  rationale for, 278
Exploitation, 131
Extra-therapy contact, 320
Eye movement desensitization and reprocessing (EMDR), 168

Facebook, 149–50
  benefits of, 150
  friend request, 149
  privacy settings, 151
  status update, 149–50
  wall, 150
False memories, 200
Family. *See also* Cheating spouses; Domestic violence
  "best interest" when dealing with, 45
  courts, 115
  sexual abuse within, 49–54, 127–35
  sexually repressive, 299
Fear of abandonment, 9–10
Federal Bureau of Prisons, policy and evaluations, 85
Federal prison hospital, 83, 88–90
Feminist therapist, 22
Fidelity, 66–67, 79, 211, 219
Filing complaint, 134
Financial compensation, 330
Fitness for duty, 340
Florida State Legislature, 328
"Foot-in-door," 200
Ford v. Wainwright, 86
Forensic(s), 3. *See also specific case studies*
  attorney with expertise in, 108
  custody, standard of, 136
Forensic evaluation
  confidentiality and, 104
  deception in, 90
  psychologist/patient relationship in, 89
Forensic psychology, 335
  capital punishment and, 85
  in death penalty litigation, 83–92
  ethical issues in, 105–6, 108
  public role of, 88
  work setting, 106–7
"For the Relief of the Parents of Theresa Marie Schiavo" (Congressional Record), 332–33
Foster care system, 252
Friend request, Facebook, 149
Friendship
  ethical issues in informal treatment, 178–79
  informal therapy in, 177–78
  in military, 175–81
  role *vs.* provider role, 177
Funeral, attending, 169

Gastrointestinal malabsorption, 167
Gaylin, William, 68
Generalizability limitations, 227
George Fox University, 273
Gifts, responding to offers of, 119, 121, 124
  case study, 9–12
  ethical issues in, 12–14

Gifts, responding to offers of (Cont'd)
  key ethical principles and standards in, 15
  work setting, 13–14
Go-no-go decisions, 2
Government service (GS) position, 209–10
  hiring board, 213
Grading experiential course, 283
Graduate student
  clinical supervision for, 275
  ethical issues of practicing, 274
  supervising in crisis situation, 269–76
  work, 281
Grey area, 239
Grisso, T., 142–43
Grodzinsky, Hayyim Ozer, 25
Group
  boundaries, 278
  dynamics, managing, 293
  here-and-now context of, 284
  leaders, effective, 280
  member, 282
  psychoeducational, design, 281–82
  psychoeducational sexuality, 299
  treatment, spiritual beliefs and, 310
Group counseling class, 278. *See also* Experiential group course
  confidentiality and, 278
  demonstrations in, 282
  effective functioning in, 281
  ethical issues, 280–81
  with experiential lab component, 277–85
  hesitation/caution in, 278
  informed consent in, 283
  multiple relationships in teaching, 282–83
  participating in required, 277–80
  potential dangers in, 282
  sharing power in, 281
  work setting, 281–82
Group process, 281
  concepts, 277, 279, 282
GS. *See* Government service
GTMO. *See* Guantanamo Bay
Guantanamo Bay (GTMO)
  confidentiality and, 186–87
  ethical principles and standards and, 187
  treatment in, 183–88
  work setting, 184, 186–87
Guardian ad litem, 111–12, 116, 131

Haldol, 209
Harm. *See also* Danger to self/others; Nonmaleficence
  avoiding, *vs.* doing good, 249–56
  avoiding/minimizing, 3
  "no harm" contracts, 37
  principle, 193
  self, 318
  self protect from, inability to, 49–54
  when clients overlap, 21
Health fair, 269–74
Health Insurance Portability and Accountability Act (HIPAA), 56
  privacy rules, 336–37
  regulations, 168–69
Heart monitoring, 331
Helplessness, 53
Hesitation in group therapy, 278
High-stakes decisions, 2
HIPPA. *See* Health Insurance Portability and Accountability Act
HIV. *See* Human immunodeficiency virus
Holistic psychology, 298
Holocaust survivors, 25–26
Hope
  in spirituality and religion, 321
  suicidality and, 39
Hospitalization
  clinician's desire for riddance and, 37
  prevention of, in HIV case, 75–76
  reliance on inpatient, 37
Human immunodeficiency virus (HIV)
  clients, 72–75, 77–79
  hospitalization prevention, 75–76
  work setting for, 76–77
Human sources, collecting information from, 197
  methods/tools without validation for, use of, 201–2
  techniques, 200
Husband, disconnect from, 317
Hypnosis, 168

Identity
  dual, 16

in spirituality and religion, 29, 320–21
Idiopathic pulmonary fibrosis, 330–31
Illegal activity, 208
IME. *See* Independent medical evaluation
Impaired clinician, 101, 290–91, 293
　ethical issues of, 291–92
　ethical principles and standards, 295
Impaired judgment, 208
Impairment, 291
Impulsivity, 208, 318
Inappropriate touch, 298
Income, volatility in, 106
Independent medical evaluation (IME), 57
Informal counsel, 299
Informal therapy, 177–78
　ethically required, 299
Information, release of rescinded, 101–5
Informed consent, 37, 72, 161, 244, 274, 298, 300, 303
　board ordered supervision and, 303
　in group course, 283
　guidelines in prison, 124
　multiple roles and, 175–81
In-house colleagues, 106
Inner city school, 249–53
Inquiries, irrelevant and offensive, 302
Insanity, not guilty by reason of, 84
Insomnia, 176
　among MHPs, 2
　self-help books related to, 177
Inspiration, in spirituality and religion, 321
Insurance constraints, 38
Intake questionnaire, 298
Integrity, 211, 219
Interaction, promotion of, 279
Intercollegiate athletics, 241–48
Internal Affairs, 338
Internal experiences
　ethics and, 264
　regulation of, 263
IQ testing, 86
Iraq, 189–96
　work setting, 194
Irrelevant and offensive inquiries, 302
Israeli National Service, 233–40
　work setting, 237–38

Job
　families, 223
　performance, below average, 337
　police psychology responsibilities, 336
　related burnout, 145
Job analysis
　confidentiality and, 226, 228
　questionnaire, 224–25
Justice, 79, 236–37

Ka-Bar, 189
Keith-Spiegel, P., 2
Koocher, G. P., 2
KSAO. *See* Common knowledge, skills, abilities and other characteristics

Labor union representation, 223
Law, 108
　confidentiality and, 55
　data privacy, 109
　ethical issues conflicting with, 59
　and ethics course, 280
　relating to mental retardation and mental illness, 86–87
Leadership, 281. *See also* Managerial/leadership positions
Leader's training, 281
Legal counsel, ethical duty of, 109
Legal qualification for execution, 86
Legislative branch, intrusion by, 328–29
Lesbian psychotherapist, 17–21
　work setting, 21–22
License, practicing without, 274
Licensing boards, 108, 293
　state-to-state variations, 109
Licensure status, 303
Life-or-death decision, 142
Life-saving treatment, 39
Life-sustaining treatments, 142
Living will documentation, 76
"Low-balling," 200
Loyalty, 66–67

Major depressive disorder, 27
Malnutrition, 290–91
　cognition and, 292
Malpractice litigation, 37
Managerial/leadership positions, 215–22
　ethical principles and standards in, 221–22

Managerial/leadership positions (*Cont'd*)
  roles of, 219
  work setting for, 219–20
Manchester Document, 184
Marginalization, 254
Marriage. *See also* Cheating spouses; Divorce
  disconnect in, 317
Meal plans, 288
  weight gain and, 289
Meaning, in spirituality and religion, 321
MEDEVAC, 193
Media
  scrutiny, 187
  sport psychology and, 244, 246–47
Medical center, case studies, 3, 141–72. *See also specific case studies*
Membership, 281
Mental coaches, 245
Mental health professionals (MHP), 1–2. *See also* Clinician
  anxiety among, 2
  competency of, judging, 133
  crisis response, 276
  insomnia among, 2
  in Iraq, 189–96
  self-care of, 13–14
Mental illness, legal contours related to, 86–87
Mental retardation, legal contours related to, 86–87
Messengers, 19–21
MHP. *See* Mental health professionals
Middlebrook, Diane, 68
Military
  Afghanistan, 202
  as client, 186
  decision making policy, 181
  friendships, 175–81
Military psychologists
  boundary crossing and, 179–80
  work setting, 179–80
Mini-Mental State Examination (MMSE), 142
Misuse of psychologists' work, 211
Mixed-agency, 186, 187
  dilemmas, 1–2
MMSE. *See* Mini-Mental State Examination
Moral distress, 145

Morality
  or client behavior, 125
  in spirituality and religion, 321
Morphine drip, 168
Move forward, 342
Multiple relationships, 178, 282–83
  managing, 3
  in school setting, 244
  social networking and, 152
Multiple roles, 3, 21, 131–32
  balancing, 181
  in group, 278, 282–83
  informed consent and, 175–81
Multiple wives, 185
Munchausen syndrome, 135
Mutism, 111–12
MySpace, 150

National Collegiate Athletics Association (NCAA), 245
National security, 3, 173–204. *See also specific case studies*
  behavioral science and, 197–203
NCAA. *See* National Collegiate Athletics Association
Needs, distinguishing/addressing, 302
Negative self-talk, 178
Neurolinguistic programming, 199
"No harm" contracts, 37
Nonmaleficence, 79, 96, 219, 263, 291
  child removal and, 236–37
Nontherapeutic interaction, 152
"No suicide" contracts, 37
Not guilty, by reason of insanity, 84
Numbness, 318
Nutrition, principles of, 291

Objectivity, 131
Obligation
  identifying, to client, 3
  to protect, 52
Obsessive-compulsive behavior, 73, 74
Office, 29–30
Old Order Amish
  community psyche, 312
  curiosity, 314
  mental health services with, 309–16
  theological views of, 310
  transportation, 314
  women, 314
Operational effectiveness, 342

Organizations, 3. *See also specific case studies*
  behavior in, 221–22
  case studies, 206–29
  ethical issues and, 218–19
  ethical principles and standards regarding psychological testing for, 213
  managerial/leadership positions in, 215–22
  police department, characteristics of, 340
  policy *vs.* ethical obligation, 207–13
  scrutiny, 245
  standards, ethical issues in, 211
Organizational psychologists
  role of, 229
  work setting, 228–29
Organs, supply of, 161
Orne, Martin, 68
Overlap, client/boundary
  case study, 17–21
  cheating spouses and, 41–48
  ethical principles and standards in, 23
  reflection, 22–23
  work setting in, 21–22

Parental alienation syndrome, 131, 135–36
Parental conflict, 116
Parental fitness examination, 134–35
Parenting, 171
  capacities, assessment of, 116
  shared, 43–44
Pastoral role
  blurred, 273–74
  psychiatric role *vs.*, 52
Patient. *See also* Client(s); Deceased patient, disclosure of information about; *specific types of patients*
  colleagues as, 294
  dangerous, 60
  in forensic evaluation, 89
  interactions, 294
  safety, 292
  self protection of, 50–54
  suicidal, 37
PCASS. *See* Preliminary Credibility Assessment Screening System
Pediatrics, 150
  psychologist, 159

Pediatric transplantation, 157–64
  ethical issues in, 160–63
  ethical principles and standards for, 164
  evaluation process for, 164
  work setting, 163–64
Peer consultation, 13–14, 163, 261–68
  as self-care, 22
Performance-based psychological life-skills, 247–48
Perpetrator, role of, 27
Personality
  change, 309–10
  testing, 112
Personal traits of profession, 293
Persuasion techniques, 200
Pique technique, 200
Police department, organizational characteristics of, 340
Police officer
  involved shooting, 337
  safety, 340
  serious use of force used by, 337
  substance abuse by, 337
  well-being of, 341
Police psychology, 335–43
  child abuse and, 337
  ethical issues in, 339–40
  ethical principles and standards, 343
  job responsibilities and, 336
  practice guidelines for, 336–37
  work setting, 340–41
Politics, 327–33
  fallout, 331
Polygraph screening form, 208
Post-traumatic stress syndrome, 27
Poverty cycles
  breaking, 251
  multigenerational patterns of, 254
Powell, Lewis, 86
Power
  differentials, between professionals, 293
  dynamics, 221
  separation of, 328
  sharing in group counseling class, 281
Prejudice against counselor, 310

Preliminary Credibility Assessment
   Screening System (PCASS),
   198, 201–2
Premature twins, 331
Priming, 200
Prison. *See also* Federal Bureau of
      Prisons, policy and evaluations
   appearance within, 123
   confidentiality within, 123
   consent guidelines in, 124
   ethical issues in, 123
   hospital, 83, 88–90
Privacy, 291
   client, 300
   confidentiality *vs.*, 292
   HIPPA rules of, 336–37
   invaded, 302
   issues, 292
   laws, 109
   limits on, 303
   settings, Facebook, 151
Private life, intrusion into, 262
Private practice, 13–14
Process discussion, over e-mail, 151
Professional boundaries, 291
   blurring of, 273–74
   ethical issues and, 292
Professional competency, 37
Professionalism, 295
Pro-life political movement, 328
Protection-of-human-participants-in-
   research protocols, 124
Provider role *vs.* friendship role, 177
Psychiatric risk, associated with GS
   candidate, 209–10
Psychodynamic psychotherapy, 288
Psychoeducational assistance, 180
Psychoeducational group
   design, 281–82
Psychoeducational sexuality groups, 299
Psycho-legalities, 108
Psychological assessment, for
   hiring GS, 210
Psychological interview, 207–13
Psychotherapist-patient privilege, 97
Psychotherapy case studies, 3, 9–79. *See
   also specific case studies*
PsyD. *See* Doctor of Psychology
Public service, 3, 327–43. *See also specific
   case studies*

Quality of life, 75–76
   for terminally ill, 71
Questionnaire, intake, 298

Racism, institutional, 251
Rage, 318
Rapport, 250
   establishing, 184–85
Rational suicide, 78
Record keeping, 300
Referral, 135
   deception about source of, 42–46
   direct management, 337–38, 340
   to police psychologist, 336
   sources, 108
Refusal of treatments, 142
   ethical principles and standards
      in, 146
Regulatory mandate, suicide and, 76
Relationship. *See also* Multiple
      relationships
   dual, 67, 126
   formalizing, 180
   psychologist/patient, in forensic
      evaluation, 89
   sexual, with client, 120
Relationship, professional
   ground rules of, 12–13
   self-care and continuity of, 29
Relaxation training, 168
Religious accomplishment, 321
Religious experience, 319
Religious life, scientific evidence of, 322
Religious settings, 3
   case studies, 309–24
Religious/Spiritual Commitments and
   Psychiatric Practice (2006), 321–22
*Religious Thought and the Modern
   Psychologies* (Browning), 322
Remedial strategies, 305
Remediation, 101
Remote wilderness therapy programs, 122
Rescinded release of information, 101–5
Research contracts, 201
Respiration monitoring, 331
Responsibility, 211, 219
   behavior, for others', 215
   deflecting, 310
   life-*versus*-death sense of, 37
   social, 269–70

Risk assessment, 57
Risk management, 37, 110
  techniques, 38
Roberts, Laura, 287
Role(s). *See also specific roles*
  clarification, 132–33
  dual, 67, 126
  friendship *vs.* provider, 177
  model, 302
  overlapping, 291, 293
  shifts, 338–40
  of victim/perpetrator, 27
Roles, multiple, 3, 21, 131, 132, 175–81, 282
  balancing, 181
  in group, 278, 282–83
Rural communities, 275
Rural psychology, 269–70

Sacrifices, psychologist's role and, 263
Safety, personal, 189–96
  of officers, 340
  of patient, 292
Sarcasm, 317
Schiavo, Michael, 327
Schiavo, Terri, 327–33
  malpractice settlement, 330
  opinions on status, 330
Schindler, Mary, 327
Schindler, Robert, 327
Schizophrenia, 191–92
School counseling
  CPS reports and, 249–56
  ethical issues in, 253–54
  ethical principles and standards in, 256
School counselor, 252
  advocacy of, 255
  compliance with policies and standards, 255–56
  legal and ethical standards for, 254
  work setting for, 255–56
Schools, 3. *See also specific case studies*
  case studies in, 232–54
Security/threat assessment process, 210, 213
Self-awareness, culture and, 315
Self-blame, 78

Self-care
  continuity of therapy relationship and, 29
  of MHP, 13–14
  peer consultation as part of, 22
Self-deprivation, 287–88
Self-determination, 292
Self-disclosure, 29–30, 122, 292
  in academic setting, 278–79
  of eating disorder history, 288
  of students, 283
Self-harm, 318
Self-help books, 177
Self protection
  ethical issues when patients fail in, 50–53
  ethical principles and standards of, 54
  work setting and patients fail in, 53–54
Self-relaxation, 177
Self-touch, as self-soothing, 112
Separation anxiety, 93
  of children during divorce, 111–12
Separation of powers, 328
Sexton, Anne, 68
Sexual abuse
  allegations of, 111–13
  of children, 111–13, 127–35
  in family, 49–54
Sexual addiction, 134
Sexual boundary violations, 297–305
  identifying contributing factors to, 299
Sexuality, embracing, 299
Sexualized behavior, troubled, 111
Sexual molesting, 310
  accepting responsibility, 310
Sexual relationship, with clients, 120
Silence, ethical, 330
Sleep
  hygiene, 177
  interfered, 49
Small world phenomenon, 339–40
Social cues, misread, 302
Socializing strategies of adolescents, 154
Social networking, 149–50
  ethical issues in, 152
  psychotherapy related to, 153
  work setting and, 153
Social responsibility, 269–70
Solo practice, 106

Soundproofing, 301
Special mission unit
    application, 207–8
    work setting, 212–13
"Special treatment," 323–24
Specialty Guidelines for Forensic Psychologists, 88
Spiritual beliefs, group treatment and, 310
Spiritual dilemmas, 317–24
Sport psychology, 241–48
    ethical issues in, 244
    ethical principles and standards in, 248
    ethical values of, 246
    media and, 244, 246–47
    work setting, 245
Standard 1.03, 221
Standard 2.04, 114
Standard 3.04, 114
Standard 9.01, 114
Standards for Educational and Psychological Testing and the Principles for the Use and Validation of Personnel Selection Procedures, 224
Starvation, 332
Status update, Facebook, 149–50
Stigma, 340
Stress management, 107, 177–78
Structured decision-making model, 14
Structured exercises to promote interaction, 279
Student. *See also* Graduate student
    as group member, 278
    informal counsel of, 299
    intern supervision, 255
    invaded privacy, 302
    self-disclosure, 283
Student issues, 249–53
Subjective grading, 283–84
Substance abuse, 269, 318
    intervention, 242
    by police officer, 337
    programs, 122
Suicidal dependence, 50
Suicidal thoughts, 33
    persistent, 73–74
Suicide
    attempts, 33
    behaviors, 33
    danger to self/others and, 72
    faith-based ideas of, 52
    as option, 39
    rational, 78
    regulatory mandate and, 76
    risk behavior, 37
    self-blame and, 78
    specific treatment plan, 38
    terminally ill and, 72–79
    training sessions, 75
    verbal threats of, 34
Suicide issues, 38–40
    case study in, 33–36
    ethical issues in, 36–37
    ethical principles and standards in, 40
    work setting, 38
Suicidoligist, 34
Supervision, 274. *See also specific case studies*
    board-ordered, 303
    clinical, 163, 275
    competency of, 303
    counter-transference and, 304
    course of, 300–304
    in crisis situation, 269–76
    ethical principles and standards of, 305
    from off-site location, 304
    range of feelings/reactions during, 305
    risks/benefits associated with, 298, 303
    of student intern, 255
Syllabus, 277
Systemic forces, awareness of, 254

Tarasoff v. Regents of the University of California, 55, 193
Team decision-making, 293
Terminally (or chronically) ill, 72–75, 77–78
    ethical issues with, 75–76
    ethical principles and standards and, 78–79
    suicidality in face of, 75–76
Termination of therapy
    anti-Semitism issues and, 25–31
    initiation of, 22
Terror, 36
Test
    administrators, 226–27
    battery, 223–28
    case, 74
    drug, 242, 244

Test (Cont'd)
  IQ, 86
  for organizations, 213
  personality, 112
  voice stress analysis, 198
Testifying, in death penalty litigation, 88
Test validation
  ethical issues in, 223–29
  ethical principles and standards, 229
THC, 242
Theology, 273
  Amish, 310
Thera-mail, 119–21
Therapeutic neutrality, 44, 45
Therapeutic relationship, 89
Therapeutic repression, 36
Third-party inquiries, 245–46
Torture therapy, 26–27
Trainees, responsibilities of, 282
Transference, 294
Transition, to new therapists, 323
Transparency, 293
Transplant
  community, 161
  decision, 163
  pediatric, 157–64
  post-, adjustment, 161–62
  post-, care, 159
  pre-, evaluation, 157–58
  team, 163
Trauma, 274
  counseling, 272–74
  memories of past, 36
  psychological/biological reactions to, 27
  treatments for victims of, 36
Twelve step culture, 122

Unconventional practices, 301
Uniform Guidelines for Employee Selection Procedures, 224
United States Navy psychologist, 175

Validity evidence, 228
Values
  capital punishment and, 84–85
  personal system of, 320
  shared, 200
  sport psychology and, 246
Victim
  deflecting responsibility to, 310
  role of, 27
  of trauma, 36
Violent client, 189–93. *See also* Danger to self/others
Visitation, supervised, 114
Voice stress analysis test, 198
Voluntary admission status, 84
Voluntary treatment, 180
Vulnerability, 36

Wall, Facebook, 150
Weapons, 194–95
Weight, 289
  excessive comparing of, 292
Well-being
  clinician's behavioral changes for, 107
  concern about subordinate, 337
  of officers, 341
Wink, 266–68
  meanings for, 266–67
Witness tampering, 134
Women
  abused, 127–36, 135
  Amish, 314
  rights of, 184–85
Work setting, 1
  in acute care setting, 170–71
  anti-Semitism and, 29
  boundary challenges and, 122–23
  cheating spouses and, 47–48
  children and, 97–98
  client/boundary overlap and, 21–22
  communication with former client and, 122–24
  confidentiality after death and, 67–68
  for death penalty litigation and forensic psychology, 88–90
  decorations/diplomas/certificates in, 29–30
  domestic violence and, investigation of allegations of, 114–15
  of eating disorder unit, 293–94
  ethical issues, context and, 126
  forensic psychology, 106–7
  gifts and, responding to offers of, 13–14
  group course and, 281–82
  GTMO, 184, 186–87
  HIV patients and, 76–77
  in Iraq and Afghanistan, 194
  Israeli National Service, 237–38

Work setting (*Cont'd*)
   lesbian psychotherapist, 21–22
   for managerial/leadership positions, 219–20
   military psychologists, 179–80
   organizational psychologists, 228–29
   overlapping roles in, 293
   patients who impose danger to self/others in, 60
   patient who fails in self protection and, 53–54
   pediatric transplantation, 163–64
   police psychology, 340–41
   for school counselor, 255–56
   social networking and, 153
   special mission unit, 212–13
   sport psychology, 245
   suicide issues and, 38
World War II, 25
Worthlessness, feelings of, 318

XO. *See* Executive officer

www.ingramcontent.com/pod-product-compliance
Ingram Content Group UK Ltd.
Pitfield, Milton Keynes, MK11 3LW, UK
UKHW022135220326
469240UK00007B/55